Practical Renal Medicine

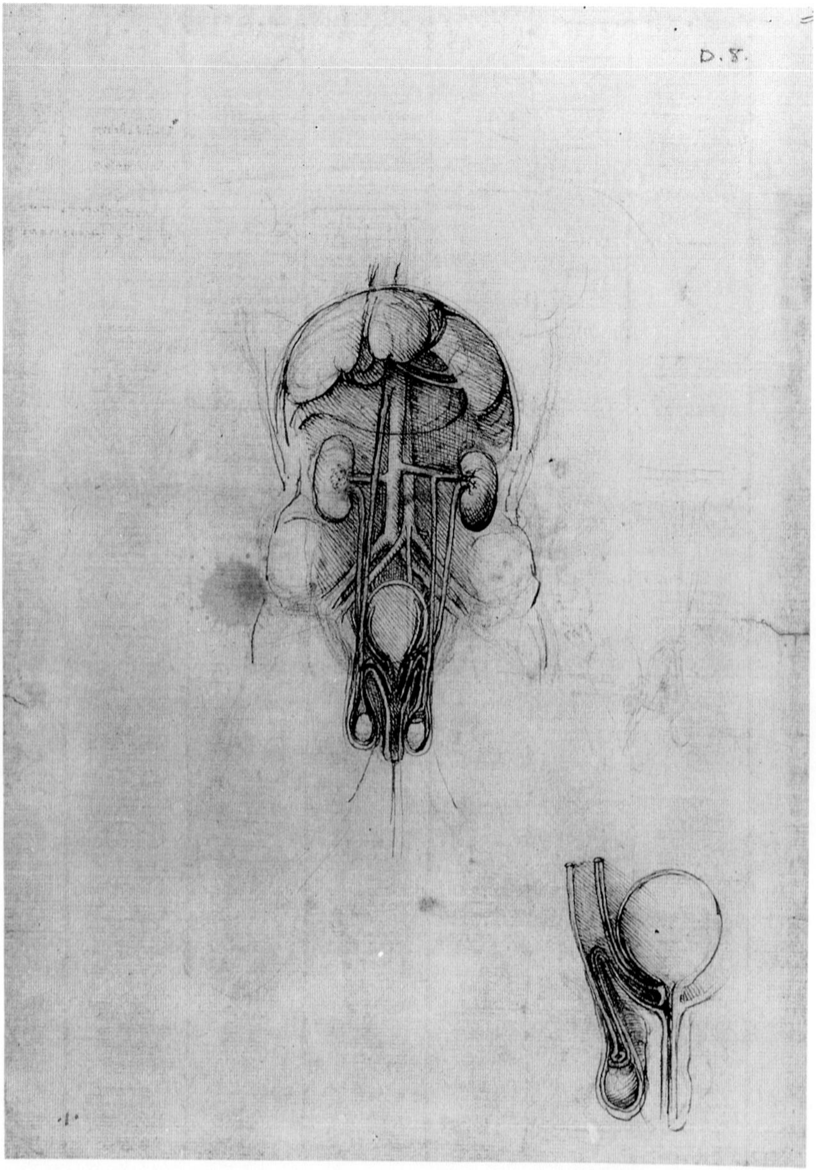

Frontispiece Leonardo, Anterior view of a male torso showing genitourinary system. Windsor Castle, Royal Library.

Practical Renal Medicine

Edited by Roger Gabriel
BA, MSc, MB, FRCP, DCH, DTM&H
Renal Physician
Parirenyatwa Hospital, Harare, Zimbabwe
and Honorary Lecturer in Medicine
Department of Medicine
University of Zimbabwe

Formerly, Renal Physician
St Mary's Hospital, London
and Northwick Park Hospital
Harrow, Middlesex

OXFORD
BLACKWELL SCIENTIFIC PUBLICATIONS
LONDON EDINBURGH BOSTON
MELBOURNE PARIS BERLIN VIENNA

Editorial Offices:
Osney Mead, Oxford OX2 0EL
25 John Street, London WC1N 2BL
23 Ainslie Place, Edinburgh EH3 6AJ
238 Main Street, Cambridge
Massachusetts 02142, USA
54 University Street, Carlton
Victoria 3053, Australia

Other Editorial Offices:
Librairie Arnette SA
2, rue Casimir-Delavigne
75006 Paris
France

Blackwell Wissenschafts-Verlag GmbH
Düsseldorfer Str. 38
D-10707 Berlin
Germany

Blackwell MZV
Feldgasse 13
A-1238 Wien
Austria

First published 1993

Set by Excel Typesetters, Hong Kong
Printed and bound in Great Britain
at the University Press, Cambridge

DISTRIBUTORS

Marston Book Services Ltd
PO Box 87
Oxford OX2 0DT
(*Orders*: Tel: 0865 791155
Fax: 0865 791927
Telex: 837515)

USA
Blackwell Scientific Publications, Inc.
238 Main Street
Cambridge, MA 02142
(*Orders*: Tel: 800 759-6102
617 876-7000)

Canada
Times Mirror
Professional Publishing, Ltd
130 Flaska Drive
Markham, Ontario L6G 1B8
(*Orders*: Tel: 800 268-4178
416 470-6739)

Australia
Blackwell Scientific
Publications Pty Ltd
54 University Street
Carlton, Victoria 3053
(*Orders*: Tel: 03 347-5552)

A catalogue record for this title
is available from the British Library

ISBN 0-632-02809-2

Library of Congress
Cataloging-in-Publication Data

Practical renal medicine/edited by
Roger Gabriel.
p. cm.
Includes bibliographical references
and index.
ISBN 0-632-02809-2
1. Kidneys—Diseases. 2. Nephrology.
I. Gabriel, Roger.
[DNLM: 1. Kidney Diseases—therapy.
2. Kidney Diseases—complications.
WJ 300 P8955 1993]
RC902.P74 1993
616.6′1—dc20
DNLM/DLC
for Library of Congress

Contents

List of Contributors

M.Z. Borok MB, BCh, MRCP, *Lecturer in Medicine, Department of Medicine, University of Zimbabwe, PO Box A178, Avondale, Harare, Zimbabwe*

E.A. Brown MA, DM, BCh, FRCP, *Consultant Physician and Nephrologist, Department of Nephrology, Charing Cross Hospital, Fulham Palace Road, London W6 8RF, UK*

D.J.S. Carmichael BSc, MB, MRCP, *Consultant Renal Physician, Southend General Hospital, Prittlewell Chase, Westcliff-on-Sea, Essex SS0 0RY, UK*

L.H. Cope MA, MB BS, MRCP, FRCR, *Consultant Radiologist, South Tyneside District Hospital, Harton Lane, South Shields, Tyne and Wear NE34 0PL, UK*

J.M. Davison MSc, MD, FRCOG, *Consultant Obstetrician and Gynaecologist, Professor of Obstetric Medicine, University of Newcastle upon Tyne, Royal Victoria Infirmary and associated Hospital Trust, Princess Mary Maternity Hospital, Great North Road, Newcastle upon Tyne NE2 3BD, UK*

K. Farrington BSc, MD, MRCP, *Consultant Physician, Lister Hospital, Coreys Mill Lane, Stevenage, Hertfordshire SG1 4AB, UK*

C. Holmes RN, RM, RNT, DipNurs, *Clinical Teacher, School of Nursing, St Mary's Hospital, Praed Street, London W2 1NY, UK*

M.J. Lynch MB, FRCS, *Research Fellow in Urology, Institute of Urology and Nephrology, University College and Middlesex School of Medicine, 48 Riding House Street, London W1P 7PN, UK*

R. Maskell DM, FRCP, *Consultant Microbiologist, Public Health Laboratory, St Mary's General Hospital, Milton Road, Portsmouth PO3 6AQ, UK*

G.H. Neild MD, FRCP, *Professor of Nephrology, Institute of Urology and Nephrology, University College and Middlesex School of Medicine, 48 Riding House Street, London W1P 7PN, UK*

M.E. Phillips MD, FRCP, *Consultant Physician and Nephrologist, Department of Nephrology, Charing Cross Hospital, Fulham Palace Road, London W6 8RF, UK*

G.A. Rose MA, DM, FRCP, FRCPath, FRSC, *Formerly St Peter's Hospital and the Institute of Urology, Cleveland Street, London W1P 7PN, and the Royal National Orthopaedic Hospital, Brockley Hill, Stanmore, Middlesex, UK*

Preface

There are many textbooks on renal medicine, the majority of which deal with academic and theoretical aspects of the discipline rather than the practicalities of the subject. *Practical Renal Medicine* has been written in the knowledge that many registrars and their seniors not experienced in renal diseases have difficulty in adequately investigating, diagnosing and treating renal conditions. The undergraduate curriculum includes little on diseases of the kidney although renal medicine occupies, perhaps, 20% of general medicine. Renal medicine is not an arcane discipline: all medical diseases and many surgical conditions have renal components.

Many of the working hours of renal unit staff are occupied by dialysis and transplantation and the complications thereof. Very little upon these topics will be found in *Practical Renal Medicine* because it has been written for a different readership. The approach to renal medicine taken in this book assumes, much of the time, that renal function has not fallen below a glomerular filtration rate of 15–20 ml/min. There is emphasis upon how to avoid iatrogenic complications of renal disease, which remain frequent.

In writing *Practical Renal Medicine* the 13 authors have concentrated upon common renal conditions. Little space has been devoted to rare disorders or syndromes. There is some emphasis on when patients should be referred to a renal physician, but many of the conditions can be dealt with adequately in the patient's local hospital.

Detailed and sometimes complex investigations are essential to making renal diagnoses, as in any other aspects of internal medicine. For this reason there are five chapters devoted almost exclusively to renal investigations and many others emphasize this aspect. No photomicrographs of glomeruli will be found for the following reasons: however good the reproduction, they bear a poor resemblance to the views obtained down a microscope. To gain an adequate appreciation of renal morphology, months of slide scanning are essential; a few pictures teach little. In glomerulonephritis the interstitium and blood vessels may contain much information which needs to be assessed to gain an adequate interpretation of overall morphology – illustrations cannot convey such a global view. Finally, photomicrographs of renal tissue remind the experienced but probably help the novice little; for these reasons they belong to a text dealing specifically with renal histopathology.

As on previous occasions, I owe my grateful thanks to Wendy Rutherford, my secretary, for dealing with correspondence, typing, word-processing and photocopying the manuscript: without her assistance these lengthy tasks would not have been completed. In particular, the long periods while the text was recast were made possible by Wendy Rutherford's indefatigable industry and secretarial expertise. Her contribution began in St Mary's Hospital, London, and was finished between power cuts in drought-stricken Zimbabwe. I cannot thank her enough. I should also like to thank the contributors to this book for their prompt contributions, the detailed knowledge of their subjects and their tolerance of my editorial activities.

I gratefully acknowledge and thank Her Majesty The Queen for permission to reproduce Leonardo da Vinci's *Anterior view of a male torso showing genitourinary system*, the original of which is housed in Her Majesty's Library at Windsor Castle. Messrs Glaxo made a generous donation to support the printing and publication of the frontispiece.

Finally, I am happy to thank Messrs Per and Peter Saugman of Blackwell Scientific Publications, from whom the idea for *Practical Renal Medicine* developed over a friendly lunch in an Oxfordshire village.

Roger Gabriel
Harare, Zimbabwe

Chapter 1
Clinical Presentation of Renal Disease

Roger Gabriel

As in other branches of medicine, many provisional renal diagnoses are rapidly made from the history before physical examination or investigations have been performed. A proportion of diagnoses rest upon precise and at times complex detailed hospital investigation, the patient having few, if any, symptoms or signs. Because there is the risk of minimizing or omitting an adequate history or examination, this book begins with a short chapter on the presentation of renal disease and some of the attendant physical signs. There is much overlap in clinical and pathological features of renal diseases. Certain renal syndromes have been recognized for centuries but have been more clearly documented and classified as renal medicine emerged as a separate discipline.

An effort has been made here to place the syndromes in approximate frequency of clinical importance in Western European hospital practice in renal medicine. They comprise:

- Chronic renal failure (CRF).
- Acute renal failure (ARF).
- Hypertension.
- Asymptomatic proteinuria and persistent urinary abnormalities.
- Nephrotic syndrome (NS).
- Urinary tract infection (UTI).
- Acute nephritis.
- Obstructive nephropathy.
- Renal stones.
- Rapidly progressive renal failure (RPRF).
- Loin pain–haematuria (LPH) syndrome.
- Renal tubular defects.

Renal syndromes

Chronic renal failure

Chronic renal failure comprises a group of overlapping syndromes which, to varying degrees, may affect any body system. It is useful to classify the functional changes of CRF into four stages (Fig. 1.1) although there are no sharp distinctions between each stage.

1 *Reduced renal reserve.* This extends from normal renal function to over 50% of loss of glomerular filtration rate (GFR). The duration of this asymptomatic period is usually measured in years but is not often documented.

2 *Renal insufficiency.* This phase correlates with a creatinine clearance of about 40 ml/min or less but may last years and is often asymptomatic. The patient may be at a risk of acute decompensation of renal function (p. 253). Serum and plasma biochemical variables begin to become abnormal.

3 *Renal failure.* The clearance is 20 ml/min or less and the majority of patients have persistent malaise. Nocturia is present in all. If the renal insufficiency phase has been very prolonged, osteomalacic bone pain may occur.

4 *Uraemia.* Patients are persistently unwell, anaemic, acidotic, hypocalcaemic, hyperphosphataemic and probably hyperkalaemic. The

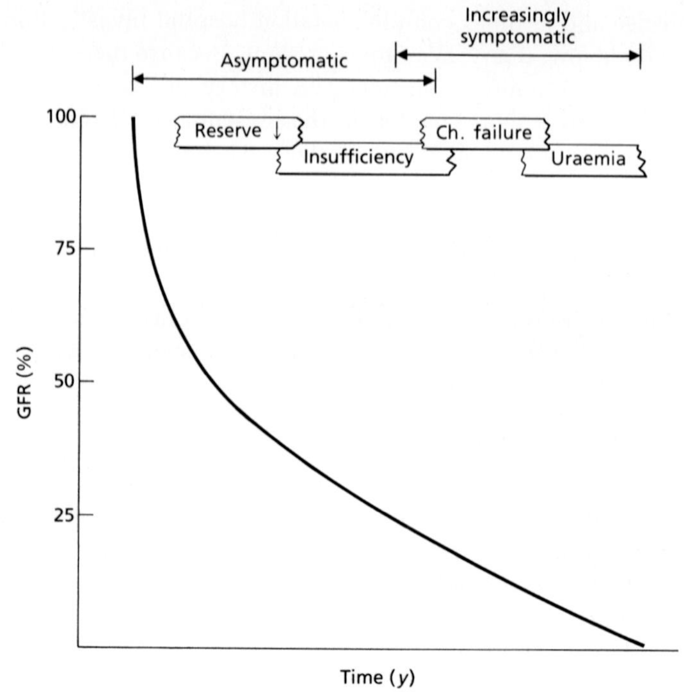

Fig. 1.1 The gradual loss of glomerular filtration rate (GFR) over years showing approximate stages of increasing renal failure with increasing symptoms. Ch., Chronic.

kidneys are 8 cm or less in bipolar length, except in the case of polycystic disease or bilateral hydronephrosis.

Causes, clinical features and management of this syndrome are described in Chapters 14 and 15, pp. 198 and 214.

Acute renal failure

Classically the clinical course of ARF is divided into onset, followed by oliguric and then diuretic phases. With correct fluid balance during the oliguric phase, the diuretic phase is much less dramatic than originally described. In polyuric ARF urine volume may not become subnormal after the onset and may be increased. This diagnosis is usually delayed because the normal or increased volume of urine gives a false impression to the clinician.

There are many different causes of ARF and there is therefore no uniform clinical picture. Patients' illnesses vary from being moderately ill to critically sick with multiple organ failure. The mortality of this latter group is considerable.

There are good data to support the following mortalities:

1	Kidneys alone involved	10%
2	Kidneys and lungs (ventilation necessary)	50%
3	Kidneys, lungs and heart (ionotropic support)	>80%
4	Kidneys, lung, heart and liver (jaundice)	>90%

Acute renal failure not infrequently occurs in patients who have pre-existing GRF. This is referred to as acute on chronic renal failure. Chronic renal failure may be first diagnosed in this circumstance or after the acute element has receded. The topic is covered in Chapter 17, p. 252.

Biochemical evidence of the diagnosis of ARF primarily rests upon a reduced and falling GFR over hours or days with, if available, evidence that the GFR was previously normal before the precipitating cause. Hyperkalaemia and acidosis frequently occur.

Causes, diagnosis and management of this often fatal condition are discussed in Chapter 16, p. 242.

Hypertension

Investigation and treatment of systemic hypertension have become a discipline in its own right. The practice of renal medicine also requires a sound grasp of hypertension because parenchymal renal disease is very frequently complicated by raised blood-pressure and hypertension itself is a cause of renal damage.

Asymptomatic proteinuria and persistent urinary abnormalities

Persistent urinary abnormalities include proteinuria (<3.5 g daily), microscopic haematuria, leucocyturia and granular casts.

Usually these abnormalities are found at routine medical or insurance examinations. There are no symptoms. Possible diagnoses include glomerulonephritis, interstitial nephritis, polycystic disease, renal tract tumour or nephrolithiasis. The finding of asymptomatic proteinuria (on two or more occasions) is an indication for investigation of the renal tract.

Nephrotic syndrome

There are three features of NS:
1 a sustained proteinuria in excess of 3.5 g/day/1.73 m^2, leading to a
2 hypoalbuminaemia of $<$28 g/L, which results in
3 dependent pitting oedema.
Hypertension, hyperlipidaemia and nitrogen retention are often also present, but are not essential for the diagnosis. Nephrotic syndrome is not a specific diagnosis. The majority of such patients require a renal biopsy for histological diagnosis.

The severity of the oedema is only very roughly related to the degree of proteinuria and of itself carries little prognostic information. The distribution of oedema in adults is largely gravitational; for example, periorbital oedema diminishes in a few hours after rising. Knee effusions in NS are common, ascites infrequent and pleural effusions uncommon. For unknown reasons, in childhood nephrotics, ascites is prominent and peripheral oedema less obvious than in adults.

There are many possible complications of NS, the most potentially dangerous being hypercoagulability: arterial or venous thromboses may occur. Renal vein thrombosis is well recognized but infrequent. It most commonly occurs in the NS accompanying membranous glomerulonephritis.

Urinary tract infection

The symptoms occurring as a consequence of lower tract infection – dysuria, frequency, strangury and urgency – are all well recognized; likewise upper tract features – fevers, urinary or bilateral loin pain, backache and dysuria – require no emphasis. Occasionally there are no symptoms from upper or lower tract infection.

Physical signs of lower UTI may or may not include suprapubic tenderness. Upper tract (renal) infection usually produces one or more of the following: fever, rigors, abdominal pain, loin tenderness and, at times, tender renal cysts. It is unusual not to find signs in a patient with renal infection.

The diagnosis of UTI depends upon culturing significant numbers of pathogenic bacteria – 10^5 or more colonies per millilitre of urine. If symptoms or signs are present and the urine sterile, infection is not excluded. Additional cultures should be set up for acid- and alcohol-fast bacilli (AAFB) and for fastidious bacteria. The topic of UTI is covered in Chapters 7 and 8, pp. 90 and 108.

Acute nephritis

The acute nephritis syndrome constitutes the renal response to acute immune inflammation of glomeruli. Quite characteristic features develop:

1 Haematuria with red cell casts.
2 Oliguria with salt and water retention and perhaps hypertension.
3 Decrease in GFR.

The severity of these events is variable and as such does not carry prognostic information.

There are three groups of conditions:

1 Postinfectious glomerulonephritis (PIGN). This is not a large group. Typically PIGN was described as developing about 10 days after infection with a nephritogenic strain of streptococci. Other bacteria have also been implicated in the pathogenesis of PIGN but it is now quite unusual to find evidence of recent infection.
2 Primary glomerular disease not known to be related to antecedent infection. This includes idiopathic mesangiocapillary and mesangioproliferative glomerulonephritides and immunoglobulin A (IgA) nephropathy.
3 Multisystem diseases. These include systemic lupus, Henoch–Schönlein purpura, infective endocarditis and mixed essential cryoglobulinaemia.

Management of these conditions is discussed in Chapter 10, p. 134.

Obstructive nephropathy

Obstruction to the renal tract is an important syndrome because recognition and correction may avoid the development of CRF. Lower tract obstruction usually presents as a reduced urinary stream, difficulty in emptying, hesitancy or overflow incontinence. These are all more common in men.

Upper tract obstruction is less straightforward to diagnose and less associated with renal colic or recurrent infection. Substantial loss of GFR is often found when a silent bilateral obstructive process is diagnosed. There are no specific symptoms, nocturia suggests renal parenchymal damage. No particular signs are present.

The diagnosis of unilateral or bilateral tract obstruction rests upon plain abdominal X-ray for stones, ultrasound to demonstrate a dilated tract and antegrade pyelography to show the level of obstruction. Computerized tomography (CT) scanning or retrograde pyelography is needed in selected patients. Obstructive nephropathy is discussed on pp. 17, 69 and 116.

Renal stones

A minority of renal stones are due to demonstrable chemical abnormalities of the urine. The long-term management is medical with urological help as required. Nephrolithiasis is discussed in Chapter 19, p. 284.

The need for pyelolithotomy and related procedures has fallen very substantially since the introduction of extracorporeal shock-wave lithotripsy. However, it is becoming clear that a proportion of patients treated in this manner develop hypertension more frequently than age-related controls. Thus continued medical assessment following lithotriptor treatment is desirable.

Rapidly progressive renal failure

The RPRF syndrome develops over days or weeks during which progressive substantial loss of GFR occurs. There is a risk of diagnosing CRF and of the need for urgent investigation and treatment not being perceived.

There is a wide range of possible diagnoses in a patient with RPRF, including arteritis, severe hypertension, toxic nephropathies, acute interstitial nephritides, acute primary and secondary glomerulonephritides and vasculitides. Systemic malaise, at times with fever, is present in some of these patients. Macroscopic haematuria tends to be prominent in patients with RPRF, which may delay diagnosis due to out-patient referral to a urologist. Figure 1.2 is a flow chart designed to assist the diagnosis of RPRF. This syndrome is discussed in detail in Chapter 11, p. 163.

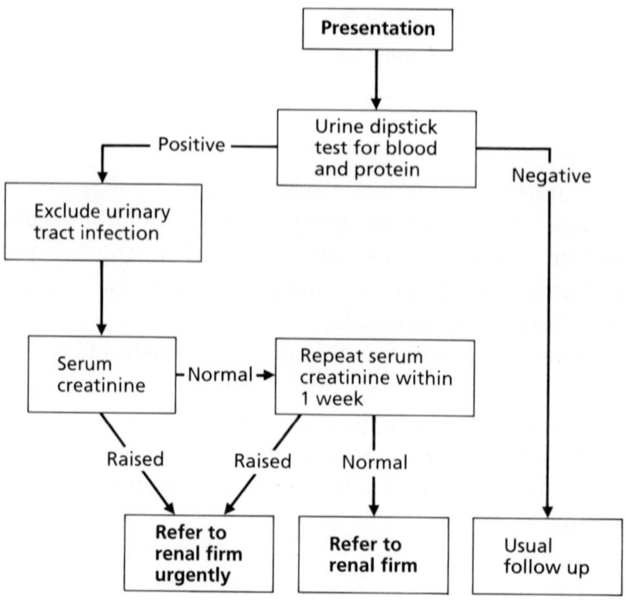

Fig. 1.2 A flow chart showing early management of a patient in whom haematuria suggests the possibility of a rapidly progressive renal failure. (From Cassidy *et al.* (1990), with kind permission of authors and editor.)

Loin pain–haematuria syndrome

The LPH syndrome is a descriptive diagnosis of patients with recurrent attacks of unilateral or bilateral loin pain accompanied by microscopic or macroscopic isomorphic haematuria where no cause can be found. It is more common in young women, and a disproportionate number of patients with LPH have direct or indirect medical connections. When malingerers are excluded and investigations are consistently negative, the label of LPH is applied. Renal function remains normal, long-term.

There is no confirmatory test. Renal histology is normal, differentiating LPH from IgA nephropathy (p. 148). Arteriography reveals very subtle changes in the finer branches of the renal circulation.

Management is long-term and not straightforward. The cause of the pain is unknown. Withdrawal of the oral contraceptive pill benefits some. Pain may be severe and persistent; such patients tend to require increasingly potent analgesics. There is therefore a risk of addiction. Renal denervation to destroy pain fibres has been used, but this usually only provides temporary relief.

Nephrectomy has been performed for those whose lives are much disrupted by pain, but pain has been described as then developing in the contralateral organ. In a small number of fully assessed patients with LPH, autotransplantation – transferring the kidney from the normal position to the iliac fossa – achieves permanent renal denervation and hence pain relief. Such surgery is only appropriate to a very small subset of LPH patients. Psychological assessment before such surgery is essential.

Renal tubular defects

Renal tubular defects are divided into two groups: anatomical and functional.

1 *Anatomical tubular defects.* These include isolated renal cysts, polycystic disease, medullary cystic disease and medullary sponge kidney diseases. Overlapping forms are recognized.

Whilst investigating an asymptomatic urinary abnormality, a UTI or a patient with hypertension, an ultrasound study or intravenous urogram (IVU) leads to, or towards, the diagnosis.

2 *Functional tubular defects.* These are rare conditions in which at onset there is a specific loss of one or more tubular functions while GFR remains normal. These defects may be subdivided into those which cause:

(a) excretion of substances which are not normally present in urine – glucose in renal glycosuria;

(b) excessive excretion of substances which are normally found in urine – cystine in cystinuria;

(c) failure of reabsorption of substances leading to an increased tubular clearance – phosphate, glucose and amino acids in Fanconi's syndrome are a good example;

(d) an inability to acidify—hydrogen ions in renal tubular acidosis.

From the above classification it is clear that there is a very wide range of possible presentations of these chronic disorders. Some are referred to in the text but, because of the rarity of many, discussion of them is only found in reference books of renal medicine.

Examination of urine

Testing of urine by the use of dipstick is essential in all new patients whether a renal disease is suspected or not. If a person is healthy and normotensive and the urine is normal in colour and clarity and negative to dipstick testing, the probability of a renal abnormality is low.

Microscopy

It is unnecessary to examine the urine of all patients microscopically. It is often difficult to find a suitable functioning microscope in a ward side-room. The indications for urine microscopy are:

1 Suspected urinary tract infection.

2 Haematuria on chemical testing: to judge whether the erythrocytes are of glomerular or non-glomerular origin.

3 With experience, microscopy of urine from a nephritic patient adds to understanding the tempo of the case.

There is disagreement as to whether or not urine should be centrifuged before microscopy. It is probably unimportant provided that the doctor or technician is practised in the observations gained after one or other technique. If centrifugation is used, it should not be prolonged because there is a danger of destroying the cellular constituents of urine.

For leucocyte microscopy it is as straightforward to count using a counting chamber as to employ a slide and cover-slip. A counting chamber gives a quantitative result: more than 2000 white cells per millilitre is pathological and often numbers are substantially in excess of this. Using a slide and cover-slip, a count of more than two cells per high-power field represents a quantitative count greater than 2000 cells per millilitre.

Urinary erythrocytes of glomerular origin are crenated and best demonstrated by phase-contrast microscopy; red cells from elsewhere are of normal configuration. It may be impossible or inconvenient to have access to a phase-contrast microscope. Coulter-counters can be used to examine urinary red cells by determining red blood cell volume distribution curves. Glomerular and non-glomerular erythrocytes can usually be easily distinguished. It is not important whether urine is centrifuged or not.

Casts

Casts form when Tamm Horsfall glycoprotein gels in tubular lumens. If excreted without the adherence of any cellular constituent, they are referred to as hyaline casts and are a normal urinary constituent. Increased excretion occurs in fever, following exercise and, in particular, after loop diuretics.

Leucocytes, erythrocytes, renal tubular epithelial cells, fat droplets, oval fat bodies and crystals, singly or in any combination, may adhere to hyaline casts, reflecting cellular and particulate excretion within nephrons. In practice, granular, red cell and white cell casts are easy to recognize. Granular casts reflect interstitial and nephron damage. Red cell casts occur in association with glomerular bleeding, which is tantamount to diagnosing a nephritis. Leucocyte casts reflect acute or chronic pyelonephritis but may occasionally be seen in the presence of acute glomerular inflammation.

Assessment of haematuria

The cause of haematuria may be suggested by symptoms which accompany it. Haematuria with colic suggests a pelvic or ureteric stone; haematuria with colic and clots suggests a neoplasm of the upper urinary tract; haematuria with dysuria and frequency suggest infection; painless haematuria may indicate a renal tract cancer or a nephritis.

If a patient reports blood in his/her urine or a dipstick is positive, the first step is to verify the presence of erythrocytes microscopically. This has the advantage that casts, if present, will also be noted. If red cells and red cell casts are both present, it is very likely that there is an underlying nephritis. If red cells alone are seen, it is essential to determine whether their origin is glomerular or non-glomerular. Differentiation of erythrocytes from these different sites has been mentioned (p. 8). The remainder of this section will assume that glomerulus-derived erythrocytes are present, as demonstrated by phase-contrast microscopy or by Coulter-counter-generated red blood cell volume distribution curves. In all patients a sample of urine should be sent for culture.

When glomerular haematuria has been demonstrated, it is necessary to determine the position, size and shape of the kidneys, using ultrasound or radiology. Small kidneys suggest a chronic glomerulonephritis or interstitial nephritis while normal or enlarged kidneys are, in these circumstances, suggestive of acute disease.

Haematuria is considered by some practitioners to be an indication for urological referral. This may lead to delay in diagnosis. An algorithm for the investigation of haematuria is shown in the next chapter, p. 15. Generally, haematuria is more actively investigated than proteinuria because more sinister causes are feared.

Assessment of proteinuria

After a second dipstick confirmation that proteinuria is present, measurement of a 24-hour excretion is necessary. Because 24-hour urine specimens are inconvenient to collect and their completeness is always suspect, use of the urinary protein:creatinine ratio (p. 50) may be substituted. The figure obtained closely agrees with the 24-hour excretion of protein. It is generally held that for the following quantities of proteinuria the appropriate management is:

< 1 g daily	observe, consider orthostatic proteinuria
1–3 g daily	culture urine, investigate tract with ultrasound
> 3 g daily	perform renal biopsy

This approach is over-simplified; the following points must be made:

1 At low concentrations of proteinuria, the quantity contributed by normal urine protein excretion (up to 200 mg daily; see Fig. 4.1, p. 49) may be clinically important and it is not possible to differentiate between these modest proteinurias in a routine laboratory. A patient excreting < 1 g of protein daily may be in the process of increasing protein excretion and hence subsequently fall into a different category. While it is true that patients with minimal-change glomerulonephritis rapidly change from having no proteinuria to 10–20 g daily, other glomerular diseases evolve less rapidly.

2 A protein excretion of 1–3 g daily is compatible with a very wide range of renal diseases. Assuming that ultrasound or IVU evaluation of the kidneys is normal, a renal biopsy is required, except in long-standing diabetes, amyloidosis and myeloma. Those diseases which have a proteinuria of 1–3 g with an associated anatomically abnormal kidney include chronic tubulointerstitial nephritis, postobstructive uropathies and analgesic nephropathy.

3 In all patients it is necessary to obtain creatinine clearance or some measure thereof. Patients with CRF (GFR < 30 ml/min) generally have a daily proteinuria of about 1–3 g despite exceptions. As increasing numbers of glomeruli become obsolescent, the amount of protein that can be excreted per glomerulus falls. Conversely virtually all nephrons that are chronically damaged are unable fully to retain all serum protein.

4 Examination of the urine sediment is desirable in all patients before biopsy; an active sediment – one containing frequent cellular casts – reflects glomerular inflammation. Sequential microscopy of sediment reflects in a general manner the activity of a nephritis or response to treatment. An active sediment in the absence of proteinuria constitutes an indication for renal biopsy.

5 Apart from clearance and proteinuria, a series of serum variables should be measured and taken into account when evaluating a patient. Such variables include plasma glucose, serum immunoglobulins, antinuclear antibodies and complement profile. Occasionally diabetes may present with proteinuria and some degree of renal failure; it is poor medicine to make the diagnosis by biopsy.

It is worth emphasizing the importance of requesting the serum concentrations of IgG, IgA and IgM. Often no information of clinical relevance is obtained but, in patients aged 60 or more years with proteinuira, myeloma is a diagnostic possibility. Having reached that diagnosis, a renal biopsy may be unnecessary. In this circumstance, the proteinuria may be the overflow type alone or may be combined with a glomerular pattern (see Fig. 4.1, p. 49).

Further reading

1 de Caestecker, M.P. & Ballardie, F.W. (1990) Unexplained haematuria. *Br. Med. J.* **301**, 1171–2.
2 de Caestecker, M.P. & Ballardie, F.W. (1992) Volumetric analysis of urinary erythrocytes: a standardized methodology to locate the source of haematuria. *Am. J. Nephrol.* **12**, 41–8.
3 Cassidy, M.J., Gaskin, G., Savill, J., Pusey, C.D. & Rees, A.J. (1990) Towards a more rapid diagnosis of rapidly progressive glomerulonephritis. *Br. Med. J.* **301**, 329–31.
4 Chin, J.L. (1992) Loin pain haematuria syndrome: role for renal autotransplantation. *J. Urol.* **147**, 987–9.
5 Editorial (1988) Is routine urine analysis worthwhile? *Lancet* **i**, 747.
6 Jordan, C.D. (1992) Normal reference laboratory values. *N. Engl. J. Med.* **327**, 718–24.
7 Marks, V. (1991) Stick testing. *Br. Med. J.* **302**, 482–3.

Chapter 2
A Urologist's View of Renal Medicine

Michael Lynch

It is important to recognize that there are occasions when, after initial history and examination, a practitioner may have difficulty in deciding whether his/her patient has a nephrological or urological condition and to which clinic the patient should be referred. This is discussed here in relation to haematuria, loin pain and deteriorating renal function.

The renal papilla appears to define the point at which the nephrologist's interest diminishes and that of the urologist takes precedence. For sister disciplines intimately involved in one small group of organs, it is surprising that there should be so few areas of overlap. Nevertheless, there is common ground, particularly in relation to stone disease, infection and renovascular hypertension.

Haematuria

Haematuria may be either macroscopic or microscopic. The distinction between the two is simply a matter of degree, although frank haematuria is more often associated with pathology in the genitourinary tract as opposed to glomerular bleeding. It does not include dipstick haematuria, which is more correctly referred to as haemoglobinuria because dipsticks detect the peroxidase-like activity of haemoglobin and not erythrocytes *per se*. Urine should be microscoped whilst fresh; red cells lyse in stale urine. The main causes of haematuria are shown in the following list:

1 *Urological*:
 (a) tumours;
 (b) trauma;
 (c) arteriovenous malformations.

2 *Renal*:
 (a) glomerulonephritis;
 (b) polycystic diseases;
 (c) renal vein thrombosis.
3 *Combined urological and renal*:
 (a) infection;
 (b) stones;
 (c) loin pain haematuria syndrome.
4 *Other*:
 (a) coagulopathies;
 (b) blood dyscrasias;
 (c) idiopathic.

Haematuria is a major symptom for a urologist, having specific implications. While painless haematuria implies a bladder tumour until proved otherwise, the presence of lower tract pain should not lead to a false sense of security: carcinoma *in situ* (a potentially curable but highly aggressive form of transitional cell cancer) was referred to as malignant cystitis because of the associated irritative symptoms and pain. Similarly, pain can occur with renal tumours, particularly if there is haemorrhage into the tumour. Haematuria, whether associated with pain or not, implies a malignancy until excluded.

Enquiries should be made regarding:

1 *Symptoms of outflow obstruction*. This is thought to be of aetiological importance because residual urine may cause an increased exposure to urinary carcinogens.

2 *Cigarette smoking*. This is a common predisposing factor to bladder tumours.

3 *Occupation*. Patients working in the rubber, petrochemical or textile industries may be exposed to bladder carcinogens; such patients may be able to claim compensation.

An interesting but unusual cause of haematuria is an angiomyolipoma. These are hamartomatous lesions made up of fat, smooth muscle and tortuous blood-vessels. Figure 2.1 shows a typical computerized tomography (CT) scan of this condition. The low density of the fatty component of these tumours helps in differentiation from malignant tumours but in some angiomyolipomas the smooth muscle element predominates making the distinction more difficult. Twenty-five per cent present with massive haemorrhage, either into the urinary tract or retroperitoneally, where they can simulate a leaking aortic aneurysm.

Investigation of haematuria

1 Microscopic haematuria must be diagnosed by microscopy. With the use of thimerosal as a preservative, samples may be analysed up to 3 days after collection. Crenated red cells, so called because of their irregular appearance in size and shape, are of glomerular origin. They are detected by phase-contrast microscopy. Isomorphic red cells are of regular size and shape and originate from sites distal to the glomerulus.

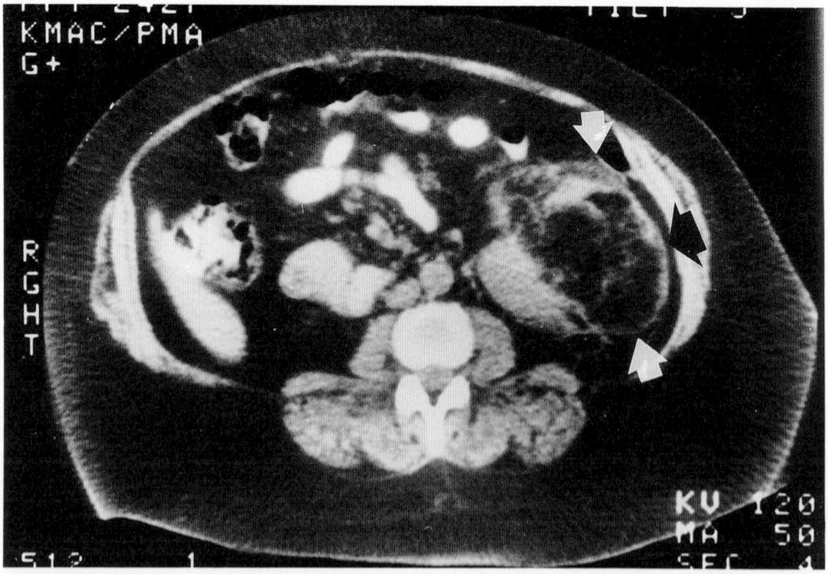

Fig. 2.1 A CT cut showing an extensive tumour (arrow) arising from the left kidney. The low-density radiological changes are characteristic of an angiomyolipoma. Despite the size of the tumour the IVU was normal.

2 A midstream urine (MSU) examination is indicated because tumours are not infrequently associated with urinary sepsis. Also an MSU is a standard investigation prior to urinary tract instrumentation to learn the sensitivities of bacteria, if present.

3 A full blood count (FBC) and film are necessary before any surgical procedure. Anaemia is rarely caused by haematuria. A sickle-cell screen will be necessary in the appropriate population groups.

4 An intravenous urogram (IVU) and cystoscopy are always required. Special precautions are necessary in patients with iodine sensitivity, asthma or myeloma and in those with impaired renal function, who should not be dehydrated (see p. 253). Intravenous contrast agents are slightly nephrotoxic and they may potentiate other nephrotoxic agents.

5 Urine cytology is most useful in identifying patients with high-grade (poorly differentiated) urothelial tumours, but gives no information on the site of the lesion. Cytological studies may fail to identify cancers but are of value when an IVU and cystoscopy are normal.

6 Ultrasound (US) is accurate at detecting exophytic bladder tumours, especially when both transrectal and transabdominal imaging is performed. Ultrasound is not likely to demonstrate small upper tract lesions.

7 If IVU and cystoscopy are normal, US may show lesions such as cysts or angiomyolipomas not diagnosed by the standard investigations. The angiomyolipoma in Fig. 2.1 produced no abnormal findings on IVU despite its large size.

8 Computerized tomography and magnetic resonance imaging (MRI) are better than US for defining lesions and are used for the same types of conditions as US. They have the advantage of being less operator- and observer-dependent than US and can be set to yield reproducible figures defining the density of the tissue being examined. The numerical data may be of value if changes are found during follow-up of patients with equivocal radiological findings. Magnetic resonance imaging has the advantage of not employing ionizing radiation, but high cost limits availability. These imaging modalities also give information about surrounding structures, such as nodal enlargement, which is not available from contrast radiography, and thus have useful advantages.

9 Renal angiography is rarely necessary in diagnosing the origin of haematuria because the rate of blood loss is usually not sufficient for

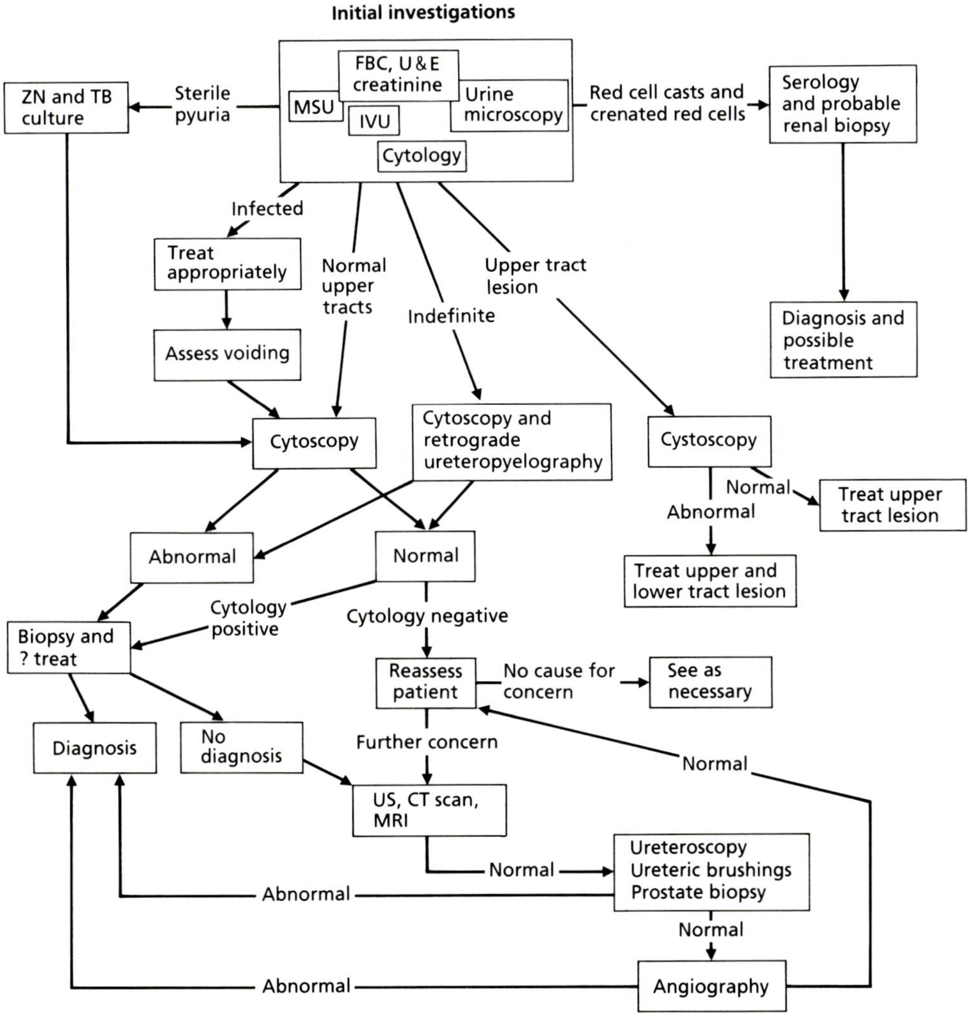

Fig. 2.2 An algorithm of the investigations of haematuria. TB, Tuberculosis; U&E, urea and electrolytes; ZN, Ziehl–Nielsen.

the bleeding point to be identified. Angiography is needed before embolizing a bleeding point where non-operative intervention is desirable; examples include continued bleeding after percutaneous surgery or renal biopsy.

10 Renal biopsy is indicated if red cell and granular casts or crenated red cells are found. This is discussed in Chapter 9, p. 125.

Figure 2.2 is an algorithm for the investigation of haematuria. This is a general guide, not a set of rules. It is worth noting that the lower tract should always be assessed even if a cause for haematuria is found in the upper tract. It is not uncommon for two pathologies to coexist, especially in adults.

Loin pain

The causes of loin pain are similar to those causing haematuria but there are more patients with stones and infections in this group. The main causes of non-renal loin pain are:

1 *Supradiaphragmatic*:
(a) basal pneumonia;
(b) pulmonary embolus.

2 *Subdiaphragmatic*:
(a) biliary colic;
(b) posterior duodenal ulcer;
(c) retrocaecal appendicitis;
(d) leaking aneurysm;
(e) pancreatitis;
(f) musculoskeletal injury;
(g) psoas abscess;
(h) herpes zoster infection;
(i) splenic infarction.

3 *Munchausen*.

Many patients will have no urinary tract pathology diagnosed. It should be remembered that in the elderly patient a leaking abdominal aortic aneurysm may produce non-specific symptoms. Malingerers may present to wards where ureteric colic is treated with opiates. These patients are very plausible and often have factitious microscopic haematuria.

Investigation of loin pain

Because loin pain is often associated with haematuria, the investigations are similar to those of haematuria except that endoscopic procedures are rarely required. Ultrasonography has a greater value in these patients because the cause of the symptoms may be extrarenal, and structures outside the renal tract can be examined.

Urine cytology is of limited value in patients with renal calculi because of false positives. Exfoliated cells in the urinary sediment of patients with calculus disease do not have the appearances of high-grade malignancy, but they may be very similar to well-differentiated transitional carcinoma cells.

An unusual and poorly understood cause of loin pain with haematuria is the loin pain–haematuria syndrome. These patients have recurrent episodes of pain with isomorphic haematuria for which no cause is found. The condition has been outlined on p. 7.

Deteriorating renal function: urological considerations

Obstruction

The most important causes of renal tract obstruction will be outlined. Patients with these conditions may present to doctors in many different branches of medicine.

1 The commonest cause is high-pressure chronic urinary retention with upper tract dilatation. Usually the presenting symptom is nocturnal enuresis in an elderly man. This is due to overflow incontinence. Diagnosis is straightforward because the distended bladder is easily palpable. Management involves drainage until renal function has improved, followed by definitive treatment of the outflow obstruction by surgery, stenting or intermittent or permanent catheterization.

2 Similar pathophysiological events occur in the neuropathic hyperreflexic bladder. The loss of descending inhibitory fibres allows an over-active reflex arc from the bladder sensory fibres back to bladder motor innervation, causing contraction of the detrusor against a closed sphincter. This leads to a hypertrophied high-pressure bladder with back-pressure transmitted up the ureters. Treatment involves either permanent catheterization or intermittent self-catheterization. Occasionally it is necessary to disrupt the bladder sphincter mechanism. Patients who develop upper tract dilatation, due to failure of conservative measures, lack of compliance or improper management, may require ureteric reimplantation in association with bladder augmentation to reduce intravesical pressure.

3 Difficult therapeutic decisions occur when an obstructive uropathy is caused by ureteric involvement by an advanced pelvic malignancy. Such tumours arise from the prostate, bladder (Fig. 2.3), cervix or rectum. Many of these malignancies are obvious on digital examination of the rectum except after an abdominoperineal resection. The guiding principle has to be whether the malignancy is likely to respond to therapy as in the case of prostatic cancer. Internal drainage is usually possible with internal stenting, using double-ended pigtail catheters, which are best placed antegradely at the time of nephrostomy. The dilated pelvicalyceal system of an obstructed kidney is easy to locate by an interventional radiologist. Where there is little chance of the tumour responding to treatment, it is best to outline the prognosis to the patient, who can then make an informed decision regarding active management, if any.

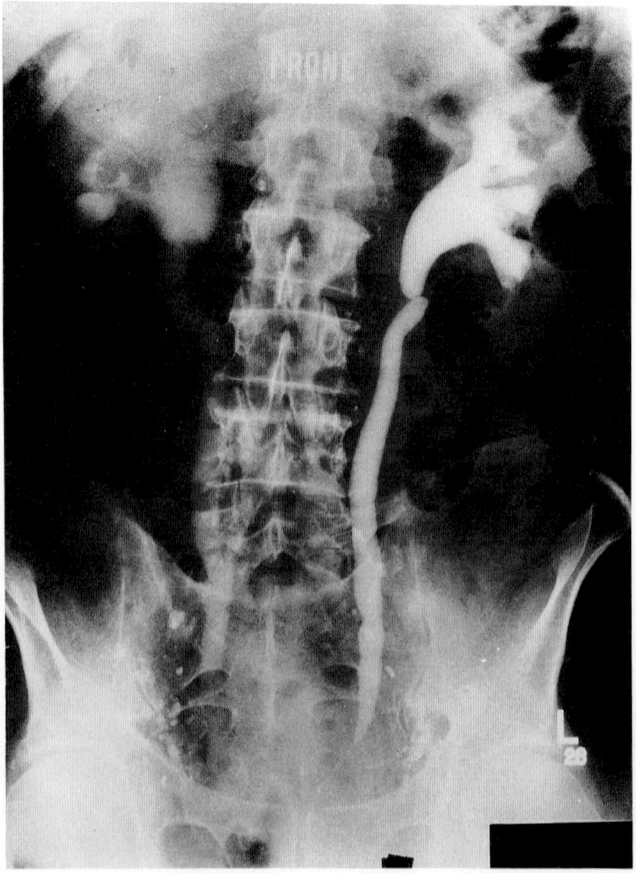

Fig. 2.3 An IVU showing bilateral hydronephrosis secondary to an advanced bladder tumour. The site of obstruction is at the trigone at the insertion of the ureters. Less contrast is excreted by the right kidney, indicating a greater degree of obstruction.

4 Obstruction to the ureters proximal to the vesicoureteric junction is rarely bilateral and consequently dysfunction of one kidney is usually compensated for by the contralateral organ. Congenital neuromuscular dysfunction of the pelviureteric junction (PUJ), often referred to as a PUJ obstruction, is bilateral in up to 33% of patients. Treatment is surgical although minimally invasive techniques are being developed.
5 Retroperitoneal fibrosis (RPF) often involves both ureters. There are four recognized types:

(a) Primary idiopathic.

(b) Secondary to an aortic aneurysm. Retroperitoneal fibrosis in this setting is thought to be due to an IgG-mediated reaction to an insoluble lipid (ceroid) that has leaked through thin-walled vessels.

(c) Due to splinting of ureters by retroperitoneal tumours (Fig. 2.4).

(d) As an unexplained complication of long-term methysergide therapy for severe migraine.

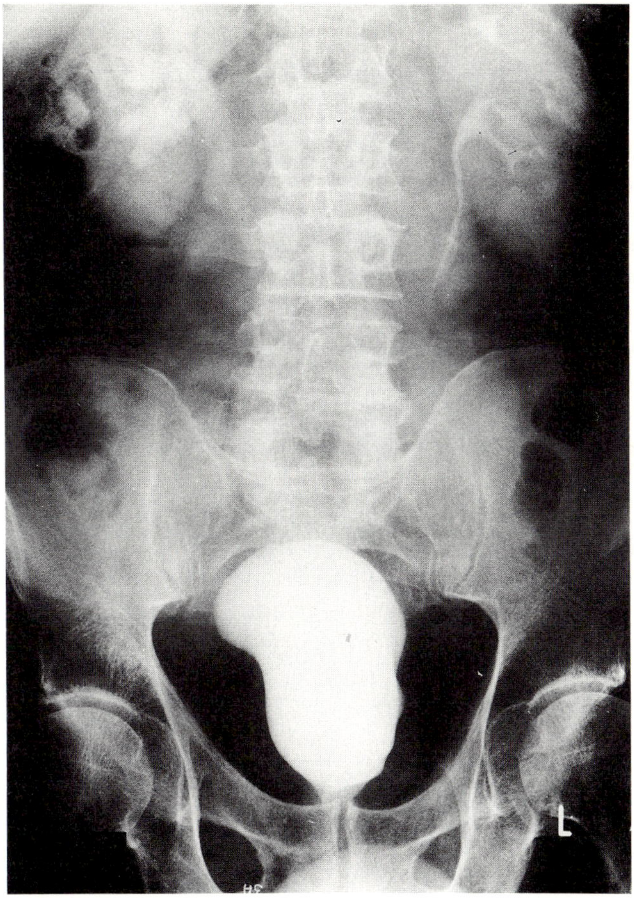

Fig. 2.4 Malignant retroperitoneal fibrosis secondary to a bladder primary. The right ureter is deviated medially by the encasing sheet of tumour. The bladder is indented on the right by lymph nodes. All aspects of the left kidney and ureter are normal.

Often the ureter is not dilated, owing to the encircling fibrosis, and may not appear particularly narrow on antegrade or retrograde ureterograms. Medial deviation of the ureters is often the best clue to the presence of RPF (Fig. 2.4). Computerized tomography may reveal the disease, although it may be difficult to distinguish fibrous plaques from malignant infiltration.

Idiopathic RPF responds well to steroid therapy but some patients may require ureterolysis, where the ureter is freed from its encasing fibrous plaque and then either wrapped in omentum or transplanted intraperitoneally, or both.

Chronic hyperfiltration

The final area of deteriorating renal function that is important to the urologist is reflux nephropathy, where renal function continues to deteriorate despite apparent adequate treatment of the primary condition. This is very disappointing for the patient, who may have undergone major surgery in the expectation that this would protect him from further loss of glomerular filtration rate (GFR).

The accepted explanation for this loss of renal function is hyperfiltration through the remaining nephrons, leading to glomerular cell proliferation and sclerosis. Patients with reflux, obstruction, recurrent infection or loss of more than 50% of GFR (serum creatinine 130–150 μmol/L, or more) should be followed up indefinitely. Regular measurement of blood-pressure, serum creatinine and proteinuria is essential. The management of such patients is discussed in Chapter 14, p. 198, and is the task of a renal physician.

Urinary infection

Urinary infection is a symptom, not a diagnosis. This important topic in urology and renal medicine is discussed at length in Chapters 7 and 8 (pp. 90 and 108, respectively) and elsewhere in the text. Nevertheless, there are additional urological points.

1 It is probably inadequately appreciated that the presence of a foreign body in the urinary tract – a stone or tumour – frequently leads to a mixed growth of organisms. These are often reported as 'contaminants' when they may well be genuine pathogens. In these circumstances, discussion with a bacteriologist is desirable to choose the most suitable antibiotic.

2 The presence of a renal stone may increase the pathogenicity of any organism present. Animal studies have shown that the presence of a silk suture reduced the infecting dose of *Staphylococcus pyrogenes* from 10^6 to 10^2 organisms by impairing local host defence mechanisms.

3 Antibiotics are rarely effective in eradicating urinary pathogens until the stone or stones are removed. Unfortunately, surgical removal or extracorporeal shock-wave lithotripsy (ESWL) may be associated with a bacteraemia or septicaemia.

4 There are a number of factors to be assessed when determining whether there is a urinary tract infection, only one of which is the colony count. Symptoms are important but are subjective and difficult to quantify. Nevertheless, the following can be quantified or identified:

(a) The number of pus cells.

(b) Bacteria detected on Gram or Ziehl–Nielsen staining.

(c) The presence or absence of obstruction, tumour, stent or anatomical abnormality.

If the same organism with the same pattern of sensitivities is recovered twice, this is strong evidence of a genuine infection. Finally, there are patients where the diagnosis of infection is based on balanced judgement rather than on conclusive proof.

5 Symptoms suggestive of cystitis can be caused by any condition that irritates the bladder. These may be either intrinsic – a stone or tumour – or extrinsic – pelvic inflammatory disease. Intrinsic abnormalities may enhance the pathogenicity of organisms present, as discussed above. Extrinsic abnormalities may produce symptoms and can result in pus cells in the urine, which may lead to the patient being wrongly diagnosed and incorrectly treated.

6 All proved cases of repeated infection in women and any single proved case in a man should be fully investigated to determine the cause. Assessment should include the following:

(a) A plain abdominal X-ray to include the whole renal tract.

(b) Ultrasound evaluation of the tract, including pre- and postvoiding bladder volumes.

(c) A urinary flow rate.

(d) Measurement of serum creatinine.

If an anatomical abnormality is found, it should be corrected if possible. Urinary infection should then not recur.

7 Tuberculous infection of the renal tract is not common. Failure to recognize the importance of sterile pyuria may allow renal function to deteriorate until dialysis is required. An IVU may be entirely normal in the presence of active *Mycobacterium tuberculosis* infection. The classical IVU changes of tuberculous disease are only found late in the course of the infection. Treatment of these patients is generally straightforward and is best supervised by a physician who is aware of the dangers of ureteric stenosis during the early months of therapy. Details are outlined on p. 122.

Urolithiasis

Urolithiasis is an area where urology and renal medicine overlap. The medical approach is fully covered in Chapter 19, p. 284. The following points represent essential surgical features:

1 Colic is the most frequent presentation of a renal stone. An emergency IVU is the diagnostic procedure of first choice. Traditionally, opiates were used for pain relief but had the disadvantages of increasing smooth muscle tone, which perhaps slowed the passage of stones, and that the availability of opiates attracted malingerers. It has been found that non-steroidal anti-inflammatory drugs (NSAIDs) reduce smooth muscle tone and are as effective in treating the pain of ureteric colic as were opiates.

2 Emergency surgical intervention in patients with renal colic is essential in two circumstances:

(a) where there is infection proximal to the obstruction, and

(b) if a single kidney is obstructed.

The preferred initial procedure is drainage by the insertion of a percutaneous nephrostomy under radiographic control. At the same stage or later, the stone can be bypassed by inserting a double-ended pigtail stent.

3 The decision to intervene in other circumstances depends on symptoms, stone size, serum creatinine or development of infection. It was held that patients with asymptomatic stones required only regular follow-up. Two major developments have modified that approach. These are:

(a) minimally invasive surgery, that is, for example, percutaneous drainage as opposed to open surgical insertion of nephrostomy tubes, and

(b) the development of ESWL. This technique allows disruption of calculi without the need for invasive surgery. Previously, exposure of a kidney and removal of stones was a major procedure with an appreciable morbidity and mortality.

While ESWL can disrupt the majority of calculi in the renal tract, because it is a new technique the indications when it is the treatment of first choice are still being clarified. Extracorporeal shock-wave lithotripsy is not without some disadvantages, including:

(a) The inception of a bacteraemia or septicaemia.

(b) The possibility of an increased chance of hypertension developing 3–5 years after treatment. Long-term studies with appropriate controls have yet to be reported. At present the patient's blood pressure should be measured at each consultation after ESWL treatment and then annually.

(c) Calculi may not be demonstrated in obese patients if the lithotriptor has only US imaging.

Decisions whether to use ESWL are made more difficult by the fact that some small stones pass spontaneously and therefore require no active treatment. Generally, stones with a diameter of less than 3 mm nearly always pass spontaneously while those over 7 mm rarely do so. As an approximate guide, for every 1 mm in maximum stone diameter the chance of spontaneous passage falls by 10%.

4 The health of the patient has to be considered. Some may be unfit for ESWL or surgery and initially require medical attention.

5 Stone consistency influences therapy:

(a) Infective stones (stag-horn struvite stones) need to be completely cleared before the urine can be sterilized. These calculi are usually debulked percutaneously and any fragments are disrupted by ESWL.

(b) Radiolucent stones, namely matrix, uric acid, cystine and xanthine, are smaller and require different approaches. Matrix stones comprise a gel-like material and do not respond to ESWL. Uric acid stones usually respond to medical treatment (p. 295).

It is possible to rid a patient of cystine stones by prolonged medical methods (p. 296) but in the non-compliant patient extracorporeal piezolithotripsy may be indicated. Because cystine and xanthine stones have a high density and hence hardness, they do not disrupt easily with lithotripsy treatment.

6 The position of the stone influences treatment because of differing accessibility via the ureteroscope by either antegrade or retrograde directions. It may be possible to retrieve a stone to the renal pelvis, where ESWL then becomes applicable. Conversely, a lower ureteric stone may be withdrawn by a ureteroscopic approach.

7 After a stone has been removed, its constituents need biochemical analysis and urine and blood need sampling for a number of variables in the hope of reaching an aetiological diagnosis (see pp. 286–290). Unfortunately, 95% of renal calculi remain idiopathic.

All stone-formers, assuming that their kidneys can excrete a water load, should be advised to make a habit of drinking at least 1.5 L of water daily in excess of their thirst requirements. Nocturia, for them, should be the norm. Such simple advice is often neglected and the chances of recurrent stones increase.

A surgeon's role in renovascular hypertension

The role of a surgeon in renovascular hypertension can be considered under four headings.

1 During some renal operations there is a risk of rendering a portion of the kidney persistently ischaemic, leading to iatrogenic renovascular hypertension. The risk is greatest when performing surgery for PUJ obstruction. During this operation the lower polar branch of the renal artery is within the operative field and thus at risk.

2 Increasingly older patients are now accepted for long-term dialysis. Thus an atheromatous population of patients have been selected for long-term management. Some with severe hypertension will be shown to have uni- or bilateral renal artery stenosis. Selection of those who are suitable for surgery is discussed on p. 218. These patients are best evaluated jointly by renal physicians and surgeons.

3 Fibromuscular renal artery stenosis is an uncommon condition, occurring chiefly in women in their 20s to late 30s. Percutaneous balloon angioplasty of the stenosis has now replaced surgical correction. One advantage of this treatment is that it can immediately follow diagnosis while the patient remains on table in the radiology department.

4 Occasionally, severe hypertension may be diagnosed in a patient with one normal and one small diseased kidney. If an excess of renin is demonstrated from the renal or adrenal vein of the small kidney, destruction of that organ may lead to cure or amelioration of the hypertension. Either nephrectomy or intrarenal arterial embolization of the kidney may be performed.

The topic of renovascular hypertension is not a large area of renal medicine, but is one where physician, surgeon and radiologist have important complementary roles.

Summary

The sister disciplines of urology and renal medicine overlap in surprisingly small areas. At times, the renal physician prepares the patient for urological intervention but the majority of urological practice stands on its own merits. Nevertheless, it is essential for practitioners in both specialities to appreciate the scope of each other's work and know when to consult over, and when to refer, their patients.

Further reading

1 Andersson, L. & Sylvén, M. (1983) Small renal calculi as a cause of renal pain. *J. Urol.* **130**, 752–3.
2 Britton, J.P., Dowell, A.C. & Whelan, P. (1989) Dipstick haematuria and bladder cancer in men over 60: results of a community based study. *Br. Med. J.* **299**; 1010–12.
3 Britton, J.P. (1993) Effectiveness of haematuria clinics. *Br. J. Urol.* **71**, 247–52.
4 Brundig, P. & Börner, R.H. (1987) Clinical results in the treatment of therapy-resistant calcium stone formers with non-steroidal anti-inflammatory drugs. *Eur. Urol.* **13**, 49–56.
5 Bullock, N. (1988) Idiopathic retroperitoneal fibrosis. *Br. Med. J.* **297**, 240–1.
6 Chin, J.L. (1992) Loin pain haematuria syndrome: role for renal autotransplantation. *J. Urol.* **147**, 987–9.
7 Editorial (1992) Loin pain haematuria syndrome. *Lancet* **340**, 701–2.
8 Elek, S.D. & Conin, P.E. (1957) The virulence of *Staphylococcus pyogenes* for man: the study of the problems of wound infection. *Br. J. Exp. Pathol.* **38**, 573–86.
9 Fernandez, J.A. & Carson, C.C. (1989) Calyceal colic: fact or fiction? *J. Urol.* **142**, 257–8.
10 Glowacki, L.S., Beacope, M.L., Cook, R.J., Pahl, D. & Churchill, D.N. (1992) The natural history of asymptomatic urolithiasis. *J. Urol.* **147**, 319–21.
11 Kass, E.H. (1956) Asymptomatic infections in the urinary tract. *Trans. Assoc. Am. Physicians* **69**, 56–64.
12 Novick, A.C., Giphaedt, G., Goz, B., Seccmuller, D. & Tubbs, R.R. (1991) Long-term follow-up after removal of a solitary kidney. *N. Engl. J. Med.* **325**, 1058–62.
13 Pode, D. & Caine, M. (1992) Spontaneous retroperitoneal haemorrhage. *J. Urol.* **147**, 311–17.
14 Riao, P.N., Dube, D.A., Weightman, N.C., Oppenheim, B.A. & Morris, J. (1991) Prediction of septicaemia following endourological manipulation for stones in the upper urinary tract. *J. Urol.* **146**, 955–60.
15 Roth, S., Renge, E. & Ratheart, P. (1991) Microscopic haematuria: advances in identification of glomerular dysmorphic erythrocytes. *J. Urol.* **146**, 680–4.
16 Schreiber, M.J., Novick, A.C. & Pohl, M.A. (1989) The natural history of atherosclerotic and fibrous renal artery disease. *World J. Urol.* **7**, 59–64.
17 Sharfi, A.R. (1991) Presentation and management of urethral calculi. *Br. J. Urol.* **68**, 271–2.
18 Watts, R.W. & Mansell, M.A. (1990) Oxalate, livers and kidneys. *Br. Med. J.* **301**, 772–3.
19 Watts, R.W., Morgan, S.H., Dunpare, C.H. *et al.* (1991) Combined hepatic and renal transplantation in primary hyperoxaluria type 1: clinical report of nine cases. *Am. J. Med.* **90**, 179–88.
20 Yokoyama, M., Shoji, F., Yomagizawa, R. *et al.* (1992) Blood pressure changes following extracorporeal shock wave lithotripsy for urolithiasis. *J. Urol.* **147**, 553–8.

Chapter 3
Nursing Care of Renal Patients

Christine Holmes

In principle, the nursing care of renal patients is no different from that of other sick people. The trained nurse will apply her/his skills and knowledge of the nursing process to develop a systematic approach to her/his patients. This will include assessment, planning, implementation and evaluation of the patients' needs. Application of nursing models to renal nursing will lead to new practical approaches to care in wards and follow-up clinics. Because renal units deal with smaller numbers of patients than a general medical unit of comparable staff members, the renal nurse has a much better opportunity to get to know individual patients. She/he is also able to help in their care over a period of years as they move through different treatments. Knowledge of personal details requires long-term confidentiality. There are many opportunities to assist in patients' psychological and social well-being. Commencing dialysis and later opting for transplantation are major events in the life of a patient with chronic renal failure. The role of the renal nurse at these times may involve acting as her/his patient's advocate, and assisting with making long-term plans. Whilst developing increasing renal failure, some patients lose a degree of independence and need nursing help to maintain an optimistic attitude in the presence of a progressive chronic illness.

Within this contemporary setting, there are essential skills which renal nursing requires. Such care is provided in hospital wards, in out-patient clinics and in the community. The nurses' role in investigation of renal function, the care of the patient with acute renal failure, including peritoneal dialysis, and the care of patients with chronic renal failure until dialysis is required are discussed. Some aspects of a patient on dialysis are covered.

The patient undergoing renal investigations

The nurse who is trained in the procedures used for assessing renal function and structure can prepare the patient more confidently, subsequently care for him/her more competently and help in interpretation of results. Some of these investigations are potentially embarrassing; careful explanation of what is to be expected helps allay fears and, by gaining co-operation, ensures greater accuracy of the results.

Examination of the urine

Examination of the urine is one of the most commonly performed investigations. A random sample of urine is collected in a clean container. Before testing with dipsticks, the colour, clarity and odour should be noted. Abnormal constituents indicate a need for further investigation.

Twenty-four-hour urine collection

It is essential that the complete volume of urine excreted during the 24 hours is collected to ensure reliable results. The patient must be told that loss of even 50 ml of urine invalidates the investigation and that particular care must be taken if defaecation occurs with micturition. If urine is to be collected at home, supplement verbal suggestions by giving the patient written instructions to read at home.

Instructions for a 24-hour collection of urine are as follows:

1 Obtain a suitable container from the laboratory. According to the variable to be assayed, preservative may be needed; urine for calcium assay is collected under acid.

2 If the in-patient is mobile, label a jug specifically for him/her and ensure he/she knows where it is kept.

3 Ask the patient to empty his/her bladder and discard that urine. Note the time on the container. This is the beginning of the save period and it is usually best begun to fit with routine ward practice.

4 Subsequent urine is collected until the same time on the second day, when the patient should micturate at 24 hours ± 5 min from beginning the collection.

5 Send urine, with the appropriate form taped to the container, to the laboratory as soon as possible. Often an aliquot is sufficient: 10 ml of well-mixed urine is sent with a total volume recorded on the laboratory form so that the technical staff can make the necessary calculations. Note that if a specimen is accidentally discarded the collection must be recommenced. In some circumstances a 12-hour collection is acceptable.

6 An accompanying blood sample is often required; this should be taped to the urine container or aliquot.

Midstream specimen of urine

If an infection of the urinary tract is suspected, a midstream urine (MSU) specimen provides urine which is not contaminated by bacteria from outside the urinary tract. The nurse must advise the patient to produce the specimen unaided; most patients are able to do so if given adequate instructions.

Instructions for collection of a midstream urine specimen

The perineal area or penis should be carefully cleansed with soap and water. Antiseptic is not required but, if used, should be throughly rinsed away with sterile water. The patient commences voiding into bedpan or toilet to flush the lower urethra of debris and skin bacteria. A specimen is then directed into a sterile container and micturition is finally completed into the toilet. The container is then sealed and labelled. If the MSU cannot be sent to the laboratory immediately, it should be stored in a refrigerator (4 °C) to prevent overgrowth of any organisms present and disruption of cellular content. (See also p. 91.)

In some units perineal or penile cleansing has been discarded before micturition in the manner described above.

Catheter specimen of urine

To collect a specimen of urine from a catheterized patient a sterile syringe and needle are used. The catheter is clamped below the self-seal port until sufficient urine (10–15 ml) has accumulated in the tubing. The port is then swabbed with alcohol and the specimen withdrawn into the syringe. The catheter specimen of urine (CSU) is transferred to a sterile, labelled container and treated as for an MSU. The clamp on the catheter tubing is then released.

The drainage system should not be broken to obtain urine for culture, because of the risk of introducing bacteria, nor should urine be obtained from the drainage bag, because this is likely to be contaminated. Catheterization of the bladder to obtain urine for culture is very rarely needed.

Renal biopsy

Renal biopsy is usually performed by using a needle biopsy in the ward or in an ultrasound unit, although very rarely an open biopsy may be performed in an operating theatre under general anaesthesia.

Details of renal biopsy are given in Chapter 9, p. 125. It is important that the patient is given a clear explanation of the procedure so that informed consent is obtained and, secondly, because this investigation is impossible without a patient's co-operation. The nurse must be ready to answer questions and give reassurance about what is to be expected. Prior to the biopsy, localization of both kidneys by ultrasound will have been performed.

Blood is sent for haemoglobin estimation, platelet count, coagulation profile and for blood group and save. Base-line recordings of temperature, pulse and blood-pressure are obtained. During the biopsy the nurse assists with preparation of equipment and gives support to the patient.

Once sufficient kidney tissue has been obtained, a dressing is applied to the puncture site and the patient lies supine overnight to reduce the chance of bleeding. Pulse and blood pressure are taken every 15 min for 3–4 hours and then progressively less frequently. The patient is encouraged to drink and urine is tested for blood. Macroscopic haematuria occurs in about 10% of patients and microscopic haematuria in all. Such bleeding resolves over 12–24 hours. If discharged the following day, the patient is advised to refrain from strenuous exercise or heavy lifting for 3–5 days.

Radiological examination of the urinary tract

Various radiological investigations are used to image the urinary tract. Details are described in Chapter 6, p. 67. The patient is prepared by explaining what to expect during the procedure. It is also useful to enquire whether an adverse reaction has occurred to any previously administered intravenous contrast. Following the injection of the contrast, observe the patient for any abnormalities, including respiratory distress, urticaria, unusual sensations or hypotension. After a contrast study, fluids should be encouraged in order to rehydrate the patient and to minimize nephrotoxicity of contrast.

If catheterization or bladder instrumentation has been performed, the patient should be observed for signs of infection and an MSU should be sent.

The patient with acute renal failure

A comprehensive nursing assessment may identify some patients at risk of developing acute renal failure. Careful monitoring of fluid balance may lead to early recognition of oliguria. Because there is no specific treatment of acute tubular necrosis, the patients' recovery depends greatly on the excellence of the nursing care received. The aim of care includes the following:

1 Prevention of infection.
2 Ensuring adequate nutrition.
3 Maintenance of fluid and electrolyte balance.

4 Supporting the patient and relatives psychologically during a very anxious time, which may last 2 or more weeks.

Prevention of infection

Patients with acute renal failure are especially susceptible to infection, and wound healing is delayed. Meticulous attention should be paid to drains, intravenous lines, wounds and all routes through which bacteria can gain access. Bladder catheters should be avoided if possible, particularly in oliguric patients. Uraemic patients may not be febrile in the presence of an infection so other signs and symptoms should be sought and blood and urine cultures sent if the clinical condition is less than satisfactory. Vigorous chest physiotherapy should be instituted with deep breathing, coughing and turning performed regularly. Chest infections are common; sputum should be sent for culture daily.

Ensuring adequate nutrition

Protein at 0.5 g/kg body-weight and a high calorie intake are necessary to prevent protein catabolism. (See Chapter 20, p. 299.) The patient with acute renal failure following surgery or burns needs protein to achieve healing. Dialysis may be employed to allow adequate intake of enteral feeds or total parenteral nutrition. Continuous arteriovenous haemofiltration obviates volume constraints (p. 246). Anorexia, nausea and vomiting are symptoms of advanced uraemia. It is good practice to serve the patient small attractive meals with high-calorie supplements, obtained from the dietitian. Antiemetics 30 min before food help achieve adequate nutrition. If an oral route fails, nasogastric feeding or total parenteral nutrition may be necessary. Repeated oral hygiene is important for comfort and to prevent stomatitis.

Maintaining fluid and electrolyte balance

During the oliguric phase, fluids are restricted to insensible losses (500–600 ml/day) plus the previous day's output of urine in order to avoid positive fluid balance. All intake, including oral and intravenous fluids, together with urine or vomitus should be accurately recorded. If possible, a patient is weighed daily, under standard conditions. Renal nurses assess for signs of dependent oedema, dyspnoea, increased central venous pressure or hypotension. When the diuretic phase is reached fluid intake must be increased proportional to urine volume to prevent dehydration.

Plasma electrolytes are measured frequently. Hyperkalaemia affects normal cardiac rhythm and therefore needs prompt attention. Emergency treatment of hyperkalaemia is discussed on p. 231. For slow control of raised plasma potassium concentrations, cation exchange resins by mouth or rectum may be used. Long-term control of hyperkalaemia can only be achieved by dialysis. If the patient has diarrhoea, hypokalaemia can occur. Sodium intake is restricted to prevent thirst.

Relief of anxiety

Emotional support to the patient and relatives is essential. Uraemia causes confusion, lack of concentration and forgetfulness. Concise, unhurried explanations must be given frequently and, if the patient is confused, orientation to time and place, in addition to precautions for his/her safety, is necessary. Convulsions occur in some, particularly in the uraemic, overloaded patient. Relatives need reassurance that this is a temporary phase having no long-term sequelae.

The management of peritoneal dialysis

For those patients in whom plasma variables and fluid balance cannot be controlled by dietary restriction, peritoneal dialysis (Table 3.1) is necessary. This is a simple procedure whereby a semirigid catheter is inserted under local anaesthetic into the abdominal cavity. Subsequently 1–2 L of warmed sterile dialysate solution is repeatedly run into and drained from the belly. The fluid is allowed to remain in the cavity (dwell time) to allow diffusion of waste substances and then drained out under gravity. This cycle is repeated using fresh dialysate until symptoms and plasma potassium are controlled. The use of a hypertonic dialysate allows the removal of excess fluid. The catheter is removed after 48 hours of use, to diminish the risk of peritonitis.

Special nursing care

1 Strict aseptic technique should be followed when changing or making addition to the bags, to prevent peritonitis. Warmed glucose solution provides an ideal growth medium for bacteria. Peritonitis causes pain, increases serum protein loss and complicates management.

Table 3.1 An example of part of an acute peritoneal dialysis chart. As dialysis proceeds an increasingly negative balance should develop

Name of patient:

Date	Fluid type and volume in	Additives	Time in	Dwell time	Drain out	Volume out	Balance	Cumulative total balance
13.1.93	2000 ml 1.36% glucose	Heparin 1000 IU	10.00–10.10	10.10–10.30	10.30–11.00	1800	+200	+200
	2000 ml 1.36% glucose	Heparin 1000 IU	11.00–11.10	11.10–11.30	11.30–12.00	2160	−160	+40
	2000 ml 1.36% glucose	Heparin 1000 IU	12.00–12.10	12.10–12.30	12.30–13.00	2090	−90	−50

2 Changing a dressing around the catheter should be performed daily, or more frequently if it becomes wet, so that infection and excoriation of the skin are prevented. Leakage of dialysate solution may be due to large volumes or too large an incision when inserting a catheter. Reducing inflow volumes or inserting a purse-string suture around the catheter may seal the leak.

3 Careful monitoring of dialysate balance is essential; the effluent should be accurately measured and charted. A small deficit is usually experienced in the first one or two cycles, but, if fluid continues to be retained after three cycles or is greater than 1 L, then medical help is required. Increasing distress will be experienced by the patient with continued inflow cycles and inadequate drainage. If the patient is fluid-overloaded, solutions with a higher percentage of glucose will be prescribed. Daily weighing at the end of an outflow cycle will indicate overall loss of fluid and should closely correlate with calculated figures.

4 If drainage is slow, check for kinks in the outflow line. If there are no kinks, try changing the position of the patient or raising the head of the bed to improve flow. If there is no improvement, the catheter may need to be repositioned to correct drainage. Slow infusion of dialysate usually implies that the catheter has become blocked with fibrin. The addition of heparin (1 ml of 1000 IU) to each bag of dialysate may help resolve this complication.

5 Each cycle of effluent should be checked: it should be pale yellow and clear. Cloudiness of dialysate or diffuse abdominal pain (or both) suggests peritonitis. If this is found, spent dialysate should be sent for urgent microscopy, cell count and culture. Intraperitoneal or parenteral antibiotics will be required if infection is present.

6 All patients should be asked to cough and carry out deep breathing exercises to prevent retention of lung secretions. A supine position for peritoneal dialysis is unnecessary and undesirable. Patients can be nursed sitting and, as they improve, it is usually possible for them to sit out of bed for short periods whilst dialysis is continued.

7 Attention should be paid to the patient's skin and pressure areas. Good hygiene and frequent changes of position will prevent skin breakdown.

8 Abdominal pain experienced by the patient may be caused by cold dialysate, hypertonic solutions or pressure from the catheter tip on a viscus. Occasionally pain may be referred to the shoulder-tip. Abdominal discomfort usually subsides very quickly and the patient should be reassured.

9 Dialysate bags should always be warmed, using dry heat, on a heating pad or in a warm cupboard.

The patient with chronic renal failure

Advanced chronic renal failure affects all body systems. Consequently, a thorough assessment of the patient's needs and fears, together with careful planning and care, is necessary if he/she is to maintain optimum health and he/she and his/her family are to cope with the many effects of the condition. The nurse should enquire about how much the patient knows of his/her disease and the consequences. When taking a social history, attempt to gain an idea of how the patient coped with previous illnesses and the support he/she expects from family and friends. This will help indicate how he/she may cope with his/her illness and what form of treatment may be the most suitable.

Gastrointestinal disturbances

Anorexia, nausea and vomiting often prompt a medical consultation. The patient's weight compared with his/her normal weight is of help in assessing overall health, although if fluid retention is present the actual weight will be obfuscated. Inspection of the mouth may reveal bleeding gums or stomatitis. Enquire if there have been changes in taste and note if there is a uraemic odour in the breath. Oozing can occur anywhere in the intestinal tract; therefore faeces and vomitus should be checked for the presence of blood.

Changes in elimination

Changes in patterns of micturition are common – nocturia, polyuria or oliguria, depending on the stage of renal impairment. A specimen of urine should be tested for abnormalities; some proteinuria is almost invariably present. If there is any possibility of an infection, urine should be sent for culture. Either constipation or diarrhoea may occur in a uraemic patient.

Condition of the skin

The skin should be examined for bruising, scratch marks or excessive dryness. Uraemic itching can become intolerable and scratches may become infected. Oedema may be present in dependent parts of the body, increasing the risk of skin breakdown and, if severe, limiting mobility.

Fatigue

Progressive anaemia causes increasing tiredness and dyspnoea of exertion. Sleep may be disturbed by 'restless legs', night cramps or nocturia. Ask if the usual work and social activities are still possible.

Mental changes

The patient or his/her family may have noticed increasing difficulty in concentration, irritability and possibly withdrawal. With advanced uraemia, confusion, fits and eventually coma ensue.

Changes in sexual function

Many patients welcome a discussion during which anxieties concerning their sex life can be frankly discussed. In uraemic men potency and fertility may be impaired and in women there is a decrease in libido, reduced fertility and, in some, amenorrhoea. These difficulties are often exacerbated by anxiety concerning treatment and prognosis.

Cardiovascular abnormalities

Blood-pressure should be measured lying, sitting and standing and the patient asked about any hypotensive medication. Headaches and dizziness may be related to high blood-pressure or hypotension. It is essential, when planning care for patients with a chronic illness, that they are involved at all times, because their co-operation is essential if a satisfactory quality of life is to be achieved. Teaching self-care is a major nursing aim.

Fluid and electrolyte balance

At first, measure and record all fluid intake and output. Then encourage the patient to undertake this for him/herself; specimens are less likely to get lost in this way. Weigh the person daily, at the same time each day. Ensure that the prescribed fluid intake is adhered to, because when the kidney loses concentrating ability it is important that dehydration and fluid overload (if urine output diminishes) do not occur. Sodium intake may be reduced, in which case the free use of other condiments, spices and flavourings to enhance the taste of food is to be encouraged (Table 3.2).

Maintaining adequate nutrition

It is well worth trying to tempt the appetite with small, attractively served meals. The mouth should be kept clean and free from infection by offering frequent mouthwashes and advising the use of a soft toothbrush to prevent bleeding gums. Cold drinks are often palatable. An

Table 3.2 Aid in planning a restricted fluid intake

1	Plan fluids to last throughout the day
2	Ask about favourite drinks, which will be the most refreshing
3	Use small cups
4	If ice-cubes are offered, count them as part of total fluid allowance
5	Offer frequent mouthwashes or clean the teeth if mouth feels dry
6	Try sucking boiled sweets or chewing gum
7	Avoid preserved foods, which increase thirst
8	If the water jug is left at the bedside, fill it only with the total daily allowance and discard an appropriate amount if other drinks are taken; this gives a visual reminder of fluid allowance remaining

intramuscular antiemetic 30 min before meals may be useful if nausea is troublesome. Calorie supplements and meal replacements should be obtained from a renal dietitian.

Maintaining personal hygiene

The oedematous person should be protected from developing pressure sores by frequent turning with protection of pressure points. Itching skin can be extremely distressing and refractory to oral antipruritics. Application of calamine lotion or bicarbonate used in the bath water can be helpful, or, if the skin is very dry, rubbing in a lotion can be soothing. The nails should be kept short to reduce the danger of excoriation when scratching.

Adequate rest and activity

Make a point of planning sufficient rest during the day, particularly if night sleep has been lost. To prevent muscle wasting and improve feelings of well-being a programme of regular exercise within the patient's capabilities should be encouraged. Severe oedema in the feet and legs can make walking difficult, particularly if shoes do not fit. Therefore the patient's legs should be raised when sitting out of bed and leg exercises encouraged. Explain to relatives and friends that patients tire easily, so that the length of visits may have to be restricted.

Blood-pressure control

It is necessary to ensure that adequate instructions are given about taking drugs, and the dangers of discontinuing therapy without medical supervision should be emphasized. The blood-pressure is taken in both the prone and erect position and postural changes are noted. The patient should be warned and moved slowly from lying to standing if there is postural hypotension. All patients should be asked to report any side-effects, which may be related to changing to a different drug. It is important that severe hypertension is not reduced too rapidly as this may have an adverse effect on remaining renal function. Therefore, junior medical staff should be made aware of the potentially harmful effects of potent intravenous hypotensive drugs (see p. 219).

Ensuring safety

It is desirable to create a safe environment for the patient. Speak clearly and slowly at all times, and particularly when giving instructions; ensure that they are understood by asking the patient to repeat the requests. This may be a time when it is desirable for the relatives to be present so that they can reinforce the information, and in addition supplementary suggestions can be given in a written form. Patients should be observed carefully for twitching or changes in level of consciousness. If fits are a possibility an airway and suction apparatus should be available by the bedside.

Preparing for the future

Give the patient and his/her family frequent opportunities to talk about the illness, and answer questions as fully as feasible. Because concentration and memory are often disturbed in ill people, information may need to be repeated. If chronic dialysis is required, it is extremely important that a decision to refer to a renal centre is taken early, because the patient will then have an opportunity to get accustomed to the fact and important decisions regarding the type of treatment can be taken whilst the patient is relatively well. This also means that the period of rehabilitation is shortened (see case histories, pp. 210 and 211). For most people replacement therapy will be considered, but, for some, age or other coexistent disease will suggest that dialysis will not give them a reasonable quality of life.

A few may decide against dialytic therapy. For them renal failure will be a terminal illness and care needs to be taken to preserve dignity and ensure comfort. Rising plasma urea may result in coma and hyperkalaemia may lead to cardiac arrest. Pain is not usually a feature of terminal renal failure.

Short-term care of the patient receiving regular dialysis treatment

Occasionally an established chronic dialysis patient will need to be housed in a general medical ward because of lack of renal unit beds or because of an emergency condition having developed whilst away from his/her main hospital. Such patients will probably have substantial knowledge of their treatment because they will have been encouraged to gain as independent a life style as possible. Because of their training, chronic dialysis patients will have clear ideas regarding fluid balance and diet and may well be suspicious of unfamiliar drugs prescribed for them. This may pose a threat to the non-specialist nurse (and doctor) when such patients are admitted to general wards or seen in accident and emergency departments. Nursing staff will need to use their expertise and maturity to gain the patient's confidence by appreciating that he/she probably knows more about some aspects of his/her condition and management than do the nurses and doctors.

Nursing assessment

The first steps are to find out which method of treatment a patient is receiving – haemodialysis or continuous ambulatory peritoneal dialysis (CAPD) – and when the next treatment is due. For the haemodialysis patient, check the vascular access site for patency and possible signs of

Table 3.3 Methods of access to the circulation for haemodialysis

	Special nursing care
Arteriovenous shunt	
Silastic tubing tied into an adjacent artery and vein and brought out through the skin. The tubing can be separated for dialysis. A dry dressing is worn over the exit sites	Observe for clotting, cold tubing, blood dark or appearing to be separating Declotting should be attempted promptly by an experienced person, which may preserve the arteriovenous shunt Avoid restricting blood flow to limb with tight clothing or identibands Change dressing aseptically, observe exit sites for infection Do not use pins on bandage in case of accidental puncturing of shunt Keep clamps easily available at all times in case of accidental separation of shunt limbs
Arteriovenous fistula	
This is a subcutaneous connection between an artery and vein which allows arterial blood to flow up the vein. Over a period of weeks the vein enlarges so that large-bore needles can be inserted	Fistulae should be observed for patency by feeling a thrill over the anastomosis and listening for a bruit with a stethoscope The limb concerned should not be restricted, the fistula should not be used for routine venepuncture or infusion, nor should blood-pressure be taken in that limb
Vein graft	
This involves insertion of a natural or an artificial vein into a thigh or forearm to connect an artery to a vein	Such a graft is treated as for an arteriovenous fistula
Subclavian catheterization	
This involves insertion of a temporary or permanent catheter into the subclavian vein	It is important to prevent infection by strict aseptic dressing techniques The catheter should never be used for drug or intravenous fluid administration After dialysis the catheter is heparinized to maintain patency

infection (Table 3.3). The CAPD catheter exit site should be checked under aseptic conditions and left under a dry dressing. Noting the weight together with lying and standing blood-pressure will give some indication of the state of hydration when compared with previous figures, which the patient or his/her relatives will probably recall. Look for ankle, sacral or periorbital oedema. Dyspnoea indicates pulmonary oedema or pneumonia, or both. Fluid overload is not uncommon, but dehydration, due to over-vigorous ultrafiltration of fluid during previous treatment or excessive fluid loss, may be encountered. Frequently, this is caused by a bout of diarrhoea and vomiting. If so, there would be complaints of dizziness, symptoms of postural hypotension and loss of skin turgor.

Normal urine output is only 200–300 ml daily and therefore the patient may well not be able to produce a sample for routine testing. If a specimen is provided, microscopy and culture potentially give more useful information than routine dipstick testing, which may be misleading if the patient is a diabetic.

During the early hours of admission of a chronic dialysis patient, it is useful to talk to one of the nursing staff of his/her unit so that:

1 specific advice can be obtained;

2 early transfer can be arranged.

Intelligent, sensitive and professional help given by a non-specialist nurse to a chronic dialysis patient temporarily under her/his care will avoid serious mistakes in clinical management.

Nursing in the renal team

Staff-to-patient numbers are the same in renal medicine as in other branches of medicine but the majority of the nursing staff are Registered Nurses, many with a diploma in renal nursing. The medical care of renal in-patients is often shared between physicians and various specialist surgeons. There are therefore many more and varied roles for nurses in renal wards than in more traditional ward work. Other members of the team include dietitians, physiotherapists, occupational therapists and counsellors. In addition, more time needs to be spent on each patient because of the detailed care many such patients require. This setting provides nurses with the opportunity to get to know their patients well.

With the application of nursing care plans and special nursing techniques, the renal nurse will be recognized in her/his own skilled right, can be creatively innovative and can develop her/his own skills and professional expertise with which to gain additional confidence and maturity. Within a renal ward, a wide range of different techniques and treatments are practised, encouraging the extended role of the nurse. Consultant ward rounds are usually held daily, which enhances a team spirit as various patient goals are planned and achieved. In this environment, the nurse is more able fully to participate in investigation, diagnosis and therapy than a comparable nurse in a less demanding setting. Further, she/he is able to devise strategies for patients who are chronically unwell so that they may enjoy reasonable health. There are important counselling roles with regard to patients awaiting dialysis and transplantation.

Renal trained nurses are essential members of teams treating patients within the whole discipline of renal medicine.

Further reading

1 Gabriel, R. (1990) *A Patient's Guide to Dialysis and Transplantation*, 4th edn. Kluwer Academic Publishers, Dordrecht.

Chapter 4
Chemical, Immunological and Histopathological Investigations

Roger Gabriel

As in other disciplines it is important in renal medicine to select the appropriate investigations and to be aware of the urgency with which the results are required and at what intervals to repeat certain tests. A list of biochemical variables is shown in Table 4.1.

Blood creatinine

The concentration of serum or plasma creatinine (which are identical in value) is the simplest approximation to glomerular filtration rate (GFR). The use of this variable is based on the assumption that, in a steady state and on an adequate diet, creatinine is produced from the skeletal muscle at a constant rate and accumulation is prevented by a constant renal excretion.

It is not widely appreciated that when the concentration of serum creatinine is a little above normal a 50% reduction in GFR has occurred.

The normal range of serum creatinine in healthy adults up to their tenth decade lies between 60 and 125 μmol/L. This range of blood creatinine is very broad and even the experienced physician has to interpret this variable in the context of a specific patient. For example, the concentration of 125 μmol/L may be normal for an 80 kg muscular

Table 4.1 Biochemical variables presented in order of frequency of clinical necessity

Plasma or serum	Urine
Often	
Potassium	Creatinine[a]
Creatinine	Protein[b]
Sodium	
Calcium	
Albumin	
Phosphate	
Bicarbonate	
H^+ ions	
Infrequently	
Urea	Sodium[c]
Urate	Potassium[c]
Osmolality	Calcium[a]
Parathyroid hormone	Osmolality[d]
	Urate[a]
Rarely	
Chloride	Concentrating ability[a]
	Ammonium chloride loading[a]
	Amino acids[a]

[a] Timed samples essential.
[b] Timed sample or random urine with variable expressed in g/L.
[c] Random samples more frequently required than timed.
[d] 'Spot' samples needed; 24-hour osmolality is uninterpretable.

manual worker but would be pathological in a small adult of 45 kg. Blood creatinine must therefore be interpreted in terms of a patient's muscle mass, which can only be judged approximately. Serum creatinine varies little with age although creatinine clearance falls as age advances. An elderly person has less muscle mass than a young adult but because production equals excretion the serum concentration remains virtually identical in healthy teenagers and octogenarians.

Sampling of blood for creatinine assay

There is no known circadian range in GFR or creatinine production; thus for routine clinical purposes blood may be sampled when convenient. Blood should not be withdrawn:

1 after strenuous activity, when serum creatinine is transiently raised;
2 for some hours after a large protein meal, when serum creatinine may be elevated to 70% above normal.

Creatinine clearance

The creatinine clearance test is the traditional measure which is clinically but inaccurately equated with GFR. Clearance is expressed by the formula

$$\frac{UV}{P} \times 100$$

Where U = urinary concentration of creatinine, V = the volume in urine in ml/min and P = plasma or serum concentration of creatinine and is expressed in ml/min. The result may be refined, by the use of tables, to ml/min/1.73 body surface area. This modification is chiefly used by paediatricians.

A clearance study is beset with difficulties:

1 Collection of urine for a set and precise period of time is essential. Such collections are frequently inaccurate even when supervised by trained renal nurses. Completeness of an out-patient collection is always suspect. Usually a 24-hour period for collection is selected; some recommend two consecutive 24-hour collection periods to compensate for errors in collection. Assuming complete bladder emptying and exact timing, a 6-hour collection period is convenient and adequate, as is a urine saved during the hours of sleep.

2 The laboratory must receive urine and blood from the patient together; this often fails.

It is difficult to accept a creatinine clearance value without knowing that the volume of urine was appropriate for the duration of the collection and urinary creatinine concentration. There is always uncertainty as to the completeness of the collection because there is no measure of its exactness.

A plot of serum creatinine against creatinine clearance is curvilinear. What is not widely appreciated is that:

1 when serum creatinine is persistently 15 μmol/L above the upper limit of normal the patient has functionally lost one kidney;

2 serum creatinine concentrations are particularly difficult to interpret when the clearance is 30–45 ml/min because further increases in blood creatinine of 30–40 μmol/L are associated with an additional 15–20% decrease in clearance. This apparent abrupt decline is explained by the curvilinear association between serum creatinine and creatinine clearance (see Fig. 1.1, p. 2).

When is creatinine clearance required?

There are three conditions in which it is essential to know the clearance:

1 When prescribing potentially nephrotoxic drugs that are renally excreted. The aminoglycosides are an excellent example of this indication (see Chapter 21, p. 318). Failure to have estimates of renal clearance if such a drug is prescribed for prolonged periods may be actionable in law if side-effects develop.

2 Functional data are essential in patients with known or suspected renal disease.

3 Likewise clearances or measures thereof are necessary in patients with systemic diseases such as systemic lupus erythematosis (SLE), polyarteritis nodosa and subacute bacterial endocarditis.

When should serum creatinine or creatinine clearance be requested?

A valid argument can be advanced that when a venepuncture is performed on any patient in one of the three groups discussed above a portion of the blood sampled is sent for assay of its creatinine concentration. Because there are often no signs with even substantial changes in GFR, it is virtually impossible to request this assay too often if there is doubt as to the stability of renal function. Blood creatinine concentration should be requested at every out-patient visit and at least twice weekly for in-patients.

A practical approach to clearance measurements

The advantages and difficulties associated with creatinine clearance have been described and the difficulties of interpretation of serum creatinine concentrations have been discussed. The possible wide differences between serum creatinine and creatinine clearance are shown in Table 4.2. Many approach serial assessments of GFR as described above (p. 40) but accurate collection of urine is always suspect and asks much of even well-motivated volunteers for metabolic experiments.

There are two manipulations whereby matters may be simplified:

1 *Linear regression plots.* It has been found by plotting the reciprocal (1/serum creatinine) against time that a linear relationship exists in patients with different diseases. This relationship appears to hold best for patients with chronic tubulointerstitial nephritis. An example of a linear regression plot is shown in Fig. 17.1 (p. 253). Once several points have been plotted, assuming that the patient has progressive loss of GFR then the time for dialysis can be predicted to within a few months. This technique has not been widely adopted, perhaps because those with experience of advancing chronic renal failure are able adequately to interpret the concentrations of increasing serum creatinine.

2 *Use of formulae.* Because the concentration of serum creatinine is closely related to skeletal muscle mass, body-weight is also related to

Table 4.2 Approximate relationships between serum creatinine and creatinine clearance

Serum creatinine (μmol/L)	Creatinine clearance (ml/min)	Degree of renal failure
60–120	120–80	Normal
130–150	80–40	Reduced reserve
160–250	40–20	Chronic failure
260–600	20–10	Uraemia
900–1500	<3	Terminal

Note the wide range of serum creatinine corresponding to different clearance values, especially when clearance is between 20 and 40 ml/min. When serum creatinine is 700 μmol/L or more, there is little need to request a clearance. Compare with Fig. 1.1, p. 2.

this variable. A person's weight can be accurately and quickly measured. This favourably contrasts with the length of time necessary to collect urine and the inherent and unknowable inaccuracies thereof.

Various formulae have been advanced which take into account the patients' age, weight, sex and blood creatinine concentration. The best to date is the following:

$$\frac{88(145 - \text{age})}{\text{Serum creatinine}} \times \frac{\text{Weight}}{70} - 3$$

where age is measured in years, weight in kilograms and creatinine in μmol/L. In women the constant 88 is replaced by 75. Results are expressed as ml/min/70 kg body-weight.

For adults of 50–75 kg body-weight, calculated clearance very closely correlates ($r = 0.95$) with a creatinine clearance of the same patient, using the same sample of blood for use in both calculations. However, the formula over-reads in adults more than 80 kg in weight and has yet to be modified for these subjects. In addition, its validation in cyesis and childhood is awaited.

Results from departments of clinical chemistry are processed and printed by computer; it is therefore easy to write a short program which can be used in the generation of calculated creatinine clearance. A final advantage is that, in principle, clearance equivalents can be available, day or night, within half an hour of sampling blood. Nevertheless, when the concentration of serum creatinine is changing rapidly, no clearance or estimate thereof is an accurate reflection of GFR because conditions are not physiological.

Conclusion

Creatinine clearance is the single most frequently required test of renal function. Unfortunately, the results reported from a laboratory are often wrong due to incomplete or over-collection of urine. Additionally, experienced physicians may have occasional difficulty in interpreting a serum creatinine value – even with knowledge of clinical circumstances. For these reasons, GFR is best assessed by the values of both creatinine and estimated clearance.

More important than the single correct figure of creatinine or creatinine clearance is whether renal function is stable or changing and, if so, at what rate. For these reasons repeated measures of serum creatinine and estimated clearance are essential to the practice of renal medicine.

Indications for measuring plasma urea

Conventionally the concentration of plasma urea is held to have a useful relationship to GFR. Unfortunately, this is a misconception because blood urea is altered by diet, fever, gastrointestinal haemorrhage, renal blood flow and urine flow rates. Urea is frequently measured because it is automatically assayed when the concentrations of plasma sodium and potassium are requested. The concentration of plasma urea is often difficult to interpret adequately. A good case can be made for abandoning the routine assay of this variable but there are two principal conditions where plasma urea concentrations remain of value:

1 In assessing the effect of, and adherence to, a reduced protein diet in stable chronic renal failure. When a patient reduces protein intake to 0.4–0.5 g/kg body-weight/day (p. 300), plasma urea should fall by about 15–20 mmol/L from concentrations measured shortly before beginning the diet. Failure to comply is easily noted.

2 Dynamic aspects of acute renal failure are usually assessed by the concentrations of plasma urea. The urea concentration together with other variables gives an indication when dialysis is required.

Plasma potassium

Because of ample renal functional reserves, plasma potassium concentrations vary modestly with dietary intake. Physical signs only develop in extremes of hyper- or hypokalaemia; hence repeated requests for this variable are necessary in many different clinical conditions.

Potassium is the major intracellular cation; total body potassium is approximately 3000 mmol in a 70 kg subject. For practical reasons, plasma potassium is the only feasible measure of potassium status, although only a small quantity of this electrolyte is available for direct sampling and there is debate as to whether plasma potassium is an adequate measure of total body potassium. There is a tendency for plasma potassium to be lower in women than men: this is unexplained.

Hypokalaemia

Low plasma potassium (< 3.5 mmol/L) is the most common electrolyte abnormality. There are a number of causes and the most important, in approximate order of frequency of occurrence, are:

1 *Renal causes*:
  (a) Diuretics – easily the most common.
  (b) Steroid therapy – common.
  (c) Hyperaldosteronism: (i) pregnancy; (ii) diuretic therapy; (iii) congestive heart failure; (iv) vasodilator therapy; (v) cirrhosis; (vi) nephrotic syndrome; (vii) accelerated hypertension.

2 *Gut causes*:
  (a) Prolonged aspiration of stomach contents or vomiting.
  (b) Prolonged diarrhoea.
  (c) Purgative addiction.

Hyperkalaemia

Hyperkalaemia is common in renal units but less so in a general medical population. Any blood potassium concentration above the upper limit of normal (5.0 mmol/L) is hyperkalaemic but the tempo at which the concentration is changing is important. There are relatively few causes of hyperkalaemia and they may be classified as follows:

1 *Renal*:
   (a) Acute renal failure (GFR < 0.5 ml/min).
   (b) Advanced chronic renal failure (GFR < 3 ml/min).
   (c) Amiloride, triamterine
   (d) Angiotensin-converting enzyme (ACE) inhibitors
   (e) Potassium supplements
   } if given in the presence of poor renal function.
2 *Acid–base disturbances*:
   (a) Metabolic acidoses such as untreated diabetic ketoacidosis and acute renal failure.
   (b) Respiratory alkaloses: hyperventilation.

A common cause of hyperkalaemia in patients with advanced renal failure is injudicious ingestion of food or fluid that has a high potassium content. Such substances include instant coffee, chocolate, chips, mushrooms, nuts, dried fruit and bananas.

Potassium and creatinine are the two most frequently required biochemical variables in the practice of renal medicine. In out-patient work with patients with stable or modestly declining function, the plasma and serum concentrations of potassium and creatinine respectively may well be the only assays needed.

Sampling of blood for plasma potassium assay

Haemolysed blood is unsuitable for analysis because it is not possible to differentiate between red blood cell potassium and plasma potassium. If there is likely to be delay in transit of the sample from ward to laboratory, plasma and cells should be separated. Unfortunately, centrifuges are rarely found in wards. Little change in plasma potassium concentration occurs if the sample is stored at room temperature for up to 6 hours. Potassium extrudes from cells at 0.5–1 mmol/hour if stored at 4 °C.

Plasma sodium

Like potassium, plasma sodium is frequently assayed and very often is normal in concentration (135–145 mmol/L). Unlike potassium, the intracellular concentration of sodium is low (*c.* 14 mmol/L). While the intravascular (4 L) and interstitial (10 L) compartments are of different volumes, the sodium concentration is identical in each. Thus the concentration of plasma sodium is a better guide to total body sodium than the potassium equivalent.

Hyponatraemia (plasma sodium <130 mmol/L) is not uncommon and is much more common than hypernatraemia. The causes of reduced plasma sodium concentrations in approximate order of frequency are:

1 *Pathophysiological*:
- (a) sweating due to fever with inadequate solute replacement;
- (b) over-infusion of dextrose or dextrose saline.

2 *Renal*:
- (a) excessive diuretic therapy;
- (b) osmotic diuresis;
- (c) syndrome of inappropriate antidiuretic hormone secretion;
- (d) advanced chronic renal failure.

3 *Gut*:
- (a) severe persistent diarrhoea;
- (b) small gut fistulae.

It is customary to classify hyponatraemia as depletional or dilutional, as shown in Table 4.3. This is a practical classification of the principal causes of hyponatraemia which leads to logical treatment, particularly if hyponatraemia is the presenting feature rather than a specific clinical diagnosis. Depletional hyponatraemia is associated with postural hypotension and a low or poorly visible jugular venous pressure (JVP). This depleted state is treated with an infusion of isotonic saline, while water and, often, salt restriction are required for dilutional hyponatraemia.

Hypernatraemia (plasma sodium >150 mmol/L) is infrequent,

Table 4.3 Depletional and dilutional hyponatraemia

Depletional hyponatraemia
1 Gastrointestinal
- (a) prolonged aspiration of gastric contents
- (b) vomiting } severe, persistent
- (c) diarrhoea } severe, persistent
- (d) gut fistulae

2 Renal
- (a) excessive diuretic therapy (sodium loss > water)
- (b) osmotic diuresis: diabetes mellitus, chronic renal failure

3 Sweat – with inadequate solute replacement

Dilutional hyponatraemia
1 Excessive intravenous 5% dextrose
2 Excess diuretic therapy (water loss > sodium)
3 Congestive heart failure
4 Decompensated cirrhosis
5 Advanced chronic renal failure
6 Nephrotic syndrome
7 Syndrome of inappropriate antidiuretic hormone secretion

Both depletional and dilutional hyponatraemia are common and usually not difficult to diagnose. Depletional hyponatraemia is treated by an infusion of isotonic saline, while water and perhaps salt restriction is required for dilutional hyponatraemia.

presumably because kidneys are very efficient in excreting sodium. The major causes are:
1 Untreated diabetic ketoacidosis (deficient water intake in an obtunded patient).
2 Injudicious total parenteral nutrition, especially if the patient has pre-existing renal impairment.
3 Treatment of infections with sodium salts of antibiotics in patients with renal failure. For example, sodium fusidate 1.5 g daily contains 40 mmol of sodium.

Calculation of sodium deficit

The amount of sodium required for plasma sodium repletion to 140 mmol/L can be calculated from the following formula:

$$Na^+ - 0.6 \times \text{lean body-weight} \times (140 - \text{plasma } [Na^+])$$

where Na^+ is expressed in mmol/L and body-weight in kg; in women, the constant 0.6 is replaced by 0.5.

The formula will not supply an accurate figure for sodium repletion if there is additional isosmotic Na^+ and water loss, as in excessive diuretic therapy or diarrhoea.

Calculation of water deficit

The volume of water required to approximately replete a patient with a pure water deficit is shown by the formula:

$$\text{deficit} - 0.5 \times \text{lean body weight} \times \left(\frac{\text{plasma } [Na^+]}{140} - 1\right)$$

where deficit is expressed in litres and body-weight in kilograms.

No more than half a calculated deficit should be given quickly, even under the control of central venous pressure measurements.

Calcium and phosphate

To avoid repetition, aspects of applied calcium and phosphate metabolism are detailed in Chapters 14, 15 and 19 (see pp. 198, 214 and 284). A formula for the correction of serum calcium concentration to that of serum albumin is given on p. 287. The value of having parathormone assayed is discussed on p. 289. Primary hyperparathyroidism is covered on p. 293 and renal failure-associated hyperparathyroidism on p. 200.

In general renal medicine, hypocalcaemia is only found in acidotic chronic renal failure and associated with the hypoalbuminaemia of nephrotic syndrome. Likewise, hypercalcaemia is not common; if detected in a patient with renal impairment, it is usually explained by an excessive dose of calcium salts, synthetic analogues of vitamin D or often the two together (p. 206). If this explanation of a hypercalcaemia is not applicable in a patient of middle or more senior years, then myeloma or another malignancy should be excluded.

Osmolality

Osmolality describes the concentration of active particles in 1 kg of solvent. Plasma or urine contains many solutes of differing activities. Osmolality is expressed in mmol/L. The figure is usually measured in a laboratory but a reasonably accurate plasma equivalent can be calculated from:

$$2[Na^+] + 2[K^+] + \text{glucose} + \text{urea}$$

where concentrations are expressed in mmol/L. Sodium is the greatest contributor to the above formula and it follows that, if plasma sodium is normal in concentration, serum osmolality will nearly always also be normal. The main exception is uncontrolled hyperglycaemia of diabetes, where plasma glucose may be elevated five to eight times above normal.

Adults eating Western European diets excrete approximately 800 mmol/day of osmotically active material, independent of urine volume. The central osmoreceptor will sense a minor increment in serum osmolality, which will lead to synthesis of vasopressin. Conversely, water intake decreases serum osmolality by 1–2 mmol/L, suppressing vasopressin release.

The indications to measure serum osmolality (normal range 285–295 mmol/L) are:

1 Occasionally in patients with diabetic ketoacidosis to help guide fluid and insulin administration.

2 In patients with acute renal failure to calculate the urine : plasma osmolality ratio (p. 237), which in health is >1.3.

3 At times to correlate with the haematocrit, usually in the course of clinical experiments.

Because osmolality is a measure of concentrating ability, urinary values are generally much more informative. 'Spot' or short-time urine samples are required; a 24-hour urine osmolality cannot be interpreted. Values vary from figures below that of serum (water diuresis or tubular dysfunction) to a maximum of four times that of serum (antidiuresis). The range is around 200–1200 mmol/L. With increasing age, the ability maximally to concentrate urine above plasma falls from 1200 in the teens to about 850 mmol/L in octogenarians.

The indications to request measurement of urinary osmolality include:

1 As an aid in interpreting nocturia. If a patient complaining of nocturia has an early morning urine with an osmolality of 700 mmol/L or more, the possibility of chronic parenchymal disease of clinical importance is excluded.

2 Together with serum osmolality to determine the U/P ratio, as described above.

3 Occasionally to learn of maximum urine osmolality after a period of water deprivation or administration of desmopressin acetate in assessment of distal tubular function.

Proteinuria

Normal urine may contain protein at a concentration of up to 0.2 g daily; more than this is abnormal but not necessarily pathological. The finding of a small quantity of proteinuria (1 g/day or less) has to be set in its clinical context. Proteinuria of 3 or more grams daily is always pathological; excretion rates of 1–3 g/24 hours usually require investigation. The caveats regarding the completeness of a 24-hour collection for protein content apply similarly to those for creatinine but less rigorously. Under- or over-collection are not particularly important because there is no clinical difference between a proteinuria of, say, 7 or 10 g. For simplicity and convenience, random urine may be obtained and the protein content interpreted, with the concentration of serum albumin from blood sampled on the same day as the urine sample. Urine protein concentrations are increased in many renal diseases.

Proteinuria is divided into five different types:

1 *Functional.* This is transient and small in quantity, occurring as a consequence of fever, exercise, lordotic posture or stress. The proteinuria is less than 1 g daily, predominantly albumin, infrequently measured and of no clinical importance.

2 *Glomerular.* This proteinuria is a result of substantial serum protein lost across glomerular capillaries in excess of tubular reabsorptive capacity. An electrophoretic pattern is shown in Fig. 4.1. Albumin is a substantial component but all classes of serum protein can be demonstrated in the urine. In nephrotic patients the serum concentrations of immunoglobulins may fall by 50% because of urinary losses.

Glomerular proteinuria ranges from 1 g to occasionally more than 30 g daily, although a proteinuria in excess of 20 g daily is uncommon. In most patients, when urine protein concentrations are persistently above 5 g daily, peripheral oedema occurs, that is, a nephrotic state has developed. The majority of proteinurias of nephrotic range are glomerular in origin. Protein excretion often varies by 2–5 g daily.

Measurement of selectivity of proteinuria is a measure of the dimensions of protein molecules crossing the glomerular basement membrane and is not indicated in adults because the information gained is of very limited benefit.

3 *Non-glomerular.* Modest (1–2 g daily) proteinuria is found in many renal conditions which do not involve glomeruli. Examples include chronic tubulointerstitial nephritis and acute pyelonephritis. Albumin is the major urinary constituent, together with larger molecules. A similar proteinuria is found in acute and chronic bacterial bladder infection.

4 *Tubular.* This proteinuria is characterized by a prominent β_2-microglobulin peak (Fig. 4.1). Lysozyme is also disproportionately prominent. Tubular proteinuria has a range of about 0.5–2.0 g daily

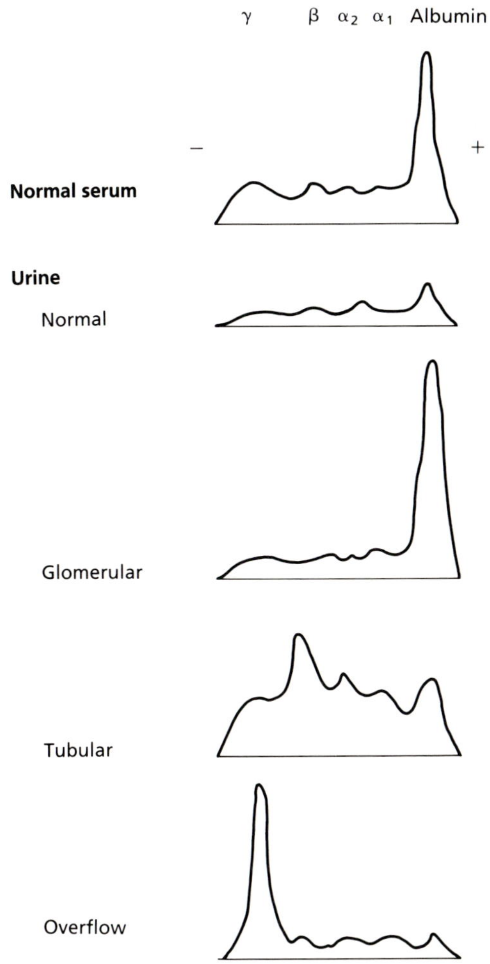

Fig. 4.1 Electrophoretic patterns of normal serum and urine proteins, together with glomerular, tubular and overflow (myeloma-type) proteinurias.

and is found in association with chronic potassium depletion, acute tubular necrosis, medullary cystic disease, Fanconi's syndrome and cadmium poisoning. It is thought that the proteinuria is secondary to impaired tubular reabsorption of low-molecular-weight proteins.

5 *Overflow.* This is a relatively common condition, due most frequently to excretion of an over-production of light chains of immunoglobulins, which occurs in myeloma. Because the molecular weight of a lambda light chain is approximately 22 kDa and tubular reabsorption is quickly saturated, the clearance is high. The amount of light chain proteinuria is often low but may exceed 10 g daily.

This proteinuria has a characteristic behaviour of precipitating and then redissolving upon heating (Bence-Jones proteinuria). It may not be detected by reagent sticks, which are often used in urine testing. An identical proteinuria is found in other monoclonal gammopathies (see

p. 184). Characterization of these disorders is by electrophoresis (Fig. 4.1) and immunoelectrophoresis.

Testing for proteinuria

The dipstick method is very convenient and is not affected by contrast material, drugs or urine turbidity. It is insensitive in that urine protein concentrations below 30 mg/100 ml are not detected, larger concentrations in a dilute urine will be 'missed' and light chains give a negative reaction.

Proteinuria is usually quantitated as turbidity measured by a nephelometer after sulphosalicylic acid precipitation. The method is only roughly quantitative because albumin is more easily precipitated than globulins. The assay report therefore tends to reflect albuminuria rather than proteinuria. Other reagents may be used to achieve total urinary protein precipitation.

Proteinuria in single voided specimens

Reference has been made to the inconvenience and frequent inaccuracy of 24-hour urine collections. It follows therefore that 'spot' urine samples potentially have an advantage. Both creatinine and protein are excreted at a constant rate. The ratio of these two variables reflects quantitative protein excretion sufficiently accurately for clinical purposes. It has been found that the protein:creatinine ratio figure is very similar to 24-hour protein excretion expressed in grams.

This manipulation has yet to be widely known but its value is considerable.

Clinical importance of proteinuria

Often the demonstration of proteinuria is the first indication of renal disease. Clinical relevance will be discussed in subsequent chapters.

Immunological investigation of renal disease

Immunological studies are classified as humoral (serological) and cellular. There are, as yet, no routine tests of cell function and such investigations will not be discussed. Transplantation immunology and tissue typing are outside the scope of this book.

Sedimentation rate and acute-phase proteins

The Westergren erythrocyte sedimentation rate (ESR) and the C-reactive protein (CRP) assay are of no diagnostic value but may indicate disease activity and response to treatment. The ESR is read at 1 hour, the upper limits being 15 mm/hour in men and 20 mm/hour in women. The upper limits rise with age, the oral contraceptive pill and the last trimester of pregnancy. The ESR is, in part, a measure of plasma viscosity and concentration of serum proteins. In patients with proteinuria of sufficient magnitude to reduce the concentration of circulating proteins, the ESR will be raised, not necessarily indicating an inflammatory process.

C-reactive protein (normal concentration less than 5 mg/L) tends to respond more to infection than to inflammation and is independent of serum protein concentrations. Used with the ESR, CRP titres may be of use when the nature of the illness is not clear in an unwell patient. Unfortunately, CRP concentrations, which are measured in a laboratory, are substantially less rapidly available than an ESR.

Serum immunoglobulins

While frequently measured, the serum concentration of immunoglobulin proteins are of little diagnostic value in renal medicine. In patients with persistent nephrotic proteinuria, the serum concentration of the three major immunoglobulins may be reduced, especially that of IgG. In long-term lupus the concentration of IgG may reach 30 g/L or more (polyclonal B cell hyperactivity).

Probably the major indication to request serum immunoglobulin assay is when myeloma involvement of the kidney is suspected.

Antibodies

Many antibodies occur in patients with renal disease. Antibodies to a few infectious agents may help in suggesting a diagnosis. The principal examples are:

1 Bacteria: streptococci; staphylococci; pneumococci.
2 Parasites: *Plasmodium malariae*; *Schistosoma mansoni*.
3 Viruses: hepatitis B; Epstein–Barr.

A single result may be difficult to interpret but rising titres (if measurable) are very suggestive of a recent infection.

Autoantibodies

Autoantibodies have specificity against a variety of components of human cells or subdivisions thereof.

Antinuclear antibodies

Antinuclear autoantibodies are most frequently found in patients with SLE. They are generally termed antinuclear antibodies (ANA). The major diagnostic ones are directed against deoxyribonucleic acid (DNA).

By an immunofluorescence test for ANA using rat liver as substrate, a wide range of antibodies to nuclear constituents have been described although they are now infrequently reported from laboratories.

A positive ANA (or antinuclear factor) not only is found in SLE but may also be detected in pregnancy, normal old people, rheumatoid

Table 4.4 Some non-organ-specific antibodies and their disease associations

Antibodies to DNA	
1 Anti-dsDNA	Highly specific for SLE
2 Anti-ssDNA	Non-specific; found in many connective tissue diseases
3 Anti-DNA histone	High titre in drug-induced SLE; non-specific at low titre
Antibodies to non-histone antigens	
1 Anti-Sm	SLE; may reflect disease activity
2 Anti-RNP	Low titre in SLE; high titre suggests MCTD
3 Anti-La	SLE and Sjögren's syndrome
Anticytoplasmic antibodies	
Anti-Ro	In ANA-negative SLE, Sjögren's

ds, Double-stranded; MCTD, mixed connective tissue disease; RNP, ribonucleoprotein; ss, single-stranded.

arthritis, chronic liver disease, organ-specific autoimmune disease, mixed connective tissue disease, scleroderma, lymphoma and other malignancies. The highest titres are likely to occur in SLE and rheumatoid arthritis.

Table 4.4 is a list of some of the nuclear antigens found in connective tissue diseases. In some settings, specific diagnoses may be made. The most useful and most frequently requested assay is that for antibodies against double-stranded DNA (dsDNA). High-percentage binding or high titres of antibody to dsDNA are of diagnostic value in SLE. Nevertheless, there are about 5% of SLE patients in whom antibodies to dsDNA never develop despite running a clinical course identical to those with detectable anti-dsDNA antibodies.

Antineutrophil-cytoplasmic antibodies

In about 90% of patients with microscopic polyarteritis nodosa, or Wegener's granulomatosis, an autoantibody is detectable in the serum which is directed against granular constituents of the cytoplasm of neutrophils – antineutrophil-cytoplasmic antibodies (ANCA). They are usually detected by indirect immunofluorescence, using normal human neutrophils as substrate.

While polyarteritis nodosa and Wegener's granulomatosis are uncommon diseases in a general medical setting, they are not infrequent in renal units. Antineutrophil-cytoplasmic antibody serology may be used in monitoring therapy and is valuable in patients who are too ill to tolerate a renal biopsy.

The ANCA test is being refined: there are more than one antibody in the current ANCA tests because serum from patients with idiopathic necrotizing or crescentic glomerulonephritis may be ANCA-positive. Nevertheless, tests for ANCA represent a major diagnostic advance.

Antiglomerular basement membrane antibodies

The antiglomerular basement membrane (anti-GBM) antibody assay is requested in the context of a stormy clinical course of a crescenteric nephritis. If positive, it is diagnostic of anti-GBM disease and can be used to monitor immunoregulatory therapy and plasmapheresis.

Complement

The complement system consists of 16 glycoproteins which are activated by an antigen–antibody complex (classical pathway) or bacterial endotoxin (alternative pathway). In renal medicine serum complement and components thereof may be measured in venous blood and are also detected in glomeruli involved in immune inflammation.

Circulating components

Many of the circulating components can be measured but for routine purposes three are usually offered as a so-called complement profile. These are the total haemolytic complement (CH) activity and the fourth and third components of the cascade (C4 and C3, respectively). These variables are usually expressed as a percentage of normal reference sera (NRS) but C4 and C3 may be expressed in mass units (mg/100 ml). Total haemolytic complement activity will be normal if all components of the cascade are normal in concentration and activity. Thus measurement of CH is a screen for the whole cascade, although partial deficiencies of complement components may only be detected by specific assay.

Complement profiles are measured in order to estimate the tempo and duration of an immunological disease. Indications for measuring activities of CH, C4 and C3 include:

1 Lupus nephritis – often in conjunction with ANA and dsDNA binding.

2 Mesangiocapillary glomerulonephritis – about 70–80% of patients with this nephritis are persistently hypocomplementaemic. This is due to the presence of C3 nephritic factor (C3 NF). C3 NF is an IgG autoantibody directed against C3 convertase; the convertase is stabilized, allowing it continuously to activate C3 such that C3 is reduced by up to 80% of NRS. Thus the typical complement profile found in this nephritis is persistent reduction in CH and C3 without altering the activity of C4 because it is not consumed. An example of this phenomenon is shown in Fig. 4.2.

3 Acute postinfectious nephritis. Complement components are classically lowered at the acute phase of this illness and return to normal with resolution of the lesion, as shown in Table 4.5. Prognosis in acute nephritis is less favourable if there is reduction in serum complement values for more than 3–4 weeks.

4 Measurement of C3 is of value in the nephritis associated with subacute bacterial endocarditis. If depressed, it represents continued activity of the glomerular lesions.

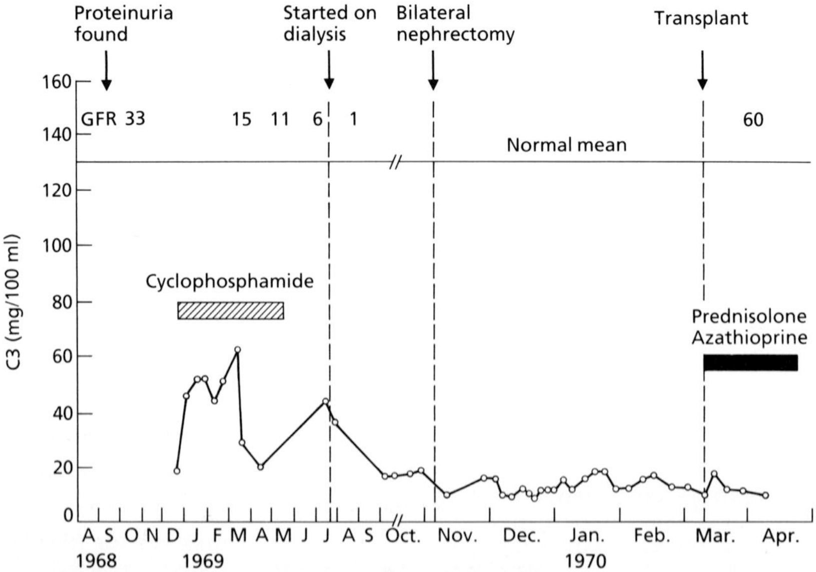

Fig. 4.2 Plasma concentrations of C3 in a patient with a mesangiocapillary glomerulonephritis. Despite differing degrees of renal function and different drugs and therapeutic strategies, the plasma C3 concentration remained very low. GFR, Glomerular filtration rate. (From Cameron, S.J. *et al.* (1970), with kind permission of authors and editor.)

Table 4.5 Clinical, biochemical and immunological variables in a girl of $7\frac{1}{2}$ years, following an acute postinfectious glomerulonephritis. Disease process considered to have begun at time 0

Time (months)	Puffy eyes	Blood-pressure (mmHg)	Haematuria	Proteinuria (g/L)	Serum creatinine (μmol/L)	ASOT (unit/ml $\times 10^3$)	CH_{50}	C4	C3	C3d	CIC
0	+	105/75	+++	1.5	88	2.4–3.2	<20	110	<20	156	Nil
0.5	–	130/80	+++	0.8	82	—	<20	120	35	177	IgG and IgM
1.0	–	100/60	+	0.3	89	1.6–2.4	65	92	39	148	—
1.5	–	90/50	±	0.1	52	—	100	110	83	122	Nil
3.5	–	120/70	–	0.0	63	2.4–3.2	105	155	145	70	Nil
5.0	–	95/65	–	0.0	64	0.8–1.2	105	135	100	58	Nil
11.0	–	80/50	–	0.0	70	<0.2	94	140	81	–	Nil

Data by courtesy of departments of chemical pathology, experimental pathology and clinical immunology, St Mary's Hospital.
CH_{50}, haemolytic complement (range 60–140%); C4, fourth component of complement (range 60–140%); C3, third component of complement (range 75–125%). CIC, circulating immune complexes. Normal range of C3d, 40–130 mU/L.

Some laboratories are able to measure cleavage products of C3, C3b or C3d or both. These breakdown products indicate utilization of CH regardless of the serum concentration of C3. Thus a low C3 in the absence of a raised C3b or C3d suggests a low synthesis rate of C3 rather than activation of the cascade.

Interpretation of the complement profile

In Type III immune disease CH is consumed; if this is substantial, serum concentrations may fall. Thus reduced haemolytic activity and reduced activity of C4 and C3 are an indirect measure of immune inflammation. During the course of a disease the complement profile should be measured on three or more occasions. When immune inflammation with complement consumption ceases, there is often an overswing in synthesis and increased concentrations result, but this is of marginal diagnostic value.

There are limitations to CH profiles in glomerular disease of immune complex origin because alterations in titres do not occur in mesangial proliferative nephritides, membranous glomerulonephritis, IgA/C3 nephropathy and the Henoch–Schönlein and haemolytic uraemic syndromes. In the presence of severe immune disease, persistent hypocomplementaemia is a measure of either insufficient or inadequate treatment.

Occasionally an apparently healthy person, such as a 'normal' control subject, is found to have continuously reduced CH activity and, upon assay of the individual cascade components, a partial or complete deficiency may be found. Such people are prone to develop SLE or mesangiocapillary glomerulonephritis. It is held that the complement deficiency renders the individual less able to eradicate infectious agents.

Tissue binding of complement components

Immunofluorescent and more recently immunoperoxidase studies upon glomeruli sampled at renal biopsy have frequently shown the presence of complement components in patients with nephritis. Usually antisera directed against C1q, C4 and C3 are employed. These complement components are generally deposited in a granular manner on glomerular capillary basement membranes and mesangium, usually indicating the presence of an electron-dense deposit. Often immunoglobulins are demonstrated in association with complement deposition. C3 is the most frequently recognized complement component but at times has to be interpreted with care because it may adhere to severely damaged tissue in a non-specific manner. Nevertheless, some patterns of complement binding are diagnostic: all tissue sampled at renal biopsy should be examined for the presence of complement components.

Conclusion

Measurement of only a few of the components of the CH cascade give some idea of the severity and duration of immune inflammation in some of the diseases of the kidney. Study of the deposition of complement components in glomeruli are essential in the diagnoses of nephritides.

Circulating immune complexes

The majority of the nephritides are believed to be mediated by immune complexes. Initially, it was thought that these complexes, composed of antigen, antibodies (immunoglobulins) and complement components, formed, circulated and became trapped in glomeruli, initiating immune inflation. Currently, *in situ* formation, that is, within glomeruli, is thought to occur and circulating complexes are of less importance because there is little correlation between the composition of glomerular complexes compared with that of circulating complexes.

Unfortunately, no nephritic process or its treatment has been shown to correlate with the presence or titre of immune complexes. It therefore appears that, at present, there is no routine need to request measurement of such complexes.

Cryoglobulins

Cryoimmunoglobulins are usually composed of mono- or polyclonal immunoglobulins which precipitate at 4 °C. If two or more immunoglobulins are present, the term mixed cryoglobulinaemia is used.

Cryoglobulins may be found in a number of conditions: collagen–vascular diseases, systemic hepatitis B infection, postinfectious glomerulonephritis, renal vasculitis, Waldenström's macroglobulinaemia and lymphoproliferative malignancies. Some are found in the absence of a systemic condition – 'essential' cryoglobulinaemia.

There are three categories of cryoglobulins:

Type I monoclonal immunoglobulins; usually IgM*; IgG or IgA.
Type II mixed cryoglobulins with monoclonal antibodies, comprising IgM with IgG* and IgG with IgG.
Type III mixed polyclonal cryoglobulins; IgM/IgG* or IgM/IgG/IgA.

Those marked with an asterisk are the most common varieties.

Cryoglobulins may produce renal damage, in addition to that of the underlying disorder, the most common feature being eosinophilic 'thrombi' in glomerular capillaries.

The titre of cryglobulins bears no relationship to immune inflammation. Having once been demonstrated, subsequent failure to detect cryoglobulins is usually taken as a measure of success of therapy. Nevertheless, there is no need to request this assay routinely.

Histopathological investigations

Renal biopsy

Indications for and techniques of renal biopsy are dealt with in Chapter 9, p. 125. A few details regarding preservatives for renal tissues are described on p. 126.

Skin biopsy

Occasionally it is necessary to sample arterioles and the dermal–epidermal junction in renal patients with a rash or a cutaneous vasculitis. Such biopsies are usually taken with a circular disposable knife. The laboratory handling such tissue uses highly specialized preservatives and techniques of cutting. It is best to discuss the planned biopsy with a pathologist before skin is sampled; in many hospitals a histopathology technician will be present at the time of the biopsy to ensure the quality of preservation.

Particulate matter in urine

Particulate matter may be recovered from the urine of patients. If the matter is soft, histological analysis may demonstrate a papilla. Such information would be of clinical importance; thus it is always worth requesting the morphology of material found in urine.

Bone biopsy

Bone biopsy is infrequently required. Whilst almost all patients with chronic renal failure have abnormal histology, a clinician can learn all that is necessary for management from serial serum biochemical variables and radiographs. The major indication for bone biopsy is either a specialist interest in renal osteodystrophy or a clinical trial of a vitamin D analogue, or both. In these circumstances, details of tetracycline labelling will be decided with the staff of the specialist laboratory before trephine biopsy of the iliac bone is performed.

Further reading

1 Appel, G. (1991) Lipid abnormalities in renal disease. *Kidney Int.* **39**, 169–83.
2 Cameron, S.J., Glasgow, E.F., Ogg, C.S. & White, R.H. (1970) Membranoproliferative glomerulonephritis and persistent hypocomplementaemia. *Br. Med. J.* **4**, 7–14.
3 Claitmans, F.H.M. & Meinders, A.E. (1990) Management of severe hyponatraemia. *Am. J. Med.* **88**, 161–6.
4 Fraser, C.G. & Fogarty, Y. (1989) Intrepreting laboratory results. *Br. Med. J.* **289**, 1659–60.
5 Gabriel, R. (1986) Time to scrap creatinine clearance? *Br. Med. J.* **293**, 1119–20.
6 Gaskin, G., Savage, C.O., Ryan, J.J. *et al.* (1991) Anti-neutrophil cytoplasmic antibodies and disease activity during long-term follow up of 70 patients with systemic vasculitis. *Nephrol. Dialysis Transplant.* **6**, 689–94.
7 Ginsberg, J.M., Chang, B.E., Matarese, R.A. & Garella, S. (1983) Use of single voided urine samples to estimate quantitative proteinuria. *N. Engl. J. Med.* **309**, 1543–6.
8 Kamel, K.S., Ethier, J.H., Richardson, R.M., Bear, R.A. & Halperin, M.L. (1990) Urine electrolytes and osmolality: when and how to use them. *Am. J. Nephrol.* **10**, 89–102.
9 Kaysen, G.A., Don, B. & Schambelan, M. (1991) Proteinuria, albumin synthesis and hyperlipidaemia in the nephrotic syndrome. *Nephrol. Dialysis Transplant.* **6**, 141–9.
10 Mustonen, J., Soppi, E., Pasternack, A. & Hallstrom, O. (1990) Clinical significance of autoantibodies against neutrophil cellular components in patients with renal disease. *Am. J. Nephrol.* **10**, 482–8.
11 Schuck, O. (1984) *Examination of Kidney Function.* Developments in Nephrology, Vol. 4, Martinus Nijhoff, Boston.
12 Scully, R.E., McNeely, R.G. & Mark, E.J. (eds) (1986) Normal reference laboratory values. *N. Engl. J. Med.* **314**, 39–49 & **316**, 1606.
13 Sterns, R.H. (1990) Treatment of hyponatraemia. *Am. J. Med.* **88**, 557–60.

Chapter 5
Acid–Base Disorders

Roger Gabriel

Large quantities of acid are produced daily. In an adult they amount to approximately 50 mM of non-volatile acid and volatile acid which comprises about 13 000–20 000 mM of CO_2. Of the CO_2, 90% momentarily generates H^+ as the CO_2 is carried in the blood to the lungs, where it is expired. These large loads of acid are generated and excreted whilst the healthy individual maintains an alkaline plasma pH.

The concept of CO_2 as an acid is unusual because CO_2 is not a proton donor nor does H_2CO_3 exist in any substantial amount in body fluids. The H^+ that result from processing metabolic CO_2 are derived from the disassociation of water, as shown in the following equations:

$$CO_2 + H_2O \leftrightharpoons H^+ + HCO_3^-$$

$$H^+ \leftrightharpoons HOH$$

$$\upharpoonleft\downharpoonright$$

$$CO_2 + OH^- \leftrightharpoons HCO_3^-$$

As metabolic CO_2 enters the blood from tissue cells the generation of H^+ (volatile acid) poses a threat to acid–base balance. The potential decrease in plasma pH is minimized by a speical property of haemoglobin as a buffer which makes non-oxygenated haemoglobin less acidic than oxygenated haemoglobin. Thus as arterial capillary blood releases O_2 it takes up large quantities of H^+ without any change in pH. At the same time CO_2 diffusing from cells combines with the OH^- of disassociated water, yielding HCO_3^-. It is chiefly in this form that CO_2 is carried to the lungs for excretion.

Apart from CO_2, other acids do not have a volatile component and they are therefore known as non-volatile or ‘fixed’ acids. Such acids are derived from the catabolism of proteins and to a lesser extent phospholipids and the partial metabolism of carbohydrates and fats, as well as the loss of HCO_3^- in stool. The acid–base balance is maintained in the presence of these acids by three lines of defence:

1 Second-by-second physiochemical buffering.

2 Second-by-second or minute-by-minute balancing by adjustment in alveolar ventilation.

3 Day-by-day buffering by the renal excretion of H^+ and renal tubular reabsorption of HCO_3^-.

The third buffer system is particularly effective in dealing with excesses or deficits of fixed acid because:

1 it involves the volatile component, CO_2, which is easily regulated by changes in alveolar ventilation; and

2 substrates for the buffer system, CO_2 and HCO_3^-, are freely available from metabolic processes.

The H^+ balance may be disturbed from either a metabolic or a respiratory origin. The relationship between pH, HCO_3^- and $P\text{CO}_2$ is shown by the Henderson–Hasselbalch equation:

$$\text{pH} = 6.1 + \log\frac{[\text{HCO}_3^-]}{0.03 \times P\text{CO}_2}$$

A metabolic change in H^+ will alter the numerator of the Henderson–Hasselbalch equation, which will tend to shift the pH in either an acid or an alkaline direction. Likewise, a respiratory change in H^+ will alter the denominator of the equation and also potentially change the pH in either direction. Primary metabolic or respiratory disturbances are acccompanied by a secondary, or compensatory, response of opposite origin, which restores plasma pH towards normal. The compensation for a primary metabolic disturbance is almost instantaneous, whereas for primary respiratory disturbances, it becomes fully effective only after 2–3 days. When primary disturbances of metabolic and respiratory origins occur together, the resulting state is known as a mixed disturbance. Such disturbances are commonplace.

Acid or alkaline loads involve not only buffers of plasma but those of interstitial fluid, cells and bone. Approximately 50% of fixed acid is buffered within cells. In contrast, buffering of more than 90% of H^+ resulting from an excess or deficit of CO_2 involves the intracellular space because these H^+ cannot be buffered by the bicarbonate system, which is the predominant buffer of the extracellular fluid (plasma and interstitium).

Acid–base disorders

Changes in plasma pH occur when renal or respiratory function is abnormal or when an acid or base load exceeds excretory capacity. The terms acidosis and alkalosis respectively refer to processes that tend to lower or raise the pH. Acidaemia is defined as a decrease in blood pH

Table 5.1 Characteristic changes of primary acid–base disturbances

Disorder	pH	$[H^+]$	Primary disturbance	Compensatory response
Metabolic acidosis	↓	↑	↓ $[HCO_3^-]$	↓ P_{CO_2}
Metabolic alkalosis	↑	↓	↑ $[HCO_3^-]$	↑ P_{CO_2}
Respiratory acidosis	↓	↑	↑ P_{CO_2}	↑ $[HCO_3^-]$
Respiratory alkalosis	↑	↓	↓ P_{CO_2}	↓ $[HCO_3^-]$

and alkalaemia as an elevation in blood pH, although these terms are not frequently used. The characteristic changes of primary acid–base disturbances are straightforward (Table 5.1). In each case the change in pH and $[H^+]$ is opposite and logical. The concentration of $[HCO_3^-]$ and P_{CO_2} always alters in the same direction.

Metabolic acidosis

In metabolic acidosis there is a fall in plasma HCO_3^- and a low pH. This is induced either by loss of HCO_3^- (as in persistent diarrhoea) or by the buffering of lactic, 3-hydroxybutyric and acetoacetic acids (diabetic ketoacidosis) or retained diet-generated sulphuric acid (as occurs in renal failure). The reduced pH stimulates ventilation, resulting in a compensatory decrease in P_{CO_2}. Restoration of pH depends upon renal excretion of the excess acid, which takes several days.

Metabolic alkalosis

Metabolic alkalosis results from a raised concentration of plasma HCO_3^- and is associated with a high pH. The disorder is produced by H^+ loss, as in chronic diuretic therapy, by loss of gastric hydrogen ions, as in persistent vomiting, or by HCO_3^- administration. Respiratory compensation leads to hypoventilation with an elevation in P_{CO_2}.

The pH can be rapidly corrected by an increase in the renal excretion of HCO_3^- but this does not occur in many patients because HCO_3^- reabsorptive capacity is enhanced, usually due to concomitant volume depletion. Here, the kidney avidly conserves sodium to maintain the effective circulating volume and cannot therefore excrete excess HCO_3^- (as $NaHCO_3$).

Respiratory acidosis

Respiratory acidosis accompanies decreased effective alveolar ventilation, leading to reduced excretion of CO_2 and an increase in the extracellular P_{CO_2}. The renal compensation consists of enhanced H^+ excretion, which raises the plasma HCO_3^- concentration. This takes 3–5 days to reach completion. Because of this delay, two different acid–base disorders may occur: acute respiratory acidosis, in which there may be a sharp fall in pH, and chronic respiratory acidosis, in which pH is relatively well protected due to the renal compensation.

Respiratory alkalosis

Hyperventilation results in a fall in extracellular $P\text{CO}_2$ and an increase in pH. The compensatory response consists of diminished renal H^+ secretion, producing HCO_3^- loss in the urine with a decrease in plasma HCO_3^- concentration. The renal compensation is time-dependent, as with respiratory acidosis, so that both acute and chronic respiratory alkalosis may occur.

Mixed acid–base disorders

Combined metabolic and respiratory acidoses are not uncommon. If the patient has a low arterial pH with a low plasma HCO_3^- concentration and a high $P\text{CO}_2$, there is a combined metabolic and respiratory acidosis. Similarly, a combined metabolic and respiratory alkalosis is present in a patient with an elevated pH, a high plasma concentration of HCO_3^- and a low $P\text{CO}_2$.

In every patient with an acid–base disorder, three questions arise:
1 What is the primary disturbance or what are the primary disturbances?
2 Is the compensatory response quantitatively appropriate?
3 What is the cause of each primary disturbance?

In many patients the clinical presentation suggests a specific acid–base disorder – acute renal failure, acute on chronic renal failure, diabetic ketoacidosis, acute exacerbation of chronic bronchitis, hyperventilation or hypoventilation. Such clinical diagnoses lead to the request for the assay 'blood gases', which comprise pH, $P\text{O}_2$, $P\text{CO}_2$ and HCO_3^-.

The normal values for the major acid–base variables in the arterial and venous blood are given in Table 5.2.

Errors in sampling

Common errors in sampling arterial blood for acid–base variables include the following:
1 The blood sample should be cooled rapidly to 4 °C. If not, at room temperature, anaerobic glycolysis by red and white cells leads to reduc-

Table 5.2 Normal values for major acid–base variables

	pH	$[H^+]$ (nmol/L)	$P\text{CO}_2$ (mmHg)	$[HCO_3^-]$ (mmol/L)
Arterial	7.37–7.43	37–43	36–44	22–26
Venous	7.32–7.38	42–48	42–50	23–27

tion of organic acids, which decreases pH and the HCO_3^- concentration.
2 The arterial sample is at risk by dilution with heparin. This may be avoided by discarding the first 10 ml of a sample so that the volume of anticoagulant is $<5\%$ of the volume of the blood sample.
3 Arterial pH may not reflect tissue pH (which may be lower) in patients with severe heart failure or in those undergoing cardiopulmonary resuscitation. In these circumstances, blood may be inadequately cleared of CO_2 in the lungs, leading to a relatively normal or even diminished arterial $P\text{CO}_2$. The low cardiac output slows the return of CO_2-containing blood from the periphery such that the mixed venous $P\text{CO}_2$ represents blood that has not entered the pulmonary circulation and may be markedly higher than in arterial blood. In severe heart failure, the mixed venous $P\text{CO}_2$ may more closely reflect cellular pH.

Measurement of pH

pH and $P\text{CO}_2$ are measured and blood drawn anaerobically into a heparinized syringe. The pH is measured by an electrode permeable only to H^+ ions and the $P\text{CO}_2$ by a CO_2 electrode. The bicarbonate concentration is then calculated by the Henderson–Haselbalch equation or measured directly.

pH and hydrogen ion relationships

There is no linear relationship between pH and $[H^+]$. The relationship is shown by the formula:

$$\log[H^+] - 9 = -\text{pH}$$

$$[H^+] = \text{antilog}(9 - \text{pH})\,\text{nmol/L}$$

Thus at pH 7:

$$\begin{aligned}[H^+] &= \text{antilog}(9 - 7)\\ &= \text{antilog } 2\\ &= 100\,\text{nmol/L}\end{aligned}$$

and for pH 8:

$$\begin{aligned}[H^+] &= \text{antilog } 1\\ &= 10\,\text{nmol/L}\end{aligned}$$

If taking an antilog is difficult, pH and hydrogen ion concentration are related as follows. For each 0.1 unit increase in pH, multiply $[H^+]$ by 0.8; thus for a pH 7.4 rising to 7.6 the hydrogen ion change is given by:

$$7.6 = 40 \times 0.8 \times 0.8 = 26\,\text{nmol/L}$$

For each unit fall in pH, multiply $[H^+]$ by 1.25; thus pH 7.3:

$$\begin{aligned}7.3 &= 40 \times 1.25\\ &= 50\,\text{nmol/L } [H^+]\end{aligned}$$

Table 5.3 Relationship between pH and H^+

pH	$[H^+]$ (nmol/L)
6.8	160
6.9	125
7.0	100
7.1	80
7.2	63
7.3	50
7.4	40
7.5	32
7.6	26
7.7	20
7.8	15
7.9	12.6

There is a fourfold change in H^+ concentration between pH 7.0 and 7.6. These marked changes are sometimes not appreciated. The relationship between pH and H^+ is shown in Table 5.3. In clinical practice, most values for pH lie between 7.0 and 7.6 (100–26 nmol $[H^+]$/L).

Estimation of bicarbonate deficit or excess

In patients with severe metabolic acidoses when the plasma HCO_3^- concentration is less than 10 mmol/L, the bicarbonate deficit (in millimoles) may be calculated from the following relationship:

$$0.7 \times \text{lean body-weight (kg)} \times (10 - \text{plasma } [HCO_3^-])$$

This formula is only applicable when the plasma $[HCO_3^-]$ is below 10 mmol/L, at which stage cell and bone buffers become responsible for almost all buffering of excess hydrogen ions. At plasma $[HCO_3^-]$ concentrations above 10 mmol/L, extracellular buffering occurs and the apparent space of distribution of HCO_3^- falls to 0.5 times the lean body-weight.

In metabolic alkaloses, the bicarbonate deficit is given by the relationship:

$$HCO_3^- \simeq 0.5 \times \text{lean body-weight (kg)} \times (\text{plasma } [HCO_3^-] - 24)$$

Compensatory responses to primary acid–base disturbances

Each primary disturbance to the acid–base balance is followed by a response that tends to restore the pH to normal. Thus, in a metabolic acidosis which decreases $[HCO_3^-]$, the compensatory response, which is in the opposite system, is alveolar ventilation. This will lower $P\text{CO}_2$

and thus tend to restore pH towards normal. In metabolic alkaloses, the compensatory response is a reverse of that described above.

In respiratory acidosis two mechanisms tend to restore the pH towards normal:

1 An immediate titration of $[H^+]$ by body buffers (p. 59). This is the rapid phase of the response.

2 A gradually developing increase in renal reabsorption of $[HCO_3^-]$ to compensate for the persistent disturbance consequent upon the pneumonia or whatever the cause of the respiratory acidosis. This is the chronic respiratory acidosis response.

The different compensatory responses to acid–base disturbances are shown in Table 5.4. The information is necessary adequately to interpret 'blood gases' in clinical practice.

A simple example of metabolic alkalosis caused by salicylate overdose is shown by the following figures:

$$pH = 7.45, \quad P\text{CO}_2 = 20, \quad [HCO_3^-] = 13$$

Alkalosis is confirmed by the slightly high pH. This is due to the low $P\text{CO}_2$, which, in the early hours of aspirin poisoning, reflects direct respiratory centre stimulation by salicylate. Later, the salicylic acid load leads to a metabolic acidosis, with a fall in $[HCO_3^-]$ and pH and with hyperventilation.

A very common pattern of acid–base changes is the following:

$$pH = 7.4, \quad P\text{CO}_2 = 60, \quad [HCO_3^-] = 36$$

These values are due to mixed respiratory acidosis (raised $P\text{CO}_2$) and metabolic alkalosis (high plasma $[HCO_3^-]$). The high bicarbonate concentration reflects long-term increased renal tubular reabsorption of $[HCO_3^-]$ in response to chronic hypercapnia secondary to chronic obstructive airways disease. If the patient received daily diuretic therapy for right heart failure, the resultant hypokalaemia might enhance the bicarbonate retention.

The normal pH together with changes in the $P\text{CO}_2$ and plasma $[HCO_3^-]$

Table 5.4 Respiratory and renal responses to primary acid–base disturbances

Disorder	Primary change	pH	Compensatory response
Metabolic acidosis	$[HCO_3^-]\downarrow$	$\downarrow$	Hyperventilation
Metabolic alkalosis	$[HCO_3^-]\downarrow$	$\uparrow$	Hypoventilation
Respiratory acidosis	$[HCO_3^-]\uparrow$	$\downarrow$	
Acute			Titration by body buffers
Chronic			Increased renal reabsorption of $[HCO_3^-]$
Respiratory alkalosis	$[HCO_3^-]\downarrow$	$\uparrow$	
Acute			Titration by body buffers
Chronic			Increased renal reabsorption of $[HCO_3^-]$

concentrations suggests a mixed disorder. If mixed respiratory and metabolic acidoses occur together, which separately would drive the $P\text{CO}_2$ in opposite directions, both $P\text{CO}_2$ and $[HCO_3^-]$ may remain normal in concentration but with a substantial acidosis. In this setting, the $P\text{CO}_2$ is inappropriately high.

Management of renal acid–base disorders

Despite the substantial academic aspects of these conditions, their clinical management is straightforward. Therapy is used to ameliorate the effects of reduced pH until healing is established or dialysis is started. Occasionally chronic treatment is needed.

Acute renal failure

A metabolic acidosis is always present. The respiratory response to severe acidosis is identical to that in diabetic ketoacidosis with a deep sighing tachypnoea (Kussmaul respiration) in an attempt to excrete H^+ as CO_2. Severe acidosis also leads to peripheral arterial vasodilatation, central venoconstriction, impairment of brain function and a fall in cardiac contractability, enhancing arrythmias. The indication for treatment of acidosis in acute renal failure is an arterial pH <7.2 or a plasma bicarbonate concentration <12 mmol/L.

A 50 ml bolus of sodium bicarbonate (8.4%) is given slowly intravenously with the aim of diminishing the severity of the acidosis but not fully to correct it. Each millimole of bicarbonate contains an identical concentration of sodium. Volume and sodium overload are risks of therapy. There is no place for oral treatment.

In acute renal failure with acidosis, hyperkalaemia is common. An advantage of bicarbonate therapy is the temporary intracellular shift of potassium which accompanies treatment. There is further discussion of the treatment of acidosis in acute renal failure in Chapter 16, p. 233.

Chronic renal failure

Acidosis invariably worsens as chronic renal failure advances but causes no symptoms until renal function is below 15% of normal. At this stage the patient should have been prepared for referral to a dialysis centre (Chapter 14, p. 209). There is probably no indication for bicarbonate therapy in chronic renal failure.

Renal tubular disorders

1 Tubular bicarbonate wasting accompanying distal disease is occasionally found in chronic tubulointerstitial nephritides. Sodium bicarbonate tablets help ameliorate the hyponatraemia and perhaps the acidosis.

2 Renal tubular acidosis, either as an inherited disorder or as part of the Fanconi syndrome, is very rare. Bicarbonate is used in both distal and proximal varieties (p. 294).

Cystinuria

Bicarbonate therapy of cystine stones is discussed on p. 296.

Further reading

1 Cogan, M.G. & Rector, F.C. (1991) Acid–base disorders. In Brenner, B.M. & Rector, F.C. (eds), *The Kidney*. W.B. Saunders, Philadelphia, pp. 737–804.
2 Rose, B.D. (1989) *Clinical Physiology of Acid–Base and Electrolyte Disorders*, 3rd edn. McGraw-Hill, New York.
3 Schrier, W. (1992) *Renal and Electrolyte Disorders*, 4th edn. Little Brown, Boston.

Chapter 6
Radiological, Ultrasound and Isotope Studies

Lance H. Cope

A wide range of radiological techniques are available which provide excellent images of the renal tract. The information obtained from the individual tests depends upon the physical principles by which the images are produced. The various techniques are complementary to one another. For example, isotope studies provide direct evidence of renal function but relatively poor anatomical detail; ultrasound demonstrates renal anatomy, from which it may be possible to make indirect inferences about renal function.

A brief description of investigations is given, explaining how the images are produced. The intention is to give a clearer understanding of the structures demonstrated by a particular test, so that the investigation of a specific clinical condition can be approached in a logical manner.

Renal ultrasound

Modern ultrasound equipment provides a high-definition, instantly moving 'real-time' image, which has greatly improved diagnostic accuracy such that ultrasound rivals intravenous urography (IVU) as the first-line investigation of the renal tract.

Renal ultrasound provides information about the texture of the renal parenchyma as well as the position, size and shape of the kidneys. Dilatation of the collecting systems and intrarenal calculi are readily shown. The renal vessels can usually be identified at the hilum and may be seen to pulsate, indicating patency. Ureters are not normally demonstrated, due to overlying bowel gas. The full bladder is very accessible, allowing study of intravesical masses.

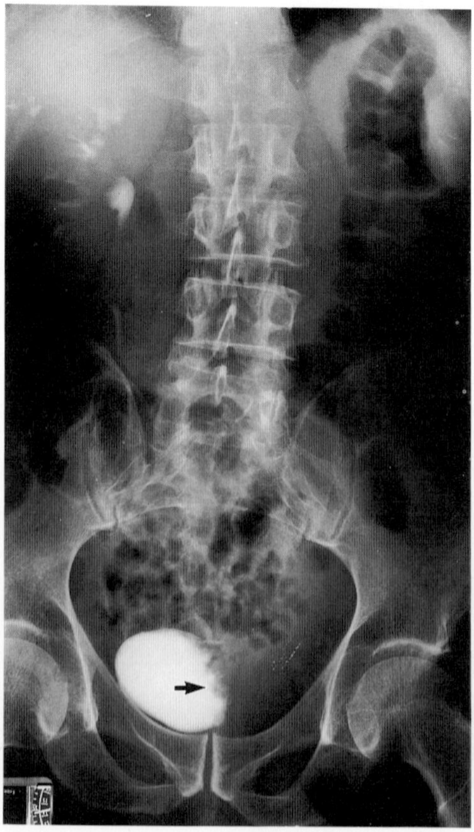

(a)

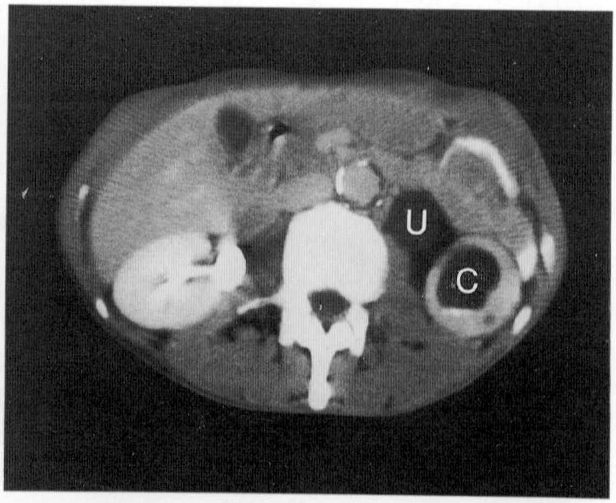

(c)

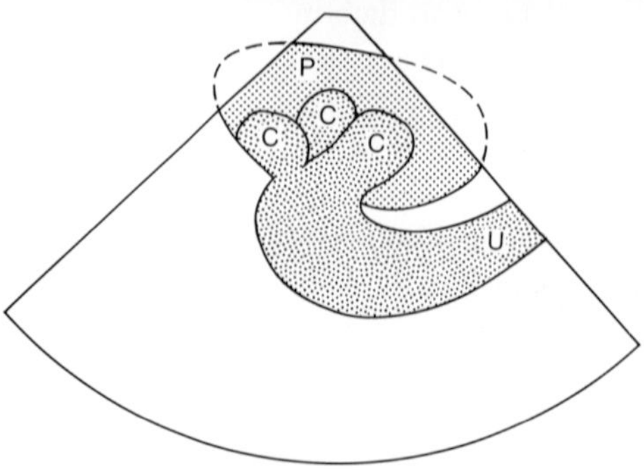

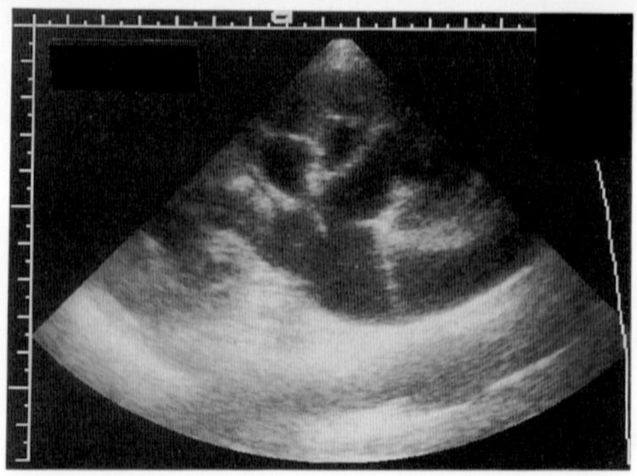

(b)

Fig. 6.1 These three images are from a patient with a left hydronephrosis due to ureteric obstruction by a bladder tumour. (a) The 90 min IVU film shows a very delayed, dense nephrogram on the left with no excretion of contrast on that side and also the tumour within the bladder (arrow). (b) A longitudinal ultrasound scan demonstrated markedly dilated calyces (C), the upper ureter (U) and shrunken parenchyma (P). (c) The CT scan shows the markedly dilated collecting system (C) and ureter (U) on the left, which remain unenhanced because of the poor renal function on that side.

Ultrasound has important advantages over conventional radiology for investigation of renal disease for the following reasons:

1 Diagnostic ultrasound is non-invasive. This is especially important in children and in pregnancy and also allows serial studies to be performed without risk.

2 The image is independent of renal function, allowing the examination of non-functioning kidneys.

3 No patient preparation is required to demonstrate the kidneys, although a full bladder is necessary to examine pelvic viscera.

4 In seriously ill patients, ultrasound can be performed at the bedside.

5 Other abdominal organs, including the liver and pancreas, can be demonstrated and may show metastases or cysts.

Indications for renal ultrasonography include:

1 Detection of obstructive uropathy. Dilated pelvicalyceal systems are readily demonstrated (Fig. 6.1b) and are nearly always apparent in chronic obstruction, providing a technically satisfactory examination is achieved (Fig. 6.2). Other causes of a dilated collecting system, such as ureteric reflux, give a false-positive diagnosis of obstruction of 10–25%. Upper urinary tract dilatation is not reliably seen in acute obstruction because it takes time to develop.

2 Investigation of renal failure, giving information about renal size,

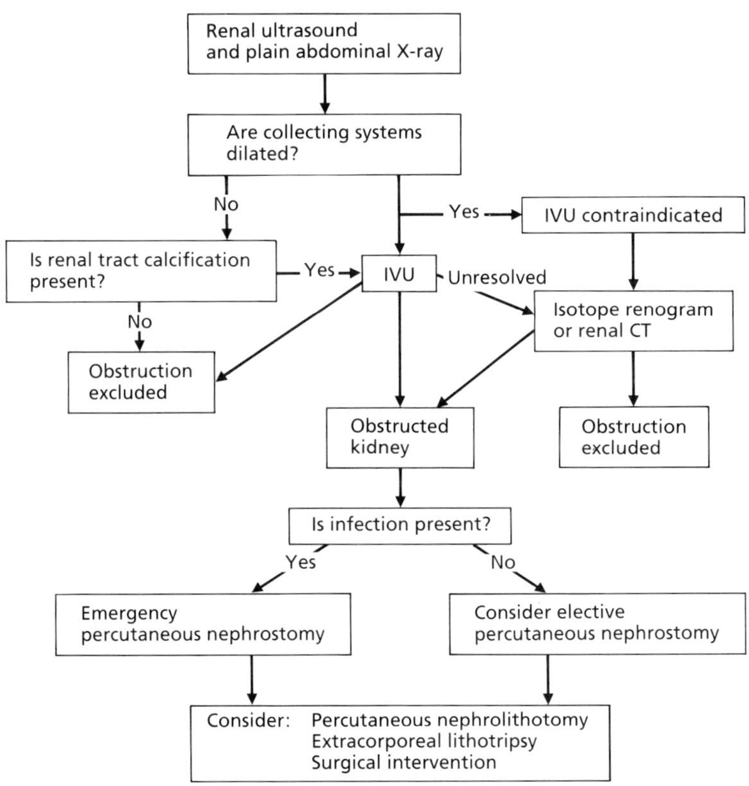

Fig. 6.2 Investigation of suspected chronic obstruction.

shape and outflow tract obstruction. A generalized increase in the echo return from the renal parenchyma occurs in glomerulonephritis, acute tubular necrosis, fibrosis and infiltrative disease such as lymphoma or amyloid.

3 Investigation of renal masses. If the appearances are characteristic of a simple cyst (Fig. 6.4b, p. 73), no further investigation is required. Tumours usually appear as solid masses of different texture (that is, a different echo pattern) from the normal parenchyma and contain areas of cystic degeneration or calcification.

4 Screening for polycystic disease.

5 Renal biopsy can be performed using ultrasonic guidance to localize the parenchyma. Likewise renal cysts may be aspirated with precision.

Intravenous urography

Intravenous urography was the most commonly requested radiological procedure and was the first investigation performed to study the urinary tract. Nevertheless, adverse reactions to contrast media occur, causing a substantial morbidity and a mortality rate of one in 40 000 investigations. With improvements in ultrasound studies of the renal tract, the number of requests for an IVU continues to fall. The subject is discussed because the quality of ultrasound studies varies and the images produced by an IVU are much easier to interpret.

The IVU provides information about the size, shape and position of the kidneys. The control film shows radio-opaque calculi in the renal tract. Over 90% of renal calculi are visible on a plain abdominal radiograph. Demonstration of a calculus depends both on its size and its radiodensity, which is directly related to the atomic weight of its chemical constituents. Thus all calculi containing calcium (high atomic weight) are clearly visible, while urate, xanthine and matrix calculi are radiolucent.

The nephrogram phase demonstrates the functioning renal tissue and may show focal or diffuse parenchymal loss. Alternatively, a space-occupying lesion produces a localized bulge in the renal outline or an area of non-opacification. The pyelogram phase demonstrates the pelvicalyceal systems, ureters and bladder. Abnormalities such as displacement, dilatation, obstruction and filling defects are demonstrated, and a crude indication of renal function is obtained.

Indications

The more common indications for IVU are the investigation of:

1 Recurrent urinary tract infections in females or single infections in males, although ultrasound may be used as the first investigation.

2 Haematuria.

3 Renal calculi or renal colic.

4 Renal trauma.

5 Before surgery: nephrectomy or pelvic malignancy.

Intravenous urography is not indicated for the detection of upper renal tract involvement in prostatic hypertrophy, as this information is more safely obtained by ultrasound.

Contraindications

There are several important relative contraindications to an IVU:

1 Pregnancy.

2 Allergy to iodine or previous adverse reaction to contrast media. Although only 10% of these patients will suffer a serious adverse reaction, other techniques, such as ultrasound or radio-isotope studies, should be used.

3 Asthmatic patients have a greatly increased risk of adverse reaction to contrast media.

4 In diabetes mellitus with associated renal insufficiency, there is a high risk of acute renal failure, which may be irreversible. An IVU should only be performed if the required information cannot be obtained by other investigations.

5 An IVU should be delayed if the patient is to have an iodine-labelled radio-isotope for the investigation or treatment of thyroid disease. The large iodine load given in the contrast medium may block uptake in the thyroid gland.

Contrast media

Water-soluble contrast media undergo glomerular filtration and are excreted unchanged in the urine. The standard contrast media are very hyperosmolar (1500–2200 mmol/L). This has the advantage of producing an osmotic diuresis, with resultant pelvicalyceal distension, but is also responsible for some of the adverse reactions to contrast media. Low-osmolar contrast media are available and should be used in patients at increased risk of adverse reactions: infants, the very old and patients with asthma, diabetes mellitus, sickle-cell disease or trait, ischaemic heart disease or impaired renal function. Uptake of free iodine from the contrast media may cause painful swelling of the salivary glands in patients with renal failure.

Radiography

A description of the radiographic technique is given, outlining specific features to aid interpretation of films.

In preparation for the procedure, laxatives are given to remove faecal residue and the patient is fasted for 6 hours to reduce nausea and vomiting. The bladder is emptied prior to the investigation. Longer periods of dehydration are not required, as satisfactory images can be produced in the hydrated patient. It is essential that patients with diabetes mellitus, myeloma and renal failure are well hydrated in order to minimize the risk of a temporary or permanent deterioration in renal function.

A control film is taken of the abdomen from the renal areas to the pubic symphysis. This demonstrates any calcification within the renal tract, which will be rendered invisible after contrast has been given (Fig. 6.3). If calcification is seen overlying the renal areas, further films, such as inspiratory or oblique films, are taken to determine whether calcification is within the kidney.

Contrast is given as a rapid bolus injection. It is pointless giving a test injection as this itself may produce anaphylaxis. The 'immediate' or '0 min' film demonstrates the nephrogram (Fig. 6.4a). At this stage, contrast is in the proximal renal tubules, producing an image of the renal parenchyma. From the nephrogram, the renal length can be measured. Normal kidneys do not differ by more than 1 cm in length and can be accurately related to the height of the lumbar vertebrae. In adults, kidneys are the same length as three lumbar vertebrae plus their intervertebral discs. Common causes of large and small kidneys are listed in Tables 6.1. and 6.2.

The '5 min' film shows excretion of contrast into the collecting systems and there may be early bladder opacification (Fig. 6.5a, p. 76). If no urinary obstruction or abdominal mass is present, abdominal com-

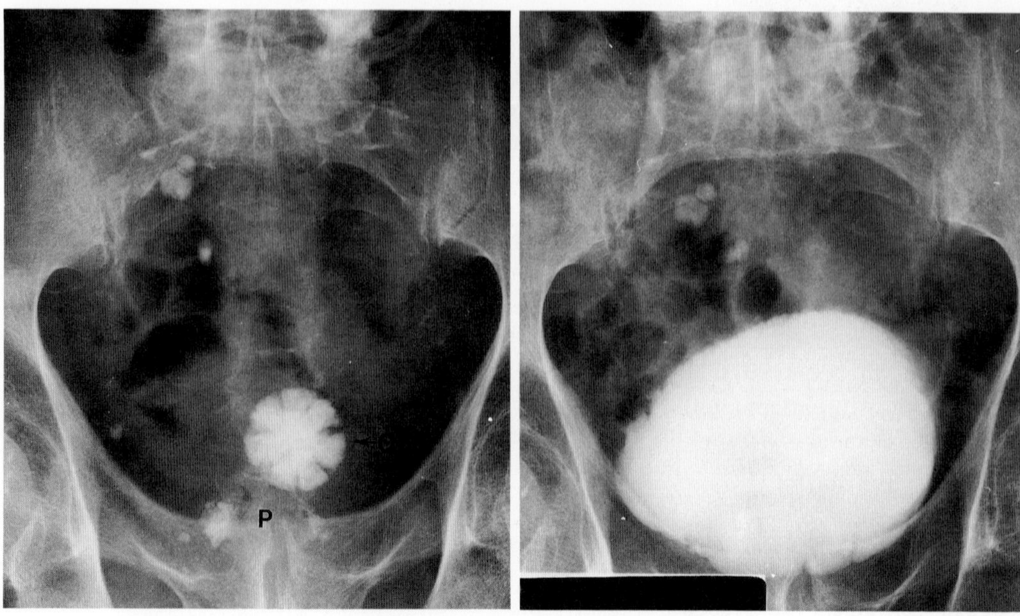

(a) **(b)**

Fig. 6.3 (a) Part of the control IVU film of a 78-year-old man showing a large stellate bladder calculus (C). There is also calcification within the prostate gland (P). (b) After contrast the bladder calculus is surrounded by contrast medium of a similar radiodensity and is no longer visible.

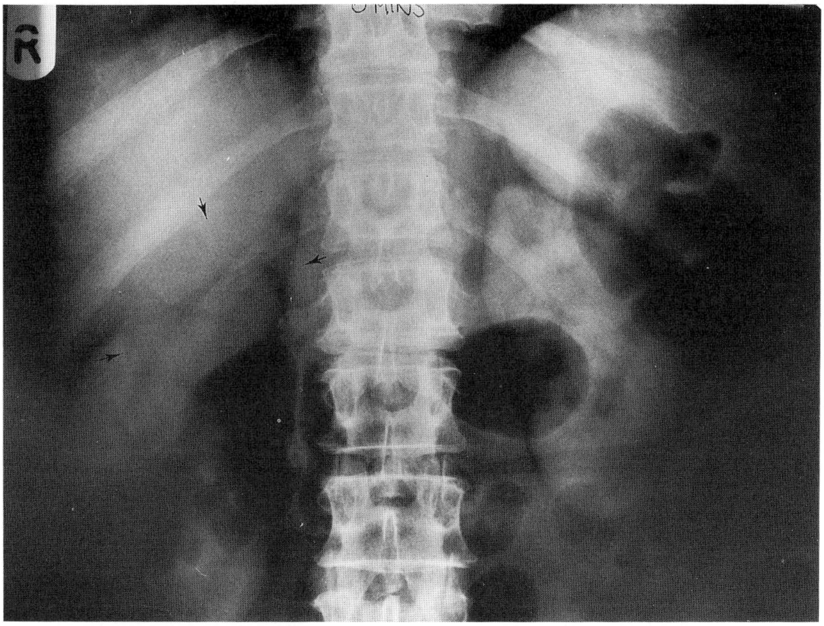

(a)

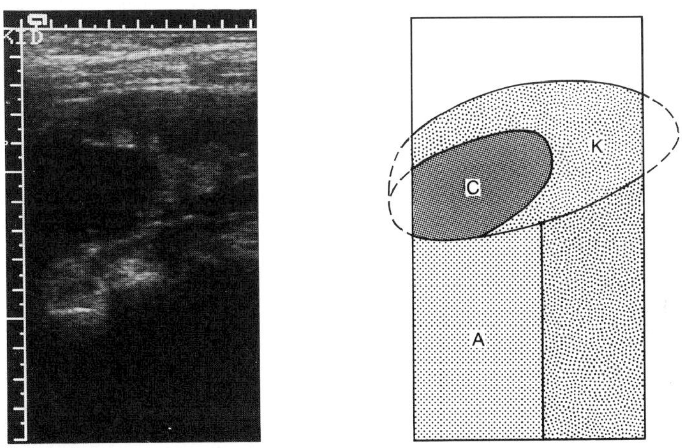

(b)

Fig. 6.4 (a) A '0' min IVU film demonstrating a nephrogram. The kidneys stand out as relatively radiodense structures because of contrast within renal tubules. There is a large simple cyst in the upper pole of the right kidney, which appears less dense than the normal kidney because no contrast is being excreted (arrows). (b) A longitudinal ultrasound section through the same kidney. It demonstrates the typical appearances of a cyst (C) in that it has a smooth 'paper-thin' wall, there are no acoustic echoes from within the cyst and, because no ultrasound energy is removed by the cyst, the echoes from behind the cyst are stronger than those from the tissue behind the normal renal parenchyma (K); this is known as acoustic enhancement (A).

pression is applied. This consists of two balloons, which are strapped behind a Perspex board and inflated to compress the ureters as they enter the anatomical pelvis. This produces distension and optimal demonstration of the pelvicalyceal system on the localized '10 min'

Table 6.1 Causes of large kidneys

Causes of unilateral large kidney	
Common	Renal cyst
	Obstructive hydronephrosis
	Duplex collecting system
	Compensatory renal hypertrophy
	Neoplasm (Wilm's tumour, clear cell carcinoma, angiomyolipoma)
	Pyonephrosis
Less common	Trauma (haematoma, urinoma)
	Acute pyelonephritis
	Renal vein thrombosis
	Polycystic kidney
	Acute arterial infarction
	Abscess
Causes of bilateral large kidneys	
Common	Polycystic renal disease
	Early insulin-dependent diabetes
	Bilateral hydronephrosis
	Bilateral duplex collecting system
Less common	Acute tubular necrosis
	Acute glomerulonephritis
	Bilateral cysts or neoplasms
	Parenchymal disease:
	Systemic lupus erythematosus
	Polyarteritis
	Wegener's granulomatosis
	Infiltrative disease:
	Lymphoma
	Myeloma
	Metastases
	Amyloid
	Acute cortical necrosis
	Acromegaly

film (Fig. 6.5b, p. 76). Tomography or oblique views of renal areas may be required further to demonstrate the renal outlines and pelvicalyceal system in patients with haematuria or suspected renal mass.

A full length '15 min' film is taken after releasing the compression to demonstrate ureters and bladder (Fig. 6.6, p. 77) and a postmicturition pelvic film if bladder outflow obstruction is suspected.

In patients with severely impaired renal function, excretion of contrast is very slow because of the low glomerular filtration rate. Nephrotomography will be required to demonstrate renal size and shape and delayed films (up to 24 hours after contrast) are taken in an effort to exclude obstructive uropathy.

Retrograde pyelography

Retrograde pyelography is indicated to demonstrate the pelvicalyceal system and ureter when the IVU images provide insufficient detail – for

Table 6.2 Causes of small kidneys

Causes of unilateral small kidney	
Common	Chronic pyelonephritis Obstructive renal atrophy
Less common	Congenital hypoplasia or dysplasia Tuberculosis Renal infarction Renal artery stenosis Radiation nephritis
Causes of bilateral small kidneys	
Common	Chronic glomerulonephritis Hypertensive nephrosclerosis Chronic pyelonephritis Ischaemia
Less common	Obstructive renal atrophy Chronic papillary necrosis Chronic urate nephropathy

example, to define a small transitional cell carcinoma, or to demonstrate the collecting system of a non-functioning kidney (Fig. 6.7, p. 78). A fine catheter is passed through the ureteric orifice at cystoscopy and advanced to the renal pelvis. Contrast medium is introduced directly into the collecting system, sharply defining the pelvicalyceal system and ureter but not demonstrating renal parenchyma.

The disadvantages of retrograde pyelography are the risk of infection (especially the conversion of a hydronephrosis into a pyonephrosis), the anaesthetic risk and the possibility of urothelial perforation by the catheter. Retrograde pyelography cannot be used as an alternative to IVU in patients allergic to contrast medium as some systemic absorption occurs.

Antegrade pyelography

The chief indication for antegrade pyelography is suspected obstructive uropathy when hydronephrosis has been demonstrated by IVU or ultrasound.

Antegrade pyelography directly demonstrates the collecting system and ureter by percutaneous injection of contrast medium into the pelvicalyceal system. It has the advantages of being performed under local anaesthesia and carrying a low risk of infection.

Using sterile technique, a fine-gauge needle is introduced into the calyceal system under radiological screening control. The needle should pass into the calyx via renal parenchyma, rather than directly puncturing the renal pelvis. This minimizes the risk of haemorrhage by avoiding the hilar vessels and also decreases urinary leakage because renal parenchyma acts as a seal. Urine, or pus, is aspirated for culture

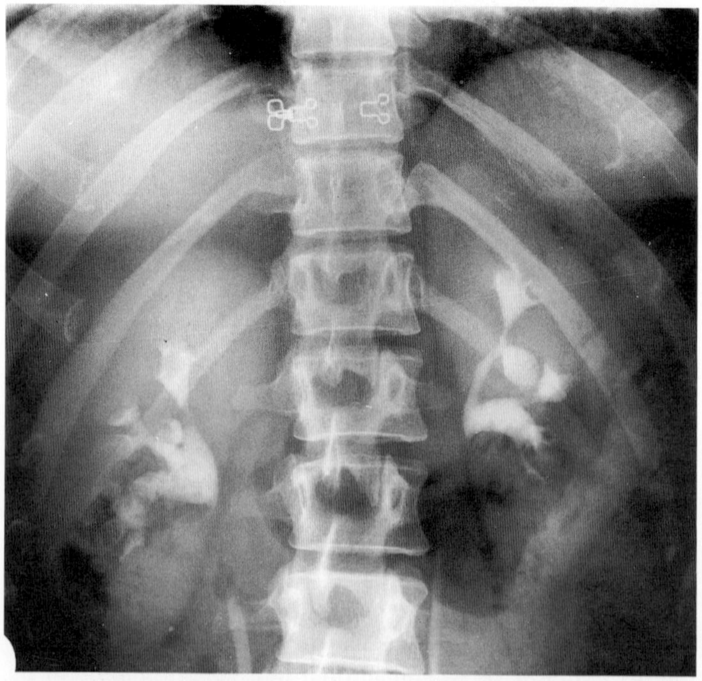

(a)

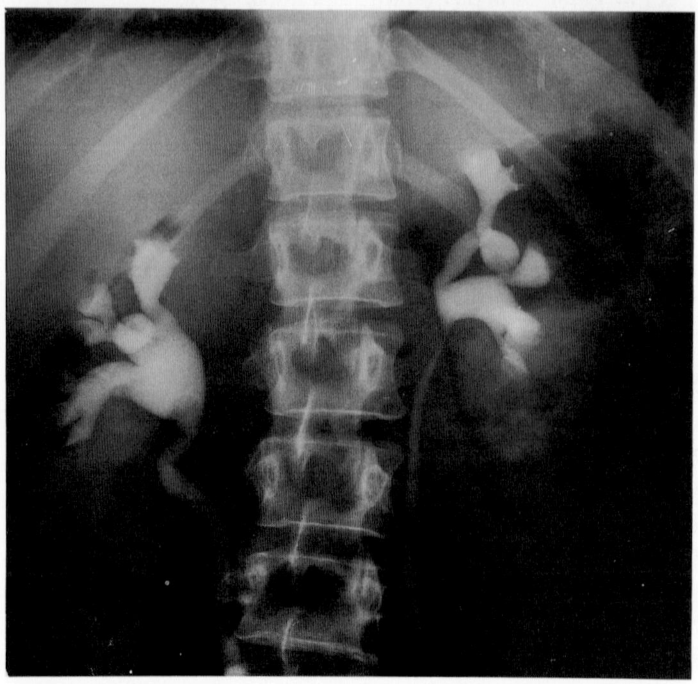

(b)

Fig. 6.5 (a) The 5 min and (b) the 10 min films from a normal IVU series. The 10 min film was taken after abdominal compression, showing distension and improved opacification of the pelvicalyceal system.

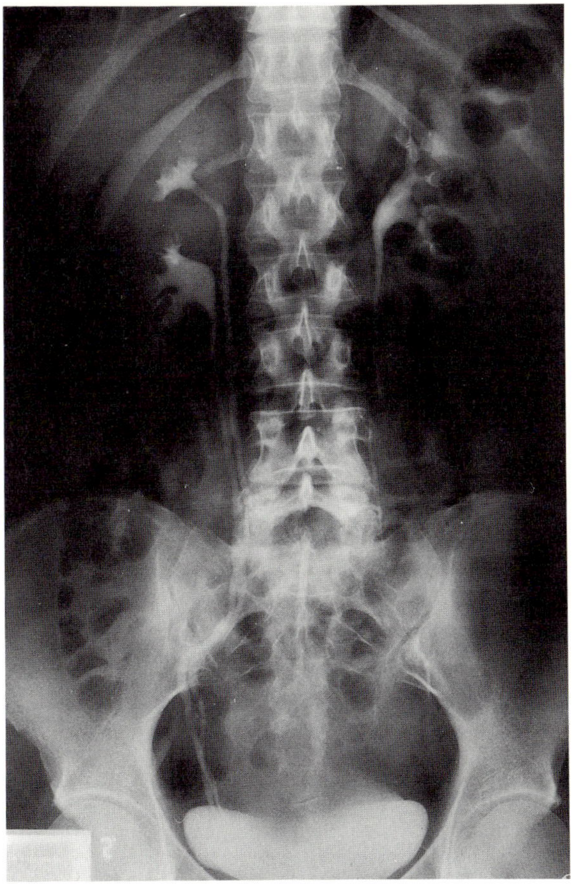

Fig. 6.6 A 15 min IVU film showing a complete duplex collecting system arising from a large right kidney.

and cytological examination. Pressure in the system is also relieved. Contrast medium is injected to demonstrate the collecting system and the level of the obstruction (Fig. 6.8, p. 79) and pressure/flow studies can be performed in equivocal cases.

The procedure may be extended to provide percutaneous nephrostomy drainage of the kidney. Because the calyces are then clearly demonstrated, a larger-calibre needle, capable of taking a guide wire, can precisely be inserted into the collecting system.

The tract is dilated, a 'pigtail' catheter inserted and the renal pelvis irrigated and allowed to drain. Continued drainage gives time for renal function to recover and sepsis to be controlled before surgery is performed.

Radio-isotope studies

Radiopharmaceuticals used in renal imaging consist of an inert compound to which a radioactive nucleus is chemically bound. The nucleus

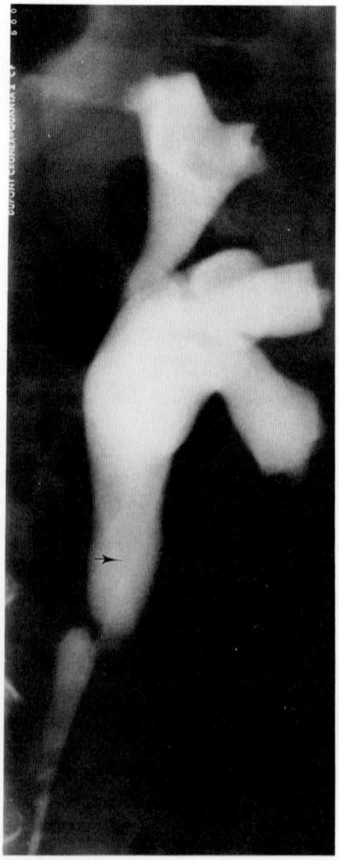

Fig. 6.7 A retrograde pyelogram demonstrating an obstructed pelvicalyceal system. The ureteric catheter is visible with its tip lying within the renal pelvis (arrow).

acts as a label by decaying and emitting radiation, which is detected by a gamma camera, showing the distribution of the molecule. The radiation dose to the patient is normally less with a radio-isotope scan than with an IVU, the gonadal dose being approximately 10% of that received during an IVU when the patient has normal renal function. However, if obstruction is present the dose to kidneys and bladder is greatly increased. The information derived from the study depends on the way the compound as a whole is handled by the kidney. The studies can be broadly divided into those providing dynamic images sequentially, demonstrating the passage of the radiopharmaceutical through the renal tract, and those providing static images of functioning renal tissue.

Gamma camera renography

Radio-isotope renography provides dynamic information about renal function, initially demonstrating renal perfusion, then the passage of

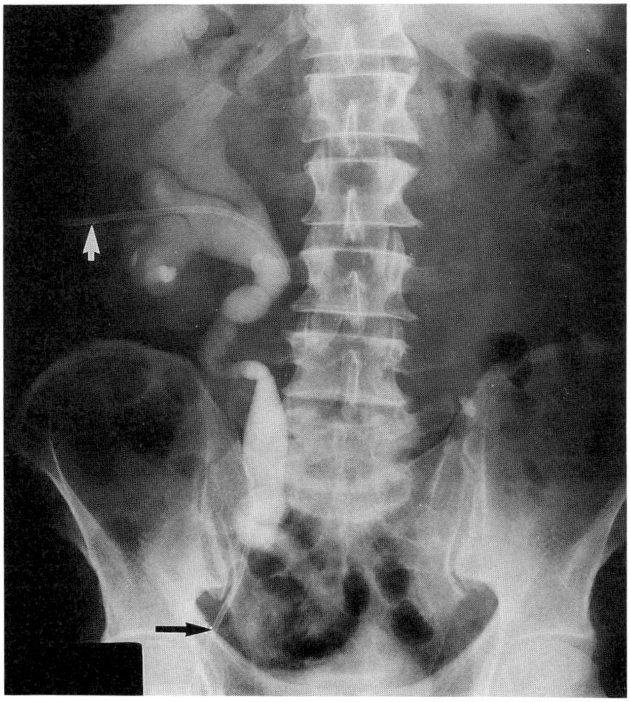

Fig. 6.8 An antegrade pyelogram from a patient with a solitary right kidney who developed renal failure. There are several ureteric strictures following an abdominoperineal resection. The nephrostomy tube (upper arrow) is shown with the 'pigtail' end of the catheter lying within the renal collecting system. There is also a haemodialysis catheter in the right iliac vein (lower arrow).

radio-isotope through the renal tubules and finally the transfer of the compound to the collecting system and bladder. The studies are quantitative, producing graphs of the counts present in each kidney against time, the renogram curve (Fig. 6.9, p. 80), but have the disadvantage of poor spatial resolution so that anatomical detail is not well shown.

Two radiopharmaceuticals are commonly used for dynamic studies:

1 *$^{99}Tc^{m}$ DTPA (diethylene triamine pentacetic acid labelled with technetium-99m.).* Diethylene triamine pentacetic acid is a chelate which is handled by the kidney in a similar way to inulin. It is filtered by glomeruli and excreted without being reabsorbed or secreted by renal tubules. Approximately 20% of DTPA is extracted from blood in a single passage through the kidney. The DTPA is labelled by chelation with technetium-99m, which is cheap, readily available and an ideal radio-isotope for imaging purposes.

2 *^{123}I Hippuran (Sodium ortho-iodohippurate labelled with iodine-123).* Hippuran is handled by the kidney in a similar way to *para*-aminohippuric acid (PAH). It undergoes both glomerular filtration and renal tubular secretion, being almost completely cleared from blood in a single passage through the kidney. Hippuran labelled with iodine-123 gives superior image quality at a lower radiation dose than

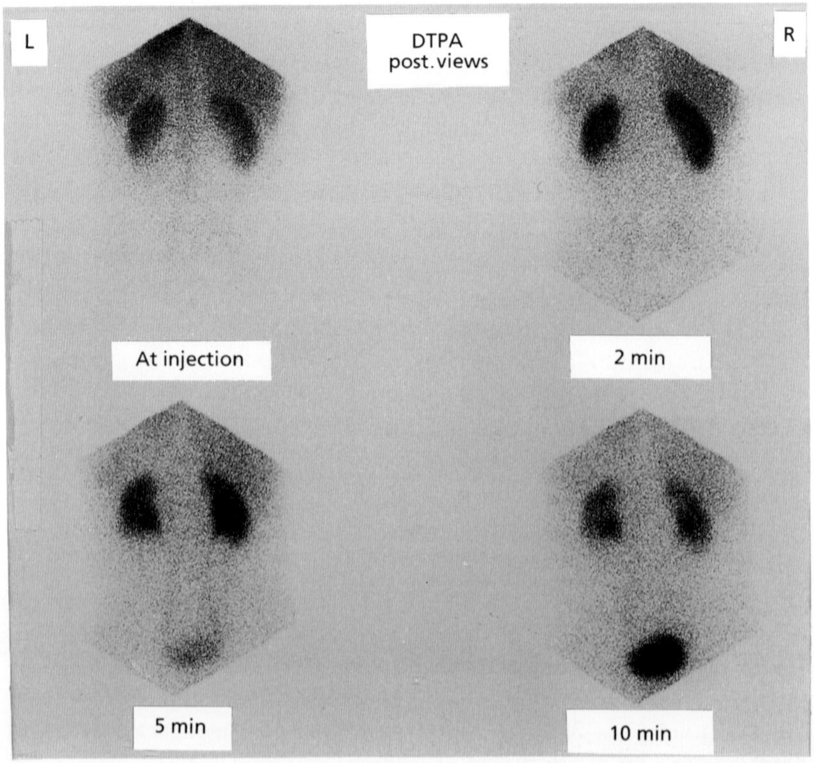

(a)

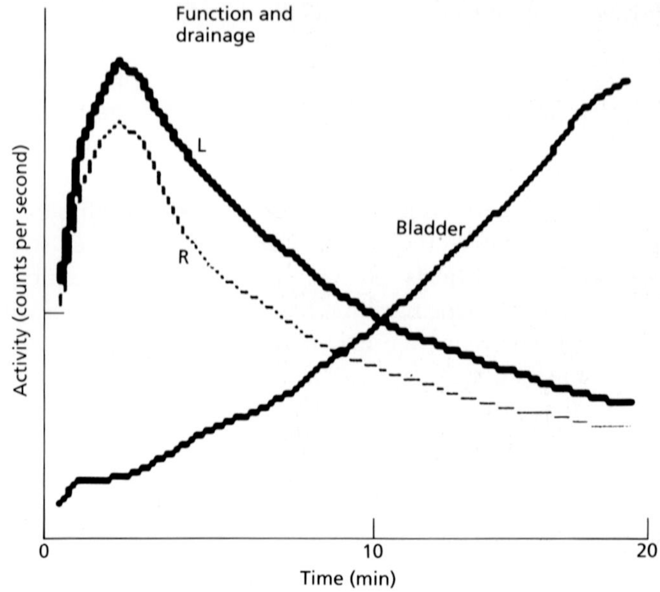

(b)

Fig. 6.9 (a) A series of images from a normal DTPA renogram. (b) The accompanying renogram curve. The peak count for a kidney should occur between 2 and 7 min (2 and 5 min with Hippuran) and the activity decrease to half the peak value within 15 min (10 min with Hippuran).

$^{99}Tc^{m}$ DTPA. Iodine-123 is expensive and of limited availability and is produced in a cyclotron.

Scans performed using different radiopharmaceuticals are not directly comparable as Hippuran is cleared more rapidly than DTPA; therefore for serial scans the same radio-isotope should be used.

Indications for radio-isotope renography include:

1 Obstructive uropathy. In acute obstruction the renogram curve rises more steeply than normal, due to a short-lived increase in blood flow, and continues to rise. A rising curve is not specific to obstruction because it is seen with low rates of urine production, with dilated collecting systems and with renal functional impairment. If a diuretic is given (frusemide 20 mg IV), this will 'wash out' the activity from a non-obstructed kidney (Fig. 6.10). If the obstruction persists, successive renogram curves will become progressively flatter due to deteriorating renal function. The radio-isotope renogram is particularly useful for serial monitoring of obstruction, as it provides quantitative information,

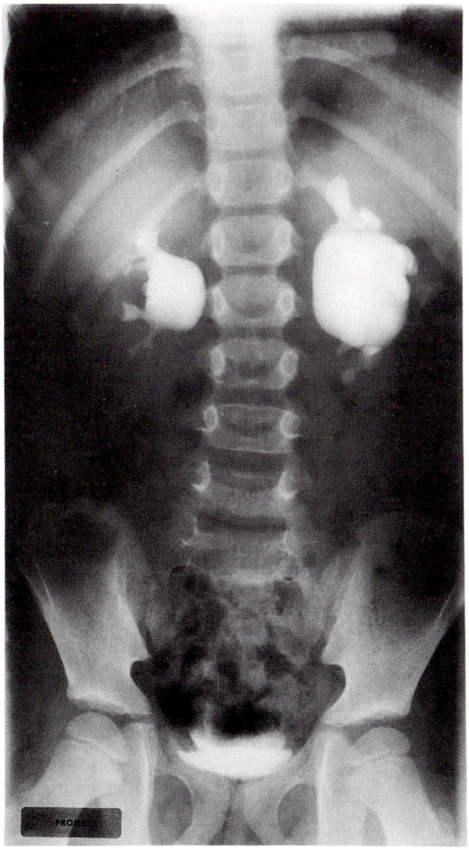

(a)

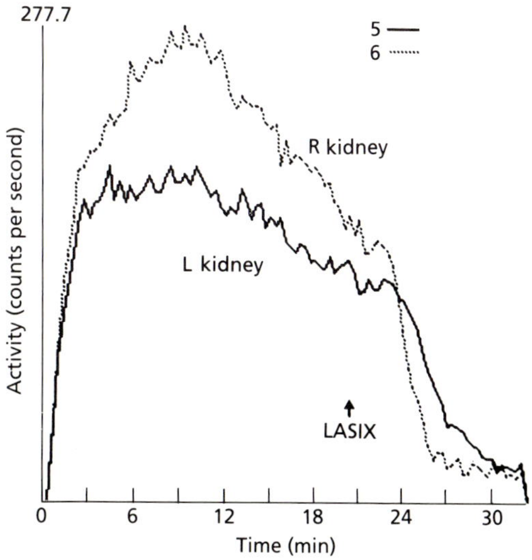

(b)

Fig. 6.10 (a) A 75 min IVU film showing a left hydronephrosis. (b) A diuretic isotope renogram on the same patient. Although the left pelvicalyceal system is dilated, the isotope activity rises and falls normally, excluding obstruction and thus demonstrating the advantage of dynamic information provided by a renogram study.

allowing early detection of changing renal function which is not available from other imaging techniques.

2 Investigation of renal failure, especially following aortic surgery. The scan will differentiate infarction, where the renal area is wholly photon-deficient, producing a ghost image (Fig. 6.11), from acute tubular necrosis, where there is an early vascular peak followed by gradual diffusion of activity from the kidney with no evidence of excretion.

3 The renogram gives an indication of the relative function of one kidney compared with its fellow. This investigation is helpful when deciding if a salvage operation should be performed on a poorly functioning kidney. A kidney damaged by reflux nephropathy is a good example. If a kidney is contributing less than 10% of total renal function, then nephrectomy may be beneficial.

4 Renal trauma. If both IVU and radio-isotope renogram are normal, clinically important renal damage is excluded and this avoids the need for arteriography or computed tomography.

5 Suspected renal artery stenosis. Renography demonstrates a slowly rising curve which may not plateau for up to 15 min, but delayed images show progressive disappearance of activity and a non-dilated

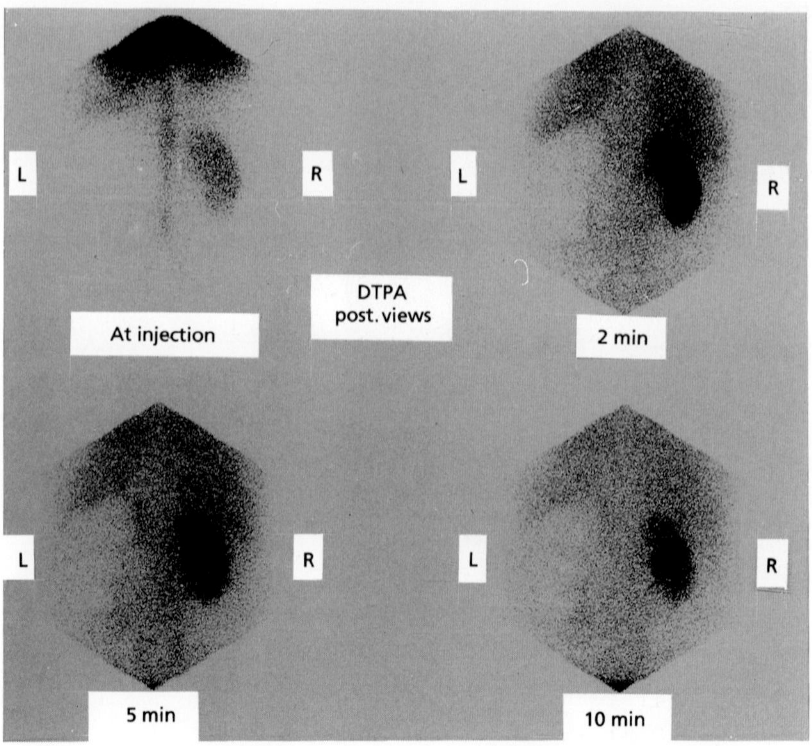

Fig. 6.11 A series of images from a DTPA scan in a patient who developed renal impairment following aortic surgery. The right kidney is avascular and is demonstrated as a totally photon-deficient 'hole' because it contains even less isotope than the normally vascularized surrounding tissues.

collecting system. Unfortunately, there is a false-negative rate of at least 10%.

Renal scintigraphy

Static images of functioning renal tissue are obtained using dimercaptosuccinic acid (DMSA). Twenty-five per cent of an injected dose is bound to proximal renal tubular cells, 25% is excreted by the kidneys and the remainder is distributed evenly throughout the body. Images of the renal parenchyma are recorded 2 hours after intravenous injection. Because DMSA is fixed, several minutes may be taken to produce a single image, allowing many more counts to be collected and a 'pinhole' collimator to be used. This results in a much more detailed and sharper image than is obtained at dynamic scanning. Dimercaptosuccinic acid scanning is particularly useful for detecting renal scarring long before an IVU abnormality becomes apparent (Fig. 6.12, p. 84) and for showing the extent of viable renal tissue following trauma. Dimercaptosuccinic acid scanning should not be performed within 6 weeks of an acute episode of acute pyelonephritis because abnormalities demonstrated in the acute stage may be reversible and not due to persistent scars.

Computed tomography

The renal tract is surrounded by fat, making it particularly suitable for imaging by computed tomography (CT). Fat has low attenuation, in that it absorbs few of the X-rays that pass through it and therefore appears relatively dark on the resultant image. Computed tomography demonstrates renal outlines; hence the cross-sectional size and the thickness of the renal parenchyma can be measured, but unenhanced CT does not differentiate renal cortex from medulla. Calyces and ureters are demonstrated as low-attenuation structures which are markedly enhanced after intravenous contrast. The retroperitoneal structures and other abdominal organs are also shown. Computed tomography cannot be performed in patients who are dyspnoeic at rest or orthopnoeic. Barium studies should not be performed in the week before CT as the high density of barium may cause image artefacts.

Indications for CT include:

1 Investigation of a renal mass where ultrasound suggests a solid lesion or is equivocal. Simple cysts can be reliably diagnosed (Figs 6.13 and 6.14, p. 85). Computed tomography will not only substantiate the diagnosis of renal tumour, but may also demonstrate metastases or extra-renal extension of the tumour, either through the capsule or into the renal vein (Fig. 6.15, p. 86). Computed tomography usually obviates the need for angiography (Fig. 6.16, p. 86).

2 Investigation of renal failure. Urinary obstruction and causes such as calculi, lymph nodes or retroperitoneal fibrosis are well demonstrated and the renal size can be measured accurately.

3 Investigation of renal trauma. Computed tomography will demon-

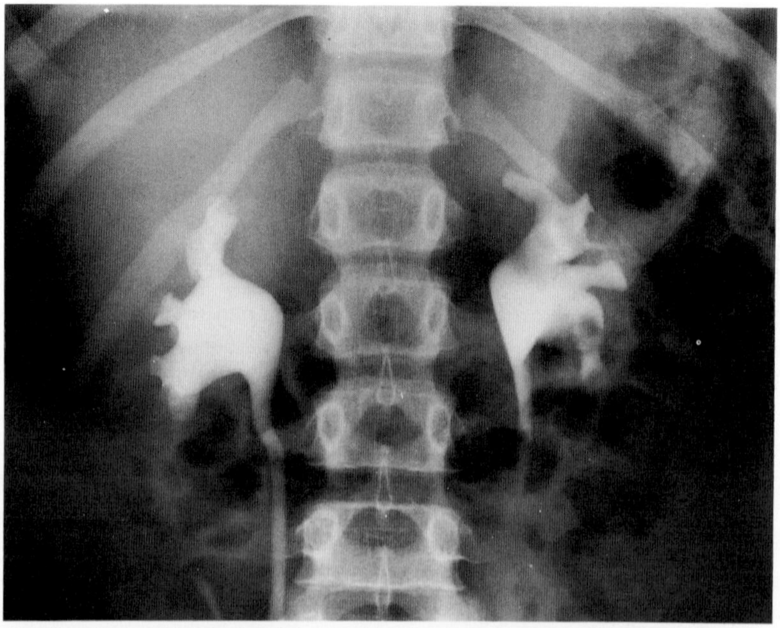

(a)

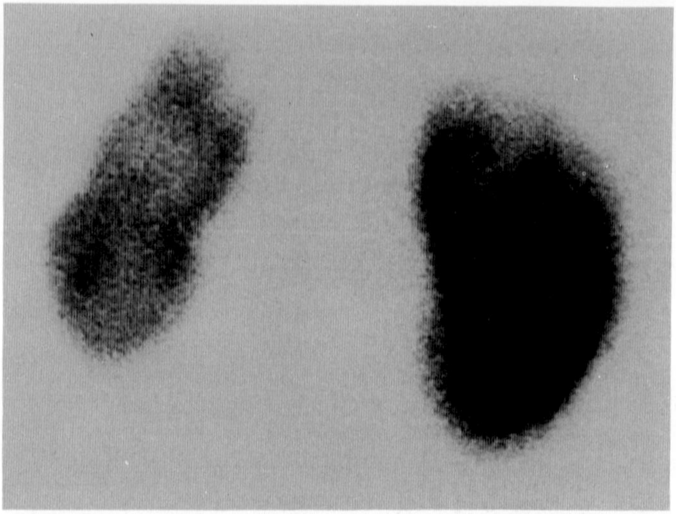

(b)

Fig. 6.12 (a) An apparently normal 10 min IVU film from a child. (b) A DMSA scan of the same patient showing severe loss of functioning renal tissue (scarring) of the left kidney and upper pole of the right kidney.

strate the renal vascular supply, excretion of contrast, haematoma formation and urinary obstruction.

Renal angiography

Renal arteriography provides the most detailed images of the renal vascular supply and is particularly useful for demonstrating intrarenal arteries. It is possible to extend the procedure to perform transluminal

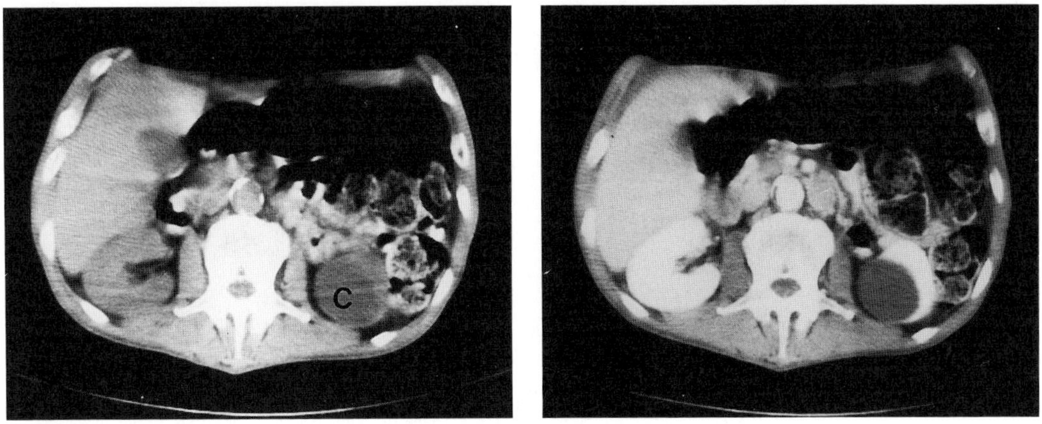

(a) (b)

Fig. 6.13 Abdominal CT scans at the same level demonstrating a simple renal cyst. (a) Before contrast the cyst (C) is seen as a smooth-walled homogeneous structure of lower density than the surrounding renal parenchyma. (b) After intravenous contrast is given, the renal parenchyma is markedly enhanced (it appears much whiter) whereas the avascular cyst is unchanged.

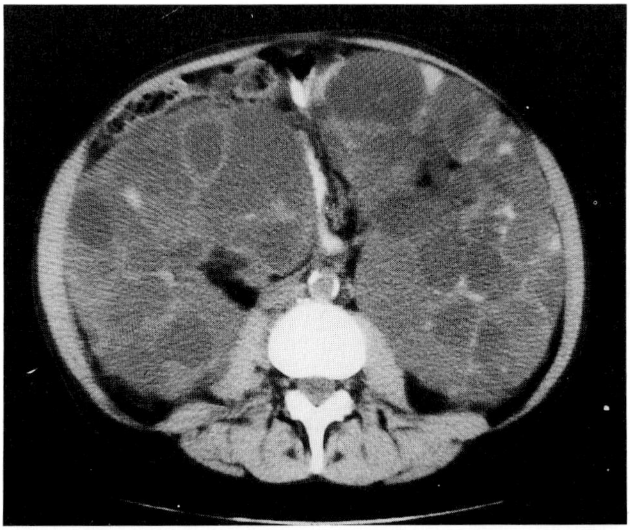

Fig. 6.14 An abdominal CT section in a patient with renal failure due to adult polycystic renal disease. Both kidneys are massively enlarged and almost entirely replaced by multiple simple cysts.

arterial dilatation or selective arterial embolization. The procedure is performed under local anaesthetic via the femoral artery. A flush aortogram is performed first, as accessory renal arteries are common, occurring in 30% of kidneys and arising anywhere from the lower thoracic aorta to the internal iliac arteries (Fig. 6.17, p. 87). Selective studies of individual renal arteries are then performed.

Indications for renal arteriography include:

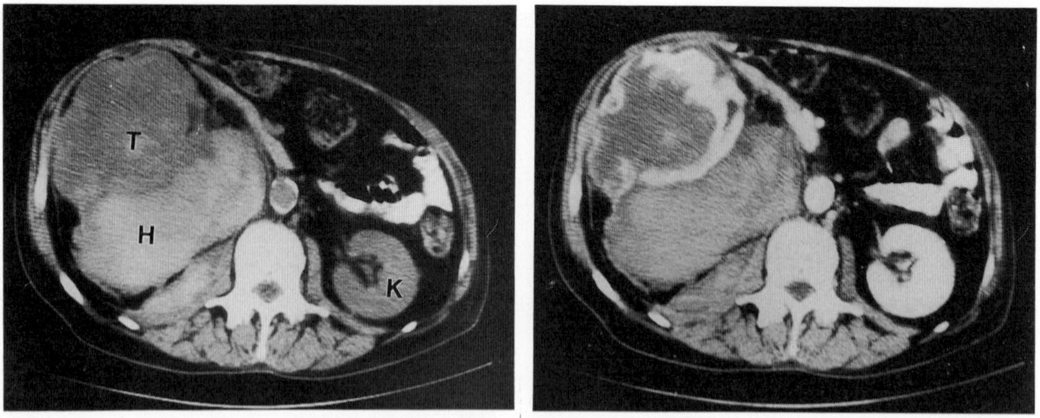

(a) (b)

Fig. 6.15 (a), (b) Abdominal CT scans at the same level demonstrating a right renal hypernephroma (T). The right kidney is displaced anteriorly by haematoma (H) and is enlarged, irregular and of variable density. The left kidney appears normal (K). (b) After intravenous contrast the vascular parts of the tumour are enhanced but the necrotic areas are unchanged.

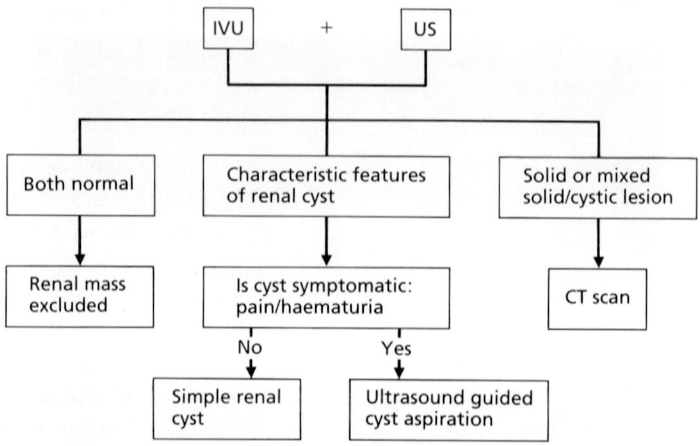

Fig. 6.16 Investigation of suspected renal mass. US, Ultrasound.

1 Renal trauma. Angiography is the investigation of choice if vascular damage is suspected.
2 Investigation of renal masses. The typical tumour circulation of a malignant lesion or vascular distortion by a cyst may be demonstrated. Ultrasound and CT have largely replaced angiography for the investigation of mass lesions.
3 Suspected renal artery stenosis.

Digital subtraction angiography

Digital subtraction angiography (DSA) produces an image of the renal vasculature by electronically subtracting a 'mask' image of the renal

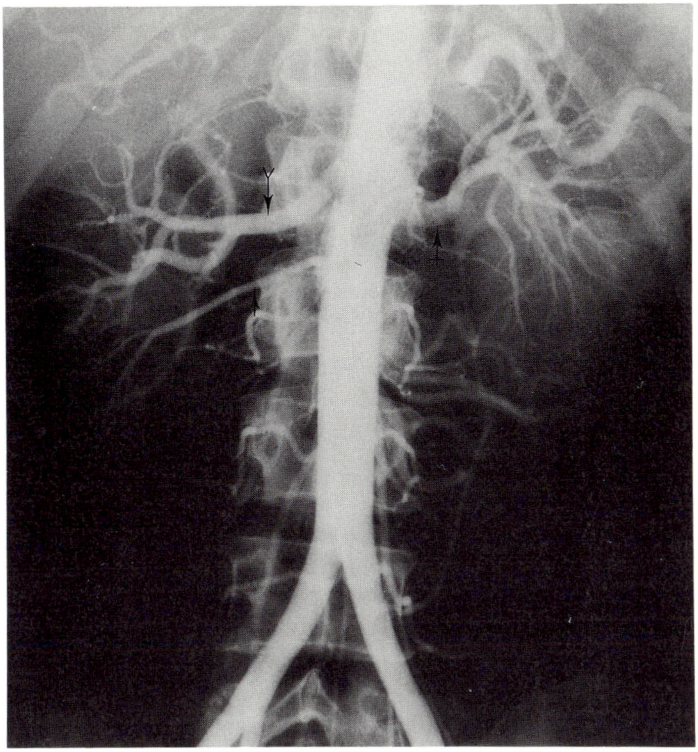

Fig. 6.17 A normal renal arteriogram of a potential renal donor. The left kidney has a single renal artery (arrow). The right kidney has an accessory renal artery (lower arrow) as well as the main renal artery (upper arrow).

area from an image produced after contrast has been injected. The contrast medium can be given either intravenously as a bolus into a central vein or intra-arterially. The intra-arterial route provides better image quality and allows selective renal arterial studies and interventional procedures to be performed but is more invasive than the intravenous route. It requires less contrast medium than conventional arteriography, allowing the use of finer-bore catheters so that procedures can be performed on an out-patient basis. Intravenous DSA is less invasive but provides relatively poor spatial resolution, such that fine anatomical detail is not shown. Intravenous DSA is indicated as a less invasive alternative to conventional arteriography where fine intrarenal detail is not essential – for example, the investigation of renovascular hypertension. Intravenous DSA is more sensitive than IVU or radioisotope studies and gives a direct demonstration of the vasculature (Fig. 6.18, p. 88).

Magnetic resonance imaging

Magnetic resonance imaging (MRI) provides images of a similar quality to CT scanning without the use of ionizing radiation but is more

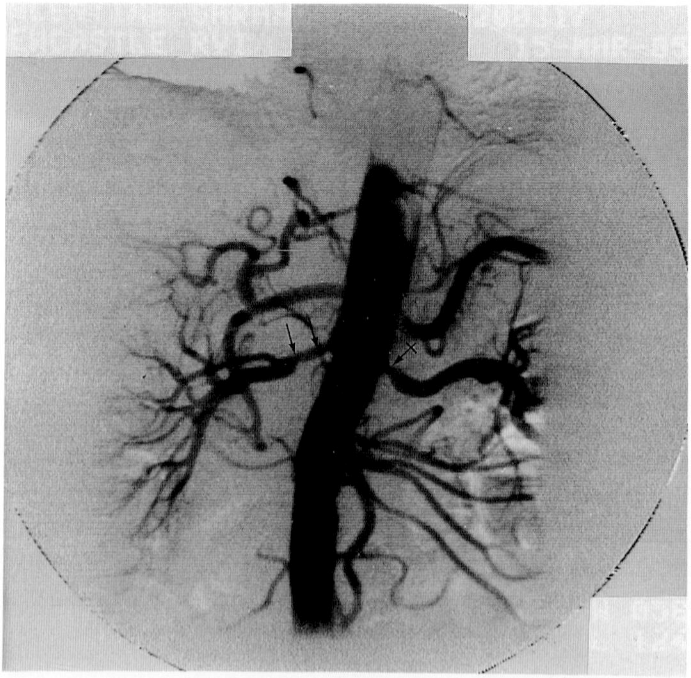

Fig. 6.18 An intra-aortic DSA image of a hypertensive patient showing a long stenosis of the right renal artery (double arrows) and a short stenosis of the left renal artery at its origin (single arrow).

expensive and not widely available. A technical limitation is the time taken to acquire data, resulting in image degradation from respiratory movement. The lack of signal from calcification complicates image interpretation and, because there is similar signal intensity between normal and abnormal renal tissue, a lesion may not be detected unless it distorts the renal outline.

The renal outlines are clearly demonstrated and the cortex and medulla are readily differentiated. The renal vessels are routinely shown but not their segmental branches. There is excellent anatomical demonstration of the collecting systems.

Magnetic resonance imaging demonstrates renal cysts, abscesses and haematomas, but has not proved more accurate than CT in these conditions. Tumour invasion of vessels, lymphadenopathy and bony metastases are readily detected, making MRI slightly more accurate than CT in the staging of renal tumours. The main clinical application of renal MRI is in those subjects who are sensitive to contrast media.

Summary

This chapter has described the radiological investigations commonly needed by the clinician investigating a patient with renal disease. Clear understanding of the information to be obtained will assist both choice of investigation and interpretation.

Further reading

1 Ansell, G.R. (1990) Adverse reactions to contrast agents: scope of problem. *Invest. Radiol.* **4**, 381–91.
2 Ansell, G.R. & Wilkins, R.A. (eds) (1987) *Complications in Diagnostic Imaging.* Blackwell Scientific Publications, Oxford.
3 Choyke, P.L. & Pollack, H.M. (1988) The role of MRI in disease of the kidney. *Radiol. Clin. N. Am.* **26** (3), 617–31.
4 Dunnick, N.R., Svetkey, L.P., Cohan, R.H., Newman, G.E., Braun, S.D., Himmelstein, S.I., Bollinger, R.R., McCann, R.L., Wilkinson, R.H., Jr. & Klotman, P.E. (1989) Intravenous digital subtraction renal angiography: use in screening for renovascular hypertension. *Radiology* **171**, 219–22.
5 Kamholtz, R.G., Cronan, J.J. & Dorfman G.S. (1989) Obstruction and the minimally dilated renal collecting system: US evaluation. *Radiology* **170**, 51–3.
6 Pollock, H.M. & Wein, A.J. (1989) Imaging of renal trauma. *Radiology* **172**, 297–308.
7 Talner, L.B., Scheible, W., Ellenbogen, P.H., Beck, C.H., Jr. & Gosink, B.B. (1981) How accurate is ultrasonography in detecting hydronephrosis in azotemic patients? *Urol. Radiol.* **3** (1), 1–6.
8 Whitehouse, G.H. & Worthington, B.S. (1989) *Techniques in Diagnostic Imaging.* Blackwell Scientific Publications, Oxford.

Chapter 7
Laboratory Investigations of Patients with Infection-related Disease of the Urinary Tract

Rosalind Maskell

Microbiological investigations are essential in the diagnosis and management of patients with diseases of the kidneys and urinary tract. They are used most commonly in connection with urinary tract infection (UTI) and its consequences, but also in dealing with other aspects of renal disease as it presents in a general hospital, for example chronic renal failure (CRF) and acute renal failure (ARF), before transfer to a renal unit. The value of such investigations is in direct proportion not only to the skill of the laboratory but also to the way in which they are used and interpreted by clinicians. Much of the laboratory work requested in hospitals is undertaken on poorly collected or incorrect types of specimens. Additionally, laboratory reports are often unhelpful to doctors because they do not provide the required information and the clinician is often uncertain what importance to attach to the reported findings. Unnecessary investigations may lead to unnecessary, and potentially harmful, antibiotic treatment. Conversely, investigations vital to the correct management of patients are frequently omitted.

In this chapter, the microbiological investigations appropriate to the diagnosis and management of patients with UTI and renal diseases will be considered. Guidance will be given about specimen collection and transport, the information that laboratories require from requesting clinicians, and ways in which communication between laboratory and clinicians can be improved so as to provide the maximum help to the patient.

Urinary tract infection

Infection is the most common disease of the urinary tract encountered in medical practice. Symptoms are troublesome and often recurrent and there are important sequelae in some patients. Referral for hospital investigation and advice about management is common. An understanding is also necessary in medical and surgical in-patient practice. Many patients admitted for other reasons will be found to have UTI. Catheterization is a predisposing factor and UTI is an important cause of fever of uncertain origin and of bacteraemia. Therefore all doctors practising in hospital should understand the correct use of laboratory investigations in diagnosis and management of UTI.

There are three essentials in the relationship between clinician and laboratory staff:

1 Send the appropriate type of specimen, correctly collected, labelled and transported.

2 Give adequate, accurate information on the request form.

3 Do not send unnecessary specimens.

Laboratory diagnosis of urinary tract infection

Specimen collection

With few exceptions, for example the patient who presents with the classical symptoms and signs of acute pyelonephritis – fever, loin pain, rigors, tender kidney and sometimes, but not always, dysuria and frequency – the diagnosis of UTI cannot be made on clinical grounds alone. Microbiological examination of a urine specimen is essential and, because the great majority of infections are caused by organisms which are commensal in the bowel or areas adjacent to the urethral orifice, specimens must be collected in such a way that the risk of contamination is minimized. Clearly, specimen collection methods vary in different types of patients; the accuracy of diagnosis and sensible use of laboratory resources depend upon a clear understanding of this by the requesting clinician.

The midstream urine specimen (MSU) is the most widely used method of urine collection for bacteriology. When carefully collected and examined within 4 hours of voiding, it provides a reliable diagnostic tool for detection of bacteriuria – the abnormal presence of organisms above the distal one-third of the urethra (which has a mixed commensal flora). After carefully washing the perineum with soap and water (boys and men should wash the penis after retracting the foreskin, if possible), the first part of the stream is discarded, and the midstream urine is collected into a sterile container. There are, therefore, two important essentials for this method: the patient must have a sufficient volume of urine in the bladder to allow the initial volume, which is assumed to wash away the urethral commensals, to be discarded, and they must have adequate voluntary control of micturition. Provided this is so,

Table 7.1 Specimen collection when midstream urine specimen is not obtainable

Old people (equivocal result from MSU)	Diagnostic catheter specimen (CSU)
Patients with neuropathic or ileal bladders Congenital abnormalities Spinal injuries Neurological disorders: multiple sclerosis Diabetic autonomic neuropathy involving the bladder	Diagnostic CSU[a]
Patients with oliguric renal failure	Diagnostic CSU[a]
Patients with indwelling catheter	CSU[a] (MSU 2–3 days after catheter removed)

[a] Only if there is a clinical indication for treatment, such as fever or loin pain.

satisfactory specimens can be obtained. The problem of perineal contamination is often exaggerated. The only patients in whom this constitutes a difficulty are elderly women, especially if they are inactive and in hospital. In these the perineum is often heavily contaminated with Gram-negative bowel organisms. In such patients and in others in whom midstream specimen collection is not possible, other methods are required (Table 7.1).

Collection of urine from elderly women by suprapubic aspiration (SPA) has been advocated, but the difficulty of retaining a sufficient volume of urine to distend the bladder makes such a procedure difficult and unpleasant for the patient. Specimen collection by careful aseptic catheterization provides a definitive answer.

Patients with urinary diversion

Organisms multiply in collection bags worn by patients with ileal bladders. Culture of urine from the bag gives misleading results and should never be requested. If investigation is indicated for clinical reasons, such as fever or loin pain, the urine should be collected by careful catheterization of the stoma.

Patients with indwelling catheters

Urine specimens from patients with indwelling catheters, whether long-term or short-term, account for much waste of time and materials in laboratories. Clinicians (or the nursing staff, who often take the initiative in the matter) generally have little understanding of the natural history of bacteriuria in such patients. An indwelling catheter provides a direct, moist connection between the bladder and the exterior, facilitating the ascent of urethral and perineal organisms. After a catheter has been *in situ* for a few days, bladder urine is inevitably colonized and culture will be positive. Antibacterial treatment given for such colonization, in response to a laboratory report, may sterilize the urine briefly, but if the catheter remains *in situ* infection will rapidly recur. The organisms will become progressively more resistant and episodes of clinical infection more difficult to treat. Therefore, urine from catheterized patients should not be sent to the laboratory unless there is a clinical indication for treatment (see below). There is no advantage in attempts to monitor the bacteriological state of the urine in such patients because the flora is usually mixed and changes constantly.

From the recognition that catheterization is an important cause of bacteriuria, it follows that an MSU should be cultured 2–3 days after removal of a catheter, and after catheterization for investigations such as micturating cystography, cystoscopy and urodynamic studies.

Urinary tract tuberculosis

Three consecutive early morning urine specimens (EMUs) are required. They should be delivered to the laboratory, each with a separate request form, as soon as possible. If this is not practicable, they may be refrigerated and delivered together on the third day.

Schistosomiasis

A terminal specimen of urine should be sent for examination for the ova of *Schistosoma haematobium*, ideally collected between 10.00 and 14.00 hours when egg excretion is maximal.

Request forms

Microbiology is an interpretative discipline. The bacteriological diagnosis of UTI is made more difficult by the fact that the causative organisms, with rare exceptions, are commensals which may contaminate urine during specimen collection. It is vital, therefore, if microscopy and culture findings are to be interpreted correctly, that the laboratory receives accurate information on request forms. The same findings can mean quite different things in a bag specimen of urine and in an SPA; in a patient who is or is not on treatment; in a patient with an indwelling catheter who is well and in one who is unwell; in men and in women.

Therefore, the following information is essential on request forms:

1 Correct name, age and sex of patient.
2 Correct nature of the specimen and the investigations required.
3 Clinical reason for the request.
4 Presence or absence of symptoms and fever.
5 Current or recent antibacterial treatment.
6 Any known abnormality of the urinary tract.

Forms should be written by the doctor who makes the decision to request the investigation. Any other system – routine requesting by nurses, for example – results in misuse of the laboratory and waste of resources. Furthermore, the findings will be interpreted in the laboratory in the light of inadequate or incorrect information and the usefulness of the report will be proportionately less. With increasing constraints on laboratory expenditure, quality can only be maintained if relevant requests are made.

Laboratory investigations

Clinicians who require laboratory examination of urine specimens should understand what tests are undertaken in the laboratory and how the results are interpreted. Technical details are inappropriate here; laboratories differ widely both in methods and interpretation.

The four commonly requested investigations for the diagnosis of UTI are detection of proteinuria, microscopy, culture and sensitivity testing.

Proteinuria

Proteinuria is not a reliable guide to the presence of infection and should not be routinely requested on all urine specimens. There is no justification for the use of 'Stix' testing for protein in laboratories – false-positive results are too common. An accurate test, usually the salicylsulphonic acid test, should be used when appropriate. Quantitative measurement of proteinuria in patients with diseases other than UTI is considered in Chapter 4, p. 48.

Microscopy

Microscopy is still undertaken in the majority of laboratories; in some, however, owing to excessive workload, it is only performed on selected specimens. The usual justification for abandoning microscopy is that infection is diagnosed on culture and that the presence of pyuria adds nothing to the diagnosis. The absence of pyuria, contrary to widely held beliefs, does not detract from the importance of bacteriuria. Unfortunately, the converse is not true; the presence of pyuria in the absence, or apparent absence (see below), of bacteriuria may be of great clinical importance and will be undetected if microscopy is omitted.

Methods of microscopy vary between laboratories. In general, when the centrifuged deposit is examined, the findings bear no accurate relationship to the concentration of cells in the urine. Methods of counting cells in whole urine are more accurate, and laboratories usually report their findings in such a way as to indicate that the white cell count is within normal limits (<10 white cells/mm^3), moderately raised (10–20 white cells/mm^3) or considerably raised (>20 white cells/mm^3).

Culture and sensitivity testing

Important considerations in urine culture are the medium or media used, the duration and atmosphere of incubation, the interpretation of the findings and criteria used for testing and reporting sensitivities to antibacterial agents.

The medium used should reliably detect the presence of all the recognized urinary pathogens and, preferably, also the Gram-positive organisms that comprise the commensal flora of the distal urethra, the presence of which suggests some contamination of the specimen.

Urine cultures are usually incubated overnight in air at a temperature of 37 °C; this enables the detection of the common aerobic pathogens and the cultures can be read the next day. This protocol leaves unexplained the symptoms of about one-half of the patients who complain of dysuria or frequency. With mounting evidence that organisms that grow slowly and require carbon dioxide in the incubation atmosphere can be isolated from the urine of such patients, it becomes necessary to consider new protocols for incubation of urine cultures. Very few laboratories provide 48-hour incubation in 7% CO_2 as a routine procedure for urine cultures as yet, but many will do so if requested by a clinician faced with a difficult clinical problem or unexplained pyuria.

Interpretation and reporting of urine cultures are particularly difficult. This stems from the very large number of urine specimens sent for culture, the traditional view that a numerical rule of thumb can be applied in interpretation, and the custom of relegating the urine work to the least skilled scientific staff.

There is now so much evidence that the urine of many patients with infections does not yield a count of 10^8 organisms/L (10^5/ml) – daytime specimens from patients with severe frequency, specimens from patients excreting a few organisms from infection stones, specimens from men with prostatitis are some examples – that there is no alternative to attempting to assess the importance of each urine culture 'on its merits'. In so doing, adequate, accurate data on the request form are essential.

In general, it is preferable that the report should tell the clinician, at least in general terms, what was isolated from the specimen. Terms such as 'no significant growth', 'moderate mixed growth' and 'no pathogens isolated' are quite unhelpful. Whoever interprets the culture in the laboratory will decide on its importance and whether to perform sensitivity tests. By the time the clinician receives the report, the culture will almost certainly have been discarded and second thoughts are not usually possible. However, it is of some help to the clinician to know that only mixed Gram-positive species were isolated, or that there was a low count of a Gram-negative organism. In the clinical context, he/she may be able to accept the former as suggesting contamination, but feel that the latter may indicate infection and therefore warrant a further MSU.

Reports of isolates considered to be 'significant' – usually a high count of a recognized pathogen in pure culture – will state the sensitivity of the organism to a variable number of antibacterial agents. These will be chosen as those most appropriate for treatment of UTI. With the satisfactory situation in Britain that the majority of urinary pathogens are still sensitive to several of the cheap oral agents, a choice of four or five of these is usually adequate. Other agents, including those that are given parenterally, should only be tested and reported for resistant organisms or for appropriate clinical circumstances. It is wise for clinicians to restrict the agents they use to those reported by the laboratory; use of other agents should first be discussed with the microbiologist.

Interpretation of the laboratory report

Many laboratory reports are misunderstood or misinterpreted by clinicians; this renders laboratory work useless and wasteful. If, after paying attention to the considerations described above, the clinician is unable to interpret reports correctly, he/she should discuss the problem with the microbiologist. The aim should be to ensure that he/she receives the information he/she needs, and that laboratory time and resources are not wasted. Improved communications may lead to increasing demand in some areas, but may be offset by a decrease in the very large number of unnecessary requests.

Urinary infection in different groups of patients

Pregnant women

Screening for bacteriuria

About 5% of women have bacteriuria in early pregnancy; the majority will have acquired it only after they became sexually active, but in a minority (1–2%) it will date back to childhood. Early diagnosis and management of UTI in pregnancy has two major beneficial effects. First, it prevents the great majority of cases of acute pyelonephritis which characteristically occur about the sixth month. The ascent of bacteria from the bladder to one or both kidneys is attributed to changes in the ureteric musculature consequent upon the hormonal changes of pregnancy, allowing reflux of infected urine from bladder to kidney. Secondly, careful questioning may detect those whose infection dates back to childhood and who are, therefore, more likely to have renal scars. Figure 7.1 gives guidelines for bacteriological screening and management of UTI in early pregnancy.

Indications for ultrasound investigation after the puerperium are:

1 Failure to eradicate infection after appropriate treatment.
2 Frequent recurrences of infection.
3 Infection with unusual or resistant organisms.
4 Urinary tract infection and hypertension.
5 Childhood history of UTI or enuresis.

If a pregnancy bacteriuria screening programme is to be effective, good communications between patient, obstetrician and laboratory are essential. If the laboratory findings are not acted upon appropriately, the procedure is costly and wasteful.

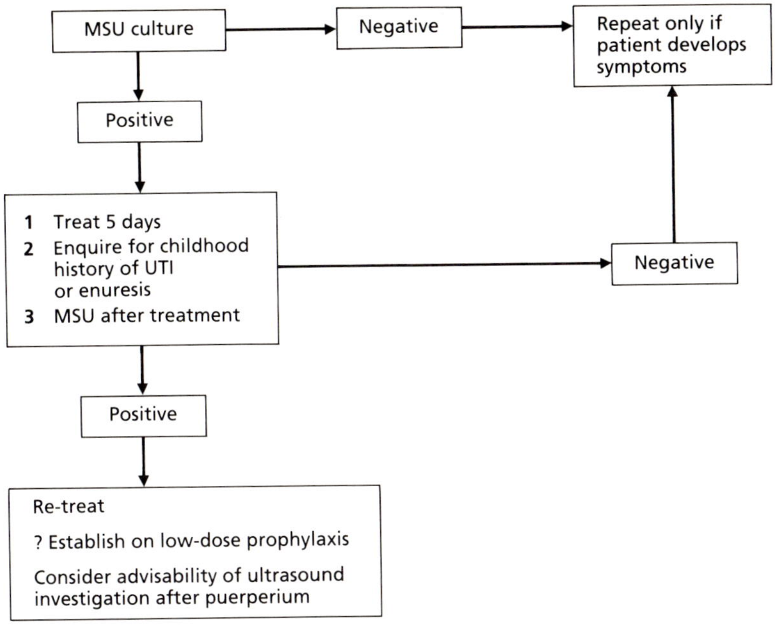

Fig. 7.1 Screening for bacteriuria in early pregnancy.

Urinary symptoms in pregnancy

Many women present during pregnancy with symptoms suggestive of UTI. Recent bacteriological advances have shown that, although some have infection with recognized aerobic pathogens, the symptoms of many others are associated with the presence of fastidious bacteria in the urine. In these women antibacterial treatment is usually contraindicated because it may distort the balance of commensal flora; alkalinizing agents may be preferable. Figure 7.2 gives guidelines for the diagnosis and management of pregnant women with urinary symptoms.

Antibacterial agents in pregnancy

Amoxycillin and cephalosporins are safe throughout pregnancy but the latter are needed only for treatment of resistant organisms. Nitrofurantoin (50 mg qds taken with food or milk) can be used safely in early pregnancy and up to the end of the eighth month. In this dose it does not cause nausea in the majority. Co-trimoxazole or trimethoprim should not be used before 12–14 weeks but may be used safely from then until the end of the eighth month.

Women who are on long-term prophylactic regimens for recurrent UTI, especially those with vesicoureteric reflux or renal scarring, should continue the regimen during pregnancy. In view of the caveats expressed above, nitrofurantoin 50 mg *nocte*, given until the end of the eighth month, is a satisfactory regimen. Women who get frequent

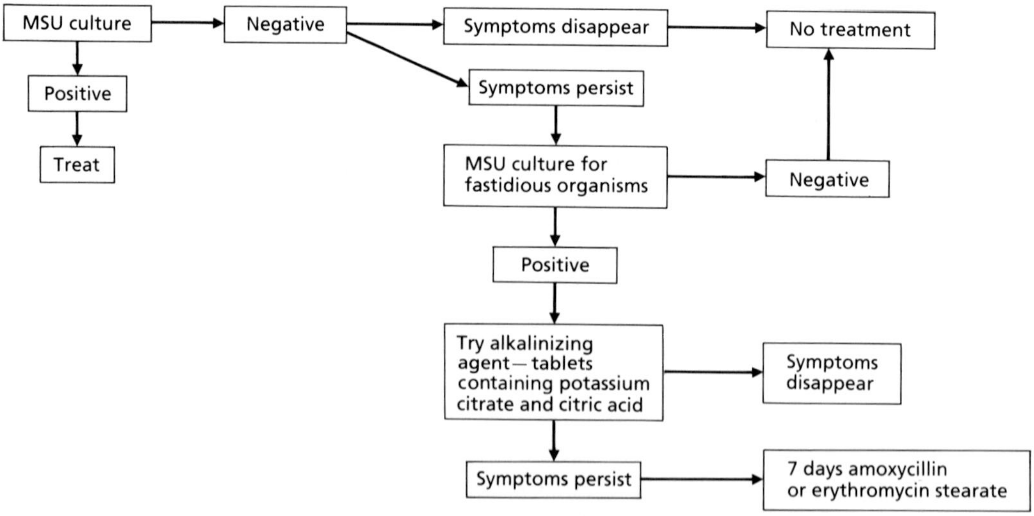

Fig. 7.2 Patients with urinary symptoms during pregnancy.

recurrences of UTI during pregnancy should also be established on a prophylactic regimen following effective treatment.

Patients admitted for gynaecological, urological or other surgery

Urinary tract infection may be an incidental finding, it may be causally related to the indication for surgery, or it may be secondary to the surgery itself or to catheterization.

Midstream urine culture is indicated for symptoms, or for any other reason to suspect UTI, and 2–3 days after removal of catheters.

Catheter specimen of urine (CSU) culture is only indicated if a catheterized patient develops a clinical indication for antibiotic treatment, for example, fever (see p. 99).

These indications apply whether or not there is an attempt to keep the urine sterile during a short period of catheterization by the prophylactic use of an antibiotic. If catheterization is likely to last 5 days or longer, antibiotics should not be prescibed because they select resistant organisms.

Septicaemia should be suspected in catheterized patients who develop fever and rigors. A CSU and blood cultures should be sent to the laboratory before 'best-guess' antibacterial therapy is started. If the patient is not already receiving antibiotics, the organism is likely to be a sensitive Gram-negative one. However, if the patient is already on treatment the likelihood of a resistant Gram-negative or Gram-positive organism should be considered and appropriate therapy discussed with the bacteriologist.

Medical and geriatric in-patients

There is no justification for the practice of sending urine specimens for culture from all patients admitted to hospital. Any such protocol should be abandoned for reasons already discussed.

The indications for urine culture from medical in-patients are:

1 Urinary symptoms.
2 Incontinence.
3 Fever.
4 Vague ill health, anaemia, in elderly people.
5 Proteinuria.
6 Hypertension.

Acute pyelonephritis with bacteraemia is an important cause of fever of uncertain aetiology; blood and urine culture should always be undertaken. Both male and female patients are subject to this condition. Furthermore, men occasionally develop bacteraemia secondary to acute prostatitis, which may present with a similar picture of fever and rigors.

The same criteria for CSU culture apply as for surgical patients. Elderly people with indwelling catheters and patients with neuropathic or ileal bladders have inevitable bacteriuria. It is important thay they are not given antibacterial treatment when they are well. Such patients are subject, from time to time, to episodes of ascending infection and septicaemia, resulting in renal damage and loss of function. If antibiotics have been withheld, the organisms will be sensitive, and these attacks can be treated immediately and effectively, minimizing renal damage. Organisms which have been rendered resistant by antibiotics given when the patient was well present a much more difficult clinical problem.

A recent advance in the management of patients with neuropathic bladders or incontinence is intermittent self-catheterization. By emptying the bladder regularly, the likelihood of ascending infection and renal damage is lessened. However, the urine of such patients is almost inevitably infected; elaborate sterile precautions do not prevent infection and are therefore unnecessary. Most of these patients remain well for much of the time, and the urine should not be sent for culture. The indications for culture and treatment are the same as those for patients with indwelling catheters. There is no place for attempts at antibacterial prophylaxis; they invariably fail and select resistant organisms.

Sterile pyuria

The problem of apparently sterile pyuria is not uncommon in hospital in-patients, especially in elderly women with long-standing cystitis and in men with symptoms of prostatitis. It should not be ignored and may indicate serious disease. An explanation should be sought by a process of exclusion, as follows:

1 Was the patient on antibacterial treatment when the specimen was collected?
2 If not, are organisms present in the urine which are not detected by conventional aerobic overnight culture (fastidious organisms)?
3 If such organisms are excluded by appropriate culture techniques and the pyuria persists, tuberculosis should be excluded (three EMUs).

The possibility that the white cells were due to contamination by vaginal discharge should be considered, but this is an uncommon explanation.

Out-patients referred for investigation and management of urinary tract infection

Except in the few hospitals where urinary infection clinics are run by nephrologists and microbiologists, such patients are referred, as appropriate, to paediatric, urological or medical out-patient clinics.

A few general guidelines for the management of such patients can be set out:

1 Microbiological proof that the patient does, in fact, have UTI is essential. If this is not available from the referring general practitioner, arrangements should be made for MSU culture at the onset of the next attack of symptoms.

2 Present resources do not allow for all patients subject to UTI to be investigated by imaging techniques. Some clinical and microbiological pointers which assist in selection of patients for these investigations are:

(a) Children, and patients with a history of UTI or enuresis in childhood.
(b) Patients who have had an attack of acute clinical pyelonephritis.
(c) Patients infected with unusual (for example, *Staphylococcus aureus, Proteus* sp.) or resistant organisms.
(d) Those in whom infection fails to respond to appropriate treatment.
(e) Patients with frequent infections or persistent asymptomatic infection.
(f) Patients with UTI and hypertension.
(g) Patients with persistent haematuria.

The investigations will provide guidance for subsequent management. A few patients, for example those with infection stones (see below) or obstruction, may require surgery.

3 The following groups of patients will benefit from long-term low-dose prophylaxis:

(a) Children with recurrent infection, reflux or renal scarring.
(b) Adults with recurrent infections and radiological abnormalities.
(c) Pregnant women with persistent bacteriuria.
(d) Women with frequent symptomatic infections.
(e) Men with recurrent prostatitis.

Other patients, provided that investigations reveal no urinary tract abnormality and their infections are infrequent, can be managed satisfactorily by advice on improving the efficiency of the bladder wash-out mechanism (good fluid intake, 2-hourly double micturition and post-intercourse micturition) and short courses of appropriate antibacterial treatment for their isolated episodes of infection.

Investigation of patients with symptoms and negative urine culture

Women

There is increasing evidence that the symptoms of many patients with negative urine culture are due to invasion by lactobacilli from either the proximal urethra or the paraurethral tissues or both. These bacteria are not detected by conventional aerobic culture methods. Their presence should be sought by appropriate techniques (see p. 95): if they are detected, many patients can be reassured by explanation supported by the laboratory findings. It seems likely that the reason for multiplication and extension of these organisms beyond their commensal site in the distal urethra is selection by antibiotics given for symptoms. Sensitive species in the commensal flora are suppressed, and resistant species multiply disproportionately – a situation analagous to *Candida* vaginitis or antibiotic-induced diarrhoea. The symptoms can sometimes be ameliorated by alkalinizing agents, but cure can only be achieved when the normal balance of the commensal flora has been restored. Repeated courses of antibiotics merely aggravate the symptoms.

A few women, in particular elderly patients with a long history of cystitis and younger women or children with abnormalities of the urinary tract, such as renal scars, in which the oxygen tension is likely to be lower than that of urine, may have infection with other fastidious species, for example *Streptococcus milleri, Gardnerella vaginalis* or *Corynebacterium* sp. Infection with such organisms should be suspected as a possible explanation of apparently sterile pyuria. Management will depend upon the results of radiology and other investigations.

Men

Symptoms suggesting UTI are far commoner in adult men than is generally believed, and they are not confined to those with urinary tract abnormalities or obstruction due to prostatic hypertophy. They are commonly due to prostatitis. About one-third of specimens from such men will yield an aerobic pathogen (quite often in a low count, reflecting prostatic infection without associated cystitis); about one-third more will yield fastidious organisms, usually streptococci, *G. vaginalis* or corynebacteria, if sought by appropriate culture. It is likely that some of the remainder are due to chlamydial or ureaplasma infection.

Antibacterial agents used to treat UTI in men should be those which achieve therapeutic levels in the prostate: co-trimoxazole, trimethoprim, tetracycline or ciprofloxacin for Gram-negative infections, with the additional possibility of erythromycin for Gram-positive infections. Other agents, for example nitrofurantoin or amoxycillin, may sterilize the urine, but organisms will persist in the prostate. The troublesome condition of chronic prostatitis may be the sequel of inadequate or inappropriate treatment of the acute attack.

Patients with renal or bladder infection stones

Bladder stones occasionally form in chronically infected bladder urine. About 10% of renal stones, characteristically the mixed phosphate stones, which may become staghorn calculi, are the result of infection. The bacteria usually associated with infection stone formation are those which metabolize urea in urine, resulting in deposition of carbonate-apatite and struvite in a friable matrix – *Proteus* sp., staphylococci and sometimes *Klebsiella* sp. Isolation of any of these organisms from urine, especially if they persist after an appropriate course of treatment, should suggest the possibility of infection stone. Management depends upon the understanding that living bacteria persist in the substance of the stones. Figure 7.3 summarizes the management of patients with infection stones. The word 'surgery' is used to include all operative procedures, including percutaneous removal and lithotripsy. The two principal adverse effects of renal infection stones are destruction of renal tissue, with consequent loss of function, and obstruction of the renal pelvis. Infection and obstruction may result in pyonephrosis and bacteraemia; unless diagnosis and treatment are prompt, the patient

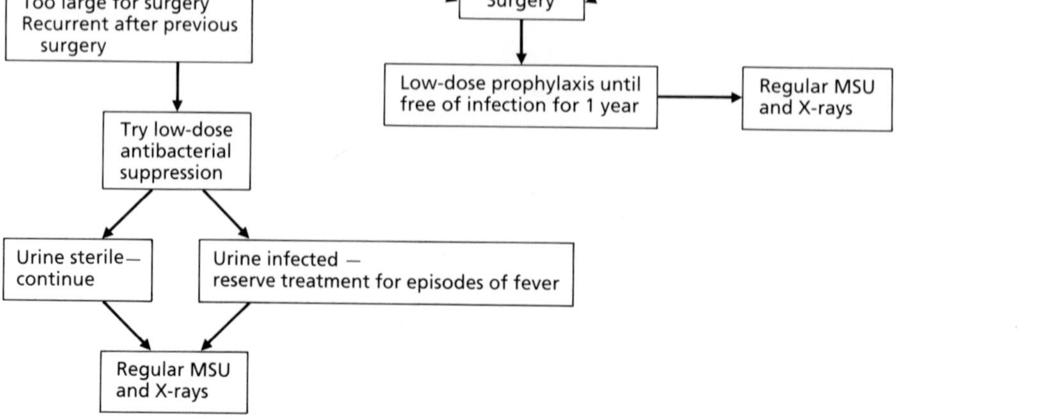

Fig. 7.3 Management of patients with infection stones.

may die. It follows that supervision of such patients should be close; if infection cannot be treated, and then suppressed by antibiotics in low dosage, antibiotic therapy should be withdrawn. The organisms will then remain sensitive and acute exacerbations of infection can be treated quickly and effectively.

Surgery, however apparently complete, is unlikely to eradicate all organisms from the kidney. After surgery, a low-dose antibiotic regimen should be established for 1 year and supervision continued after it is stopped.

Renal diseases other than urinary tract infection

Predialysis chronic renal failure

Urinary tract infection, whether or not it is the primary cause of CRF, may have a deleterious effect on already impaired renal function. Regular monitoring of the bacteriological state of the urine of such patients and correct treatment when needed are important. Diabetics in early renal failure should be supervised particularly carefully; neurological changes may affect the efficiency of bladder emptying and thereby increase the likelihood of UTI.

Acute renal failure

Causes and diagnosis

Table 7.2 shows the infective and infection-related causes of ARF. The causes listed in the upper half of the table are those most frequently encountered; those in the lower half are much less common. Acute renal failure may be related to infection and should be borne in mind in:

1 Abdominal operations in the presence of sepsis.
2 Septicaemia secondary to infection of urinary, biliary or intestinal tracts.
3 Patients who have recently returned from abroad.
4 Patients receiving nephrotoxic antibiotics.

In some of these conditions, for example tetanus and leptospirosis, the diagnosis is made or strongly suspected on clinical grounds. In others, some of the diagnostic tests are not microbiological, for example chest and abdominal X-rays for *Mycobacterium tuberculosis*, examination of thick and thin blood films for malarial parasites or *Borrelia* and examination of renal biopsy material for acute parenchymal disease. The appropriate microbiological tests for diagnosis are:

1 Blood cultures: septicaemia, subacute bacterial endocarditis (SABE), typhoid, *Clostridium welchii*.
2 Urine for microscopy and culture: acute on chronic pyelonephritis, infection stone, red cells in SABE, *Salmonella typhi*, *Schistosoma haematobium*, sulphonamide crystals.

Table 7.2 Infection and infection-related causes of acute renal failure

Prerenal	Antimicrobial drug nephrotoxicity	Interstitial nephritis	Acute glomerulonephritis	Obstruction
RELATIVELY COMMON				
Septicaemia Gram-positive Gram-negative	Aminoglycosides	Leptospirosis	Postinfectious glomerulonephritis	Infection stone (bladder or single kidney)
Falciparum malaria	Amphotericin B	Septicaemia (bacterial)	Subacute bacterial endocarditis	
Haemolytic uraemic syndrome (enteropathogenic *Escherichia coli*.)		Acute on chronic pyelonephritis		
Enteroviruses		Immune response to: penicillins sulphonamide rifampicin		
Fluid loss: cholera, typhoid				
RELATIVELY VERY UNCOMMON				
Clostridium welchii	Polymyxin B	*Mycobacterium tuberculosis*	*Streptococcus pneumoniae*	Renal papillary necrosis (secondary to diabetic renal disease)
Clostridium tetani	Colistin	*M. leprae*	*Salmonella typhi*	*Schistosoma haematobium*
Rickettsial diseases	β-lactams	*Candida*	*Neisseria gonorrhoeae*	Sulphadiazine crystals
Viral haemorrhagic fevers	Antituberculous drugs		*Treponema pallidum*	
Borrelia burgdorferi (Lyme disease)			*M. leprae*	
			Viruses: Epstein–Barr Echo influenza	

3 Stool culture hypovolaemia due to: *Clostridium difficile*, enteropathogenic *Escherichia coli* in haemolytic uraemic syndrome, viruses.
4 Throat swab: acute postinfectious glomerulonephritis, viruses.
5 Serum concentrations of nephrotoxic antibiotics.
6 Serology: leptospirosis, ASO titres, viruses, rickettsiae.

The diagnosis of virus infection is usually made by serological tests. Some viruses may be isolated from stools or throat swabs and a few, such as cytomegalovirus, can be seen on electron microscopy of the urine. Correct transport of specimens for virological investigation is essential and advice from laboratory staff should be sought.

Acute peritoneal dialysis

Patients with ARF may require dialysis: in hospitals without renal units this usually takes the form of intermittent peritoneal dialysis. Provided that obsessional sterile precautions are followed, bacterial peritonitis is a rare complication. If skin infection at the catheter entry site occurs, swabs should be sent for culture. Peritonitis is indicated by a cloudy appearance of the effluent; small numbers of organisms, most commonly staphylococci, are present in large volumes of fluid and may not be detected in the laboratory if only fluid is sent for culture. Five to ten millilitres of effluent should be inoculated into a good blood culture medium and subcultured at daily intervals. The organisms which most commonly cause peritonitis in patients on peritoneal dialysis are those of the commensal flora of the skin. The clinician should discuss the patient with a bacteriologist, ensuring that the presence of *Staphylococcus epidermidis* (*albus*) or corynebacteria (diphtheroids) in the effluent from patients with clinical infection or cloudy effluent is reported and appropriate sensitivity tests are carried out. If the peritoneal effluent is clear, it should not be sent for culture.

Catheters in patients with acute renal failure

Bladder catheters should be avoided whenever possible. Catheterization is sometimes necessary for diagnostic reasons at the onset of ARF, but the supposed advantage of precise monitoring of urinary output is heavily outweighed by the disadvantage of the infection which inevitably occurs after a few days (see above). Distension of the bladder during the recovery phase can be diagnosed by regular clinical examination of the abdomen. Intravenous catheters are increasingly used in the management of severely ill patients. Infection is a common complication and staphylococci are the commonest infecting organisms. If infection becomes established because of delayed or inappropriate treatment, the catheter may become colonized irretrievably and must be removed. Careful supervision of catheter sites, swabs and blood cultures taken promptly at the first suspicion of infection, and early treatment with a 'best-guess' antibiotic will ensure the maximum usefulness of the catheter.

Antibiotic treatment of patients with impaired renal function

Most antibiotics and their metabolites are excreted at least partly by the kidney; therefore regimens must be adjusted in treating patients with renal insufficiency (see p. 121). If a patient is treated with an aminoglycoside, blood must be regularly taken for assay for the concentration of the drug, both to ensure that a therapeutic concentration is attained and to avoid toxicity resulting from accumulation. Pre-dose and post-dose serum should be sent to the laboratory, the request form stating the doses given and serum creatinine concentration.

Nitrofurantoin should never be used in patients with impaired renal function, however slight; accumulation of metabolites causes peripheral sensory neuropathy. Likewise, nalidixic acid and related substances should be avoided because of the accumulation of metabolites and the rapid emergence of resistant organisms. Ampicillin, amoxycillin, co-trimoxazole and trimethoprim may be given in normal doses for treatment of UTI in the presence of mild renal insufficiency. Dosage interval should be increased in patients with advanced renal failure. Tetracyclines, other than doxycycline, have antianabolic effects in patients with renal failure and should be avoided. Doxycycline may be used if there is a valid indication for treatment with a tetracycline, for example prostatitis.

Vancomycin is used increasingly for staphylococcal infections of peritoneal dialysis fluid or intravenous catheters in patients with renal failure. High concentrations are ototoxic and occasionally nephrotoxic; measurement of serum concentrations is advisable.

Summary

The clinician who uses the laboratory for help in the diagnosis and management of patients with renal or urinary tract diseases should:

1 Request only appropriate investigations.
2 Ensure that specimens are collected and transported correctly.
3 Give accurate relevant information on request forms.
4 Familiarize him/herself with the reporting methods used in the laboratory and ensure that he/she places the correct interpretation on them.
5 Use only those antibiotics to which the laboratory reports sensitivities.
6 Seek the advice of the microbiologist in the investigation of unusual conditions or suspected virus infections.

Further reading

1 Asscher, A.W. & Brumfitt, W. (eds) (1986) *Microbial Diseases in Nephrology*. John Wiley and Sons, Chichester.

2 Barr, J.G., Ritchie, J.W.K., Henry, O., El Sheik, M. & Eldeeb, K. (1985) Microaerophilic/anaerobic bacteria as a cause of urinary tract infection in pregnancy. *Br. J. Obstet. Gynaecol.* **92**, 506–10.

3 Fairley, K.F. & Birch, D.F. (1989) Detection of bladder bacteriuria in patients with acute urinary symptoms. *J. Infect. Dis.* **159**, 226–31.
4 Garrod, L.P., Lambert, H.P. & O'Grady, F.W. (1990) *Antibiotic and Chemotherapy*, 6th edn. Churchill Livingstone, Edinburgh.
5 Maskell, R. (1988) *Urinary Tract Infection in Clinical and Laboratory Practice.* Edward Arnold, London.
6 Maskell, R. (1989) Urine microscopy and culture in the selection of patients for urinary tract investigation. *Br. J. Urol.* **63**, 7–10.
7 Maskell, R. (1989) A new look at the diagnosis of infection of the urinary tract and its adjacent structures. *J.* Infect. **19**, 207–17.
8 Papapetropoulou, M. & Pappas, A. (1987) The acute urethral syndrome in routine practice. *J. Infect.* **14**, 113–18.
9 Payne, S.R., Timoney, A.G., McKnoving, S.T. *et al.* (1988) Microbiological look at urodynamic studies. *Lancet* **ii**, 1123–6.
10 Shanson, D.C. (1988) *Microbiology in Clinical Practice*, 2nd edn. Wright PSG, Bristol.
11 Wilkie, M.E., Almond, M.K. & Marsh, F.P. (1992) Diagnosis and management of urinary tract infection in adults. *Br. Med. J.* **305**, 1137–41.
12 Wilkins, E.G.L., Payne, S.R., Pead, P.J., Moss, S.T. & Maskell, R. (1989) Interstitial cystitis and urethral syndrome: a possible answer. *Br. J. Urol.* **64**, 39–44.

Chapter 8
Urinary Tract Infections in Hospital In-patients

Edwina A. Brown

Different types of urinary tract infections in hospital in-patients will be discussed, using case histories to illustrate particular features. In many instances, infection of the urinary tract was the principal reason for admission to hospital, either for general care or for administration of parenteral antibiotics. In some patients, severe urinary tract infection complicates bladder catheterization.

Infections of the urinary tract can be divided into those involving the lower urinary tract and those involving the upper urinary tract. Lower urinary tract infection – 'cystitis' – is not usually associated with systemic symptoms and is rarely a cause for admission to hospital except very occasionally for cystoscopy. Conversely, patients with upper urinary tract infections often have systemic manifestations such as pain and fever and may well require hospital admission. Furthermore, upper urinary tract infections are often associated with underlying renal disease and may cause deterioration in renal function. In diabetics, any infection can cause deterioration in glycaemic control and may possibly lead to diabetic ketoacidosis.

Clinical management of urinary tract infection

All types of urinary infection may be completely asymptomatic. The clinical features of upper urinary tract infections are shown in Table 8.1. Such infections may be associated with septicaemia. The key investigations in all patients with suspected urinary tract infection is to examine the urine, macroscopically and microscopically, before culture. Ideally, a midstream specimen of urine (MSU) should be obtained. This is not always possible if the patient is unconscious, uncooperative or catheterized or has a nephrostomy or an ileal conduit. One then has to accept a catheter specimen. To avoid bacterial contamination, the specimen should be taken direct from the catheter and not from the drainage bag (see p. 27). It is also possible to take specimens direct from the bladder (suprapubic aspiration), using a 10 ml syringe and a needle, but only if the bladder is full and therefore palpable.

Urine may be macroscopically normal in patients with urinary tract infection but more commonly it is turbid and may even be thick and contain particulate material. Blood-staining is common, although gross haematuria is an unusual feature. In addition, urine may have a 'fish-like' odour.

Microscopy of such urine will show white and red cells. For a urinary infection to be 'significant' there should be more than 10 white cells per cubic millimetre. Culture of urine is essential to determine the organism causing the infection and establish antibiotic sensitivities. Blood cultures should be taken in febrile patients. Most microbiology laboratory staff will only screen urinary pathogens initially against a limited number of antibiotics. They usually include ampicillin, co-trimoxazole, trimethoprim, nalidixic acid, nitrofurantoin and cephalexin. In many in-patients, a more potent antibiotic is required, either because the patient is very ill or because previous urine cultures have shown that the organism grown is resistant to common antibiotics. To avoid waiting an extra day for the laboratory to determine additional antibiotic sensitivities, it is wise to request extra sensitivities in advance.

As well as specific urinary investigations, patients requiring admission for urinary infection should have various base-line blood tests performed at the start of antibiotic treatment (see Table 8.2).

It is essential to have a measure of renal function because the dose of antibiotic given may have to be adjusted appropriately. Urinary in-

Table 8.1 Clinical features of urinary tract infection

Lower urinary tract	Upper urinary tract
Symptoms	
Dysuria	Fevers
Frequency	Loin pain (unilateral or bilateral)
Urgency	Back pain
(None)	Dysuria
	Haematuria
	(None)
Signs	
Suprapubic tenderness (occasionally)	Pyrexial
	Loin tenderness
Pyrexial (rarely)	Kidney, if palpable, is tender
None (commonly)	None (rarely)

Table 8.2 Investigation of patients with urinary tract infection

Urine
MSU/CSU:
microscopy
culture
Early morning urine:
Lowensheim–Jensen culture
Blood
Urea, creatinine
Plasma Na^+, K^+ and bicarbonate
Haemoglobin
White cell count and differential
Glucose
Blood cultures and blood gases (in 'toxic' patients)
X-rays
Plain abdominal X-ray
IVU
Renal ultrasound
Micturating cystogram
Antegrade pyelogram
Retrograde pyelogram
CT scan
Isotope
Renogram
White cell scan
Gallium scan

fection may cause a deterioration in renal function in the presence of underlying renal disease, especially in patients sensitive to fluid depletion. Thus serum creatinine and plasma urea, sodium, potassium and bicarbonate should be measured repetitively during the early days of severe infections. Urinary infection can be the presenting feature of, as well as a complication of, diabetes mellitus; therefore blood glucose should be assayed in all new patients.

Total white cell and differential counts can give a useful indication of the severity of infection, but it should be noted that, in patients with renal failure, there is often no marked leucocytosis.

After admission and beginning appropriate antibiotics, it is important to provide adequate analgesia and hydration, to watch for and treat any complications and to establish the presence or absence of any underlying renal disease.

The major complications of urinary infection are shown in Table 8.3. The patient may be septicaemic with hypotension or have high fevers and there may be bacteraemic involvement of other organs. Commonly, fluid depletion occurs in patients whose fluid intake is limited or in

Table 8.3 Possible complications arising in patients with urinary infection

1	Septicaemia
2	Fluid depletion Hypotension, low cardiac output Deteriorating renal function
3	Obstruction of urinary tract Pyonephrosis Deteriorating renal function Continued infection despite antibiotics
4	Exacerbation of diabetes

patients who are unable appropriately to reduce urinary sodium or water excretion. This is most frequently found in the elderly, patients who have been treated with diuretics or those with 'salt-losing renal disease' such as reflux nephropathy, analgesic nephropathy or chronic obstruction. 'Salt-losing renal disease' and 'salt-losers' are jargon phrases describing specific groups of patients in whom disease has damaged the distal tubules and collecting ducts such that they are unresponsive to antidiuretic hormone (ADH). Such patients are therefore unable adequately to conserve sodium and there is a persistent high obligatory loss of sodium and chloride. The management, in part, comprises oral sodium chloride capsules. In some, potassium supplementation is also necessary. Fluid depletion in such patients not only can result in hypotension and poor peripheral perfusion but also can cause decreased renal perfusion, thereby further compromising renal function.

Very occasionally, ureteric obstruction occurs secondary to calculi or a sloughed papilla. Sometimes ureteric obstruction can be caused by plugs of 'pus'. If obstruction occurs in the presence of infection, pyonephrosis can result, with local symptoms such as loin pain or tenderness, together with continuing fever despite antibiotics.

At some stage in the management of patients with urinary tract infection, investigations should be performed to determine whether there is any structural abnormality of the renal tract. If a patient has an uncomplicated acute pyelonephritis which responds rapidly to antibiotic treatment, then ultrasound should be delayed for about 6 weeks so that any intrarenal oedema can resolve. If there is suspicion from the presentation or progress of the patient that there may be some underlying renal condition, an ultrasound study should be performed promptly.

The main radiological procedures used in the investigation of urinary infection are listed in Table 8.2. A plain abdominal X-ray may show calculi within the urinary tract or nephrocalcinosis and, depending on the quality of the film, renal size may also be determined. More information about the size of the kidneys, the site of possible calculi and the presence or absence of obstruction can be obtained from an

IVU. Renal ultrasound is not so useful in the investigation of urinary infection, despite its accuracy at determining renal size and the presence of obstruction, because ultrasonography may not detect calculi or renal scars. Ultrasound demonstrates cysts and polycystic disease very well.

Having performed an IVU, it may be necessary to proceed to more specialist renal investigations. A micturating cystogram may show ureteric reflux. Antegrade (percutaneous) pyelography may be required to reveal the actual site of obstruction, especially in the presence of renal failure, when the ureters may not be well opacified by an IVU. There is a limited role for CT scanning: abscesses are well demarcated (see p. 83).

Isotope investigations are not often required in the management of in-patients with urinary infection. A diethylene triamine pentacetic acid (DTPA) renogram may be used to exclude obstruction and to determine the differential renal function of each kidney if nephrectomy is being considered to prevent recurrent infection. Iridium-labelled white cells or gallium scans are used to localize infection to one kidney and occasionally are of value.

Urinary tract infection and pre-existing renal disease

Many types of renal disease predispose to recurrent urinary tract infection (Table 8.4). These infections are usually symptomatic and can result in deterioration in renal function, either by fluid depletion, especially since many of these patients tend to be 'salt-losers', or by causing further renal damage. Because the management of patients with renal disease and urinary infection must depend somewhat on the nature of the underlying renal disease, each category will be discussed separately and will be illustrated by case histories.

Table 8.4 Types of renal conditions predisposing to urinary tract infection

1 Renal calculi
2 Nephrocalcinosis
3 Papillary necrosis
Analgesic nephropathy
Diabetes
Sickle-cell disease
4 Reflux nephropathy
5 Polycystic kidneys
6 Obstruction
Bladder neck
Ureteric
7 Renal transplantation

Renal calculi or nephrocalcinosis

Any calculus or area of calcification within the kidney may act as a nidus of infection: antibiotics penetrate calculi only poorly. Persistent infection, especially if due to *Proteus*, will often encourage further growth of calculi.

Case 1

A 26-year-old woman presented with severe right loin pain radiating to the groin and complained of urinary frequency without dysuria. There was fever of 38 °C and right loin tenderness. An IVU performed 2 years previously had shown the presence of a medullary sponge kidney on the right, associated with many intrarenal calculi. She was admitted for pain relief and was treated with oral amoxycillin. An MSU taken on admission subsequently grew *Escherichia coli* sensitive to ampicillin. A renogram performed the day after admission showed no evidence of obstruction. The pain rapidly settled and the patient was discharged after 3 days to continue at home a 10-day course of amoxycillin. Renal function remained normal throughout the course of the infection.

The important feature in this case history was the need to exclude obstruction in a patient with known renal calculi. A calculus lodged in one of the ureters can exacerbate loin pain and add a further predisposing factor to urinary infection. Renal ultrasound could have been used to exclude obstruction but might have failed to detect early minor dilatation of the calyces if the obstruction had only recently occurred. A renogram was chosen because it can be done quickly, has much less morbidity than an IVU and, in the presence of normal renal function, will detect early acute obstruction before there has been much calyceal dilatation.

Although a short course of antibiotics will control the acute infection in a patient with renal calculi, often a prolonged course of prophylactic antibiotics is needed to prevent further infection. This patient was treated with a nightly dose of trimethoprim for 6 months and remained free of infection for 3 years.

Papillary necrosis

Papillary necrosis is a feature of many different types of renal disease, such as diabetes, analgesic nephropathy and sickle-cell disease. It can predispose to recurrent urinary infections because it is difficult to eradicate bacteria from the relatively avascular papillae. Many of these patients, therefore, should be given long-term prophylactic antibiotics. It is important to remember that patients with papillary necrosis are usually ‘salt-losers’ and become volume-depleted when they develop an infection. This often results in deterioration of renal function, which should return to the previous level with adequate rehydration.

Case 2

A 71-year-old woman had had insulin-dependent diabetes for 35 years. She also had retinopathy and autonomic neuropathy. Proteinuria had been present for some years and she was known to have a plasma urea of 16 mmol/L and a serum creatinine of 150 μmol/L. She presented with rigors, fevers and lower abdominal pain for 12 hours, during which she had had a severe attack of left loin pain. There was no dysuria or frequency. On admission, she had a temperature of 38.5 °C and mild left flank tenderness. Plasma urea was 21 mmol/L and serum creatinine 210 μmol/L. She was treated with intravenous cefuroxime and her temperature settled. *Escherichia coli* was subsequently grown from urine and blood. An IVU performed 2 days later showed papillary necrosis of the left kidney, not present when investigated 2 years previously. There was no evidence of obstruction. It was presumed that the left loin pain which had occurred immediately before admission had been caused by a sloughed papilla, causing transient obstruction. She has subsequently been treated with prophylactic antibiotics and has had no further urinary infections; renal function is stable, with a serum creatinine of 180 μmol/L 3 years later.

Reflux nephropathy

Recurrent urinary infections associated with ureteric reflux and causing renal scarring is a condition arising in the first 2 years of life. As adults, some of these patients continue to have reflux and this, together with the presence of relatively avascular renal scars, predisposes to recurrent urinary infection. These infections rarely result in further renal scarring and do not often contribute to additional decline in renal function. Hypertension secondary to renal scars may lead to some loss of glomerular filtration rate (GFR). Chronic renal failure occurs in those patients who develop proteinuria and focal glomerulosclerosis. Such patients tend to be 'salt-losers' and are prone to fluid depletion and hence decline in renal function during the course of an infection. Renal function should return to its previous level after adequate hydration. This is illustrated in Case 3.

Case 3

A 25-year-old woman was known to have reflux nephropathy for 6 years: she had presented with recurrent urinary tract infections. Intravenous urography at that time had shown bilaterally scarred kidneys compatible with previous reflux. During follow-up she had developed heavy proteinuria and in out-patients 1 month before admission her serum creatinine had been 200 μmol/L. She was admitted with a 2-day history of dysuria, frequency and fever. Her temperature on admission was 39 °C, her blood-pressure was 90/60 mmHg, and her weight had fallen from 65 to 61 kg. On admission, serum creatinine was 400 μmol/L.

She was given 4 L of intravenous saline over 12 hours and intravenous cefuroxime. *Escherichia coli* sensitive to cefuroxime was grown from MSU and blood cultures. The pyrexia settled within 24 hours and by discharge, 5 days later, her serum creatinine had returned to 200 µmol/L. She was continued on oral cephalexin for a further 5 days.

Many patients with reflux nephropathy acquire recurrent urinary tract infections, the majority of which are not severe enough to require admission. These patients require long-term prophylactic antibiotics. This patient had a further infection 2 months later, since when she has taken 250 mg cephalexin each night for 3 years with no further infections. Although her urine has been kept sterile, her serum creatinine has risen to 600 µmol/L.

There has been much debate as to whether ureteric reflux should be corrected in these patients by surgical reimplantation of the ureters into the bladder. Unfortunately, this appears to have no effect on progression into renal failure, although in some instances ureteric reimplantation may decrease the number of urinary infections.

Polycystic kidneys

Urinary infection involving polycystic kidneys can cause substantial morbidity, occasionally requiring nephrectomy, because of poor penetration of antibiotics into infected cysts. The infection often spreads haematogenously from one kidney to the other; the kidneys can also become a secondary site of infection from a septicaemia, as illustrated in Case 4.

Case 4

A 20-year-old woman was admitted with a 1-week history of suprapubic pain, fever and haematuria. Her mother had polycystic kidneys and was receiving haemodialysis. On admission, serum creatinine was 131 µmol/L and the urine contained numerous white cells and grew *E. coli* sensitive to ampicillin. Renal ultrasound confirmed the diagnosis of polycystic kidneys. She was treated with ampicillin, the pyrexia rapidly settled and she was discharged home after a few days.

One month later the patient was readmitted because of right loin pain, and an MSU at this time grew *E. coli* and *Pseudomonas aeruginosa*. She was treated with intravenous ampicillin and tobramycin. Two weeks later, she was still febrile, with fever up to 39.5 °C, and she developed tobramycin toxicity, with serum creatinine rising to 410 µmol/L. An MSU at this time showed numerous white cells but was sterile. A gallium scan showed increased concentration of isotope in both kidneys, the right more than the left – evidence of continued renal infection. She was treated with intravenous ticarcillin and ceftazidime for 1 month. The temperature settled after 2 weeks and she was discharged 2 weeks later; serum creatinine had then fallen to 160 μmol/L.

This case demonstrates the difficulty that can be encountered in eradicating infections in polycystic kidneys. Presumably the tobramycin did not penetrate well into the cysts. Studies have shown that, whereas cephalosporins and penicillins are detected in fluid aspirated from cysts, aminoglycosides are not. This patient also illustrates the potential nephrotoxicity of aminoglycosides if not adequately monitored when given to patients with renal failure.

Case 5

A 45-year-old woman with polycystic kidneys had been on home haemodialysis for 1 year. She presented one evening with a history of fevers and rigors for 24 hours. Her temperature was 39.7 °C. The Scribner shunt exit sites appeared to be infected and her abdomen was generally tender, but her large kidneys were not particularly tender. She was treated with intravenous cefuroxime and tobramycin. The MSU on admission showed no white cells and was sterile. The infected shunt was removed. *Staphylococcus aureus* sensitive to cefuroxime and tobramycin was grown from blood cultures.

Despite continued antibiotics she remained febrile. Two weeks after admission, she suddenly developed severe left loin pain and gross haematuria; her haemoglobin fell from 8 g/dl to 4 g/dl. Two days later, because of continuing fevers and severe loin pain, she underwent bilateral nephrectomy. The left kidney was more inflamed than the right, but pus was found in the cysts of both kidneys. Fever settled over the next 2 days: she made a slow, uneventful recovery.

This case history demonstrates how polycystic kidneys may become the site of secondary infection by bacteraemia spread.

Obstruction

Obstruction of the urinary tract, partial or complete, at any site or from any cause, will predispose to urinary infection because of poor urine flow and hence poor drainage. Obstruction of the urinary outflow tract does not usually lead to irreversible renal damage, and renal function completely recovers even after a few weeks of unrelieved obstruction. Nevertheless, if infection occurs behind an obstruction, leading to pyonephrosis, rapid irreversible damage to that kidney occurs. Treatment of urinary infection in the presence of obstruction therefore not only involves use of antibiotics but also drainage of the urinary tract, either by catheterization for urethral obstruction or by nephrostomy tubes for ureteric obstruction. Unfortunately, catheterization itself predisposes to further urinary infection, as demonstrated in Case 6.

Case 6

A 72-year-old diabetic controlled by diet was known to have chronic renal failure, the serum creatinine concentration being 360 μmol/L. He was admitted to his local hospital with acute urinary retention and was catheterized. Further treatment was not carried out because it was felt that he was unfit for surgery. One month later, he was transferred to a renal unit; he was still catheterized and serum creatinine had risen to 430 μmol/L. *Pseudomonas aeruginosa* was grown from the urine and was eradicated by a 1-week course of intravenous ceftazidime. He then had a urethral dilatation and the catheter was removed: he subsequently passed urine normally.

One week later, he was again admitted in acute urinary retention; he was mildly febrile and had some suprapubic and right loin tenderness. He was recatheterized and treated with intravenous ceftazidime. *Pseudomonas aeruginosa* was again cultured. Over the next few days, urine output declined and serum creatinine rose. Peritoneal dialysis was begun. A renal ultrasound performed 2 days later, when he was clinically more stable, showed a small left kidney and a large right hydronephrosis. A nephrostomy tube inserted into the right kidney drained pus from which *Streptococcus faecalis* was isolated. A nephrostogram showed blockage at the distal end of the right ureter. He was treated with trimethoprim while continuing ceftazidime. Over the next 2 weeks, urine flow from the nephrostomy tube decreased while bladder drainage increased: renal function steadily improved. All tubes were then removed. One month later an ultrasound confirmed the absence of obstruction to the right kidney; serum creatinine at this time (off dialysis) was 460 μmol/L.

This case shows the importance of investigating any unexpected decline in renal function associated with obstruction. Although never confirmed, it was thought that the obstruction at the distal end of the right ureter was due to a collection of pus and debris, which cleared with treatment. If long-term drainage of an infected obstructed kidney is not feasible, it may be occasionally necessary to remove or resect part of a kidney to prevent recurrent infections. Such a decision is made easier if the affected kidney contributes little to the overall renal function, as judged by an isotope study (see p. 82).

Urinary tract infections in diabetics

Urinary tract infections are perhaps more common in diabetics than in the normal population, for various reasons:

1 An autonomic neuropathy may lead to impaired bladder emptying.
2 There may be structural renal damage such as papillary necrosis.

Urinary tract infection is not infrequently the presenting feature of diabetics. It is perhaps more than coincidental that four of the nine patients with urinary infections described in this chapter were diabetic.

As with all infections in diabetics, urinary infection can increase insulin requirements, which, if not recognized and treated, leads to persistent hyperglycaemia and perhaps diabetic coma. The hyperglycaemic osmotic diuresis results in fluid depletion and deterioration in renal function. This is illustrated by Case 7.

Case 7

A 64-year-old diabetic had been well controlled with tolbutamide for many years. He presented with severe renal failure secondary to prostatic obstruction. Following catheterization and a subsequent prostatectomy, renal function improved, with serum creatinine concentrations stabilizing at 500 μmol/L. Two months later he was readmitted with a history of dribbling and general malaise for a few days. He had lost 8 kg in weight and there was postural hypotension – blood-pressure 150/70 mmHg lying and 80/40 standing. The urine was cloudy. By admission, serum creatinine had risen to 920 μmol/L. A diagnosis of urinary infection was made and he was given saline, insulin and cefuroxime intravenously. *Pseudomonas aeruginosa* was grown from the urine and ceftazidine substituted. Ten days later, his diabetes was again well controlled on oral tolbutamide and the serum creatinine concentration had returned to 500 μmol/L.

Urinary tract infection and catheterization

A bladder catheter strongly predisposes the patient to a bladder infection (see also p. 92). Bacteraemia and pyelonephritis may develop after any manipulation, such as recatheterization or cystoscopy. To minimize the chance of introducing an infection, the catheter should be inserted in as sterile a manner as possible, the patient should have a good fluid intake to maintain a urine flow rate above 2 ml/min and the drainage bag should be emptied at least twice daily. When urine flow rates are low, as in the presence of volume depletion or hypotension, urinary infection due to the presence of a catheter is almost inevitable. Thus, unless the patient is unconscious and still passing urine, the bladder catheter should be removed at the earliest possible opportunity. When the catheter is removed, neomycin or noxythiolin (Noxyflex) may be instilled into the bladder to try and prevent infection.

Case 8

A 44-year-old man was admitted with acute renal failure secondary to rhabdomyolysis caused by an embolus to his right iliac artery. During his stay on the intensive care unit he was ventilated for a number of days and a urinary catheter was left *in situ*. Urine volume was about 50 ml daily. After 45 days pus was being drained from the bladder; cultures grew *E. coli*. The catheter was removed and he was treated with trimethoprim via a nasogastric tube. Urine was subsequently collected by using Paul's tubing. The urine cleared over the next 3 days.

Repeated brief catheterization to drain residual urine on alternate days is much preferable to an indwelling catheter in such patients. If it is essential for a patient to be on continuous drainage, it can be extremely difficult to treat the infected urine. It can be argued that such infections are best left untreated unless there is evidence of infection of the upper urinary tract systemic infection. Antibiotics often fail completely to eradicate infection and merely promote the emergence of resistant strains and colonization by bacteria such as *Klebsiella* and *Pseudomonas* (see also p. 93). Over-enthusiastic use of antibiotics may also result in fungal infections.

Case 9

A 70-year-old man, who had been diabetic for 10 years and was controlled on glibenclamide, was admitted after a fall fracturing his 12th thoracic vertebra. Shortly after admission, he went into acute retention and had to be catheterized. There was a history of prostatic symptoms for 6 years. Over the next week he became progressively drowsy, irritable and febrile. *Klebsiella* was grown from blood and urine cultures; renal function deteriorated, plasma urea rising to 43 mmol/L and serum creatinine to 550 μmol/L. He became volume-depleted and was treated with intravenous fluids and cefuroxime. An IVU excluded obstruction. After the infection had cleared, the catheter was removed, but it had to be replaced because of incontinence.

One week later, still catheterized, *Pseudomonas* was grown from the urine. Because of continued renal failure (creatinine 300 μmol/L), he was treated with ticarcillin (prior to the availability of third-generation cephalosporins or ciprofloxacin). Two weeks later, *Pseudomonas* was still present in his urine so the catheter was removed. Renal failure supervened and after 3 days he passed heavily contaminated urine. He was therefore recatheterized and given a 2-week course of tobramycin, the dose being regularly changed according to trough blood concentrations of the antibiotic. Prostatectomy was considered but not performed because of a myocardial infarct 2 months previously. A further trial of removal of the catheter was attempted successfully. Urinary infection did not recur.

This case history illustrates three features: first, the difficulty in eradicating infection in the presence of a bladder catheter; secondly, that the use of antibiotics in a catheterized patient encourages the growth of *Klebsiella* or *Pseudomonas*, both of which are difficult to eradicate; and, thirdly, the value of tobramycin in the treatment of *Pseudomonas* species. Aminoglycosides may be used in patients with renal failure; they are safe if the dose is appropriately reduced and blood concentrations are frequently measured to judge subsequent doses.

Treatment of urinary tract infection

From the above histories, the main principles of treatment of urinary infection are:

1 Appropriate antibiotic treatment.
2 Intravenous fluids.
3 Drainage of the urinary tract.

Antibiotic treatment

There are two aspects of antibiotic treatment of urinary tract infection:
1 The presenting infection must be treated with an appropriate antibiotic as judged by the results gained from culturing urine and blood.
2 If the patient has suffered from recurrent urinary infection, he or she should, after the urinary tract has been rendered sterile, be treated with low-dose oral antibiotics at night for at least 6 months.

If treating a severe infection, it is necessary to start the patient on an antibiotic before the culture results are available. It is always useful to check the case notes for results of previous urine culture because there is often a consistent pattern of organism and of antibiotic resistance in an individual patient. If treating 'blind', it is sensible to start treatment with an antibiotic to which most of the common organisms are sensitive. This will depend on whether the infection is acquired as an in- or out-patient and also on local patterns of antibiotic resistance. Generally, urinary pathogens are becoming increasingly resistant to ampicillin, which should therefore be avoided in the absence of sensitivity reports. Whether an oral or parenteral antibiotic is chosen depends on the result of cultures and the clinical condition of the patient. Often an antibiotic is given parenterally for the first 1–3 days until the patient is afebrile and then the same or a similar antibiotic can be given orally to complete a 7–10 day course. Prophylactic treatment, if indicated, could then be given with the same oral antibiotic. For 'blind' therapy, ciprofloxacin, trimethoprim or cephalexin are appropriate oral drugs and ciprofloxacin or cefuroxime if a parenteral antibiotic is indicated.

It is essential that the concentration of serum creatinine be measured before an antibiotic is administered, because renal impairment is a common feature of urinary infection. Table 8.5 shows the antibiotics most commonly used in the treatment of urinary infection and appropriate dose reduction in the presence of renal failure. It is unwise to use nalidixic acid or nitrofurantoin. Other antibiotics, particularly aminoglycosides, are potentially nephrotoxic. In renal failure, peak and trough concentrations must be measured repeatedly.

Unfortunately, many urinary pathogens, particularly *Proteus*, *Klebsiella* and *Pseudomonas*, are becoming resistant to the safer antibiotics. *Pseudomonas* was particularly difficult to treat until the introduction of ciprofloxacin. Until recently, aminoglycosides were the only

Table 8.5 Antibiotics commonly used in the treatment of urinary tract infection: administration in renal failure

Antibiotic	Dosage[a] recommendation (GFR < 10 ml/min)	Comments
Oral		
Amoxycyllin	Max 250 mg tds	
Cephalexin	Max 500 mg daily	
Ciprofloxacin	Reduce dose	
Nalidixic acid	Avoid	Nausea, photosensitivity
Nitrofurantoin	Avoid (GFR < 50)	Peripheral neuropathy
Co-trimoxazole	Max i bd	Rashes, blood dyscrasias
Trimethoprim	Max 100 mg bd	
Parenteral		
Aminoglycosides: tobramycin, gentamicin	Reduce (GFR < 50)	Measure serum concentrations Ototoxic, nephrotoxic
Ceftazidine, ceftizoxime	Reduce dose	
Cefoxitin, ceftizoxime, Cefuroxime		
Ciprofloxacin	Reduce dose	
Azlocillin, mexlocillin, ticarcillin, piperacillin	Reduce dose	

[a] Rough guide only: check dosages suggested on clinical data sheet of drug before prescribing.

available antibiotics. Piperacillin, ciprofloxacin and third-generation cephalosporins are useful anti-*Pseudomonal* agents and are much less toxic than aminoglycosides. Ciprofloxacin is particularly useful because it can be given orally. Aminoglycosides are still the most potent and should not be avoided because of pre-existing renal failure. If dose is adequately reduced, and blood concentrations regularly measured aminoglycosides are very effective, safe antibiotics. Improperly used, worsening renal failure and ototoxicity are serious risks.

Fluid management

Fluid depletion is a frequent feature of urinary tract infection, particularly if there is obstruction or an underlying 'salt-losing' state such as papillary necrosis or reflux nephropathy. It is therefore essential that the hydration of the patient when first seen should be fully assessed. This can usually be done clinically by: (i) weighing; (ii) judging skin turgor; and (iii) demonstrating postural hypotension. The patient is not fluid-depleted if the jugular venous pressure is easily visible. Rarely, a central venous pressure line may be needed. Fluid depletion will cause deterioration in renal function and as a result plasma urea will rise more than serum creatinine.

If there is evidence of fluid depletion the patient should be given an adequate fluid intake, usually intravenously. Because sodium and water have been lost, the correct fluid to give is intravenous normal (0.9%) saline. If the patient is 'in shock', it may be necessary to infuse purified protein fraction, which increases circulating volume.

A careful fluid balance chart should be kept on all patients, who should also be weighed daily under standard conditions. As fluid depletion is corrected, the patient's weight will rise daily. Several litres of fluid may be required over the first 2–3 days to correct dehydration. Creatinine clearance should be measured repetitively until renal function becomes stable.

Drainage of the urinary tract

The presence of obstruction impairs or prevents eradication of infection. Prostatic obstruction is easy to diagnose, either historically or best by ultrasonography. Obstruction at other sites in the urinary tract must be demonstrated by ultrasound or radiologically (see pp. 69, 81 and 83). If obstruction is present, a bladder catheter or percutaneous drainage to allow a free flow of urine is essential before infection can be treated adequately.

Tuberculous infection of the renal tract

About 10% of new cases of tuberculosis are extrapulmonary: the renal tract is a common site. There is usually a latent period from infection to clinical manifestation of 10–15 years. There may well be no evidence of active pulmonary infection. Tuberculosis occurs more frequently in people of Indian or Asian origin.

Typically the patient presents with recurrent bacterial infections. In the minority, frequency and dysuria do not occur: non-specific symptoms lead to a diagnosis of renal of functional impairment and the renal tract is investigated. Occasionally, the diagnosis is made by chance.

Excretion of acid- and alcohol-fast bacilli (AAFB) is probably intermittent and thus three to six early morning urine specimens (EMUs) should be sent in the hope of obtaining a positive culture and later sensitivities. Renal tract tuberculosis is an important cause of the inaccurate phrase 'sterile pyuria'. Proteinuria of 1–2 g/day is present in many. An ultrasound assessment or an IVU may be normal in an early case and is rarely pathognomic. Only gross changes – strictures, cavities and calcification–are distinctive.

Treatment involves three drugs for 2 months and then isoniazid and rifampicin for a further 7–10 months. In the first 4–6 weeks of treatment, it is essential to assess the patient weekly with isotope or ultrasound studies to be sure that stricture of the ureters does not occur. If a stricture is diagnosed, percutaneous drainage and later stent insertion are indicated. Overall management is chiefly medical but reconstructive surgery or removal of necrotic tissue may be needed.

Summary

Patients admitted because of urinary tract infection are likely to have involvement of the upper tract. They need admission because of the systemic manifestations of the infection such as fever and pain, because of deteriorating renal function or for the administration of parenteral fluids and antibiotics. Urine and blood cultures should be performed on all such patients before antimicrobial therapy.

All patients requiring admission to hospital for urinary infection should be investigated in detail because a further renal lesion is often present. If obstruction is found, it is necessary to relieve this in order to eradicate the infection. Some renal diseases associated with urinary infection are 'salt-losing'; these patients tend to become very fluid-depleted in the presence of infection. There is a consequent deterioration in renal function and large volumes of normal saline are required before renal function improves.

Diabetics are thought to be prone to urinary infection, especially if they also have underlying renal disease. Infection in such patients increases insulin requirements and may impair glycaemic control. An osmotic diuresis and deterioration in renal function occur.

Bladder catheterization predisposes to urinary infection, particularly in the presence of oliguria. Catheterization should therefore be avoided if the 24-hour urine volume is less than 300 ml. Infection in this circumstance is very difficult to eradicate unless the catheter is removed.

Reduction of antibiotic dose in the presence of renal failure is essential.

Further reading

1 Asscher, A.W. (1980) *The Challenge of Urinary Tract Infections.* Academic Press, London.
2 Asscher, A.W. & Brumfitt, W. (eds) (1975) Urinary tract infection: a symposium. *Kidney Int.* Suppl. 4.
3 Bennet, W.M., Elzinga, L., Pulliam, J.P., Rashad, A.L. & Barry, J.M. (1985) Cyst fluid antibiotic concentrations in autosomal-dominant polycystic kidney disease. *Am. J. Kidney Dis.* **6**, 400–4.
4 Cox, C.E. (1974) Urinary tract infection and renal lithiasis. *Urol. Clin. N. Am.* **1**, 279–97.
5 de Wardener, H.E. (1985) *The Kidney*, 5th end. Churchill Livingstone, London.
6 Gower, P.E. (1976) A prospective study of patients with radiological pyelonephritis, papillary necrosis and obstructive atrophy. *Quart. J. Med.* **45**, 315–49.
7 Jones, V.E., Velosa J.A., Holley, K.E., Kelakis, P.P., Stickler, G. & Kurtz, S.B. (1980) The progression of vesico-ureteral reflux nephropathy. *Am. Intern. Med.* **92**, 776–84.
8 Marsh, F.P. (1985) Infection of the urinary tract. In Marsh, F.P. (ed.), *Postgraduate Nephrology*. Heinemann Medical Books, London, pp. 296–324.

9 Sussman, M. & Asscher, A.W. (1979) Urinary tract infection. In Black, D. & Jones, N.F. (eds), *Renal Disease*. Blackwell Scientific Publications, Oxford, pp. 400–36.
10 Savanborg, C., DeMan, P. & Sandberg, T. (1991) Renal involvement in urinary tract infection. *Kidney Int.* **39**, 550–6.
11 Zucchelli, P. & Gaggi, R. (1991) Reflux nephropathy in adults. *Nephron* **57**, 2–9.

Chapter 9
Renal Biopsy

Roger Gabriel

Renal biopsy is one of the major diagnostic procedures of renal medicine. The information gained has led to the classification and clarification of the natural history of glomerulonephritis, together with a number of other parenchymal renal diseases.

Indications

The majority of renal biopsies are performed in adults. The following indications are also applicable to some children.

1 Persistent asymptomatic proteinuria of more than 1 g daily, provided that renal cortex is not scarred as judged from an intravenous urogram (IVU) or dimercaptosuccinic acid (DMSA) scan. In the presence of lesser degrees of proteinuria and provided that there is no systemic condition, a renal biopsy usually does not provide information of clinical importance.

2 Chronic renal failure. This is a common indication. Provided that creatinine clearance is 20 ml/min or more and that the bipolar length of the kidneys is not less than 10 cm, useful information may be gained as to prognosis, possible treatment and the likelihood of transmission of the nephritis to a graft kidney.

3 Recurrent haematuria in adults; a neoplasm of the urinary tract must be excluded prior to biopsy. The finding of crenated red blood cells (phase-contrast microscopy; glomerular haematuria) or red cell casts or both indicates renal parenchymal disease. Paediatric renal physicians may adopt a more conservative approach.

4 Nephrotic syndrome in all teenagers and adults. A biopsy is also indicated in childhood nephrotics who have non-selective proteinuria. If a diabetic becomes nephrotic, a biopsy is needed if haematuria is also present (see p. 194).

5 Lupus glomerulonephritis. Renal tissue should be examined in all patients to help estimate the type and duration of therapy.
6 Acute renal failure. About 20% of patients with this condition require a tissue diagnosis. Indications are discussed in Chapter 16, p. 224.
7 Suspected polyarteritis nodosa or Wegener's granulomatosis. A biopsy of the kidney in either of these uncommon diseases may well be diagnostic and will help in deciding upon appropriate therapy.
8 Natural history of renal parenchymal conditions. Only a few patients require more than one biopsy because much is known of the natural history of many nephritides and to a lesser extent interstitial nephritides. Thus, once a diagnosis is made, the clinical course is usually predictable. Second or third renal biopsies are occasionally necessary if the clinical picture becomes atypical, or if a patient was biopsied early in the evolution of a condition before a specific morphology had developed or to assess effects of treatment—as in lupus nephritis (see pp. 152 and 155).

Contraindications to renal biopsy

There are four circumstances when a percutaneous biopsy should not be performed:
1 Coagulation defect or bleeding diathesis.
2 Obstructive uropathy.
3 Uncontrolled severe hypertension.
4 Lack of patient co-operation. This occurs occasionally as a consequence of premedication.

Single functioning kidneys may only be biopsied if they are graft organs.

Preparation for renal biopsy

It is prudent to develop a routine that suits the operator and is then maintained unchanged. This helps nursing staff, reduces the stress of the procedure upon the operator and is beneficial to the patient. The major matters to be considered are the following:
1 The physician should arrange that the renal biopsy pack contains the items that he/she requires based upon his/her experience. A gallipot, sponge forceps, a scalpel with a no. 15 blade, swabs and sterile orange-sticks are necessities.
2 A supply of fixatives should be kept on the renal ward so that urgent biopsies can be performed at any time. Most pathologists prefer tissue to be preserved in 10% formaldehyde for fixation for light microscopy and 1–2 mm segments of cortex cut and placed in 4% glutaraldehyde prior to preparation for electron microscopy.

In addition it is desirable that one or two 5 mm lengths of cortex be snap-frozen in liquid nitrogen. This has the following advantages: there is a reserve of tissue for extra histological examination if required;

immunofluorescent microscopy can be performed (although immunoperoxidase staining of paraffin-embedded tissue has largely replaced immunofluorescence); and finally further tissue is available for future studies should they prove necessary.

3 A dissecting microscope is of considerable value. Direct inspection of cores of kidney is possible, which ensures that cortex is placed in glutaraldehyde. In addition, with experience an informed guess can be made as to morphology – especially in patients with acute renal failure, rapidly progressive glomerulonephritides and the haemolytic uraemic syndrome.

4 The Tru-Cut needle is almost universally used. The 11.5 cm length is adequate for most patients but in large men the 15 cm one may be required. There is also a 7.5 cm Tru-Cut for paediatric use.

5 A variety of techniques have been suggested for localization of the kidney. Ideally, the crescent of the inferolateral pole of left or right kidney is biopsied. It is now routine to locate the position and depth of the kidneys either by real-time ultrasound or by a radiologist marking the area for biopsy.

6 Before biopsy, a platelet count and prothrombin time should be measured and the patient's blood group determined.

7 Written consent is obtained after explaining the procedure to the patient to gain his confidence.

8 It is essential to know that the patient has two functioning kidneys before the biopsy is performed. This is determined by an ultrasound study or a diethylene triamine pentacetic acid (DTPA) scan. A single kidney (other than a transplant) should not be biopsied percutaneously.

Procedure

The procedure is most simply explained stepwise:

1 A premedication of omnopon with stemetil or oral diazepam is given $1-1\frac{1}{2}$ hours before the procedure.

2 Prior to the procedure, both kidneys are imaged by ultrasound with the patient lying prone. At the height of inspiration, a cross is drawn over the inferolateral border of each kidney. The importance of taking deep breaths when requested can be emphasized at this stage if the operator performs his/her own pre-biopsy imaging. Otherwise the required breathing pattern must be explained separately.

3 The patient is positioned supine with a firm sandbag under the abdomen, placed so that it is between pelvis, inferior ribs and bed. If a sandbag is not available, a pillow rolled longitudinally will suffice.

4 The bed is raised so that the top of the patient's back is about horizontal with the operator's umbilicus. This saves stooping and is comfortable. The operator puts on mask, sterile gown and gloves. The patient's skin is prepared by painting with an antiseptic solution.

5 One per cent lignocaine is infiltrated from the skin down to the kidney. A long flexible needle is necessary in some; up to 20 ml of anaesthetic is required.

6 A 5 mm incision is made, using a no. 15 blade. The Tru-Cut is advanced down to the lower pole; this should be painless but the patient needs to be told that a pushing sensation will be felt.

7 With the patient holding his/her breath in full inspiration, the physician takes a comfortable stance, often leaning against the bed with elbows at sides, advances the trocar into the kidney, flicks the cannula over the trocar and removes the needle. The patient is then asked to breathe normally. In practised hands the Tru-Cut is within the renal substance for less than 1 sec.

8 The core of tissue is transferred to an orange-stick and placed upon the stage of a dissecting microscope. At a magnification of about × 20, cortex and medulla are easily differentiated. The orange-stick is placed on the trolley and two blocks are cut off and placed in glutaraldehyde; the remaining tissue is preserved in formalin.

9 Step 7 is repeated at least once: it is essential to obtain sufficient tissue for the histopathologist to examine approximately 15–20 glomeruli and surrounding structures.

10 Renal tissue may not be obtained at the first attempt. One then considers whether the kidney is deeper than expected or whether the incision site was incorrect. To test the depth of the kidney, the Tru-Cut is reinserted into the perirenal fat until resistance of renal substance is felt. The sensation can only be learnt by experience. A fairly common error is to insert the biopsy needle too low or too lateral or both. Most adult kidneys can be reached if the incision is 10 cm from the midline and just below the twelfth rib. Steps 5–9 are then repeated.

11 After adequate tissue is obtained, a dry swab it placed over the incision and taped in place. The dressing may be removed the next day. A very small scar is left, which will indicate the correct site for further biopsies.

Often, if the biopsy is correctly performed, the patient will ask at the end of the procedure when it is going to begin. Failure to obtain tissue is exceptional.

Post-biopsy care

After the procedure the patient is asked to drink 200 ml of fluid and given a tablet of bumetanide or frusemide, the dose being proportional to glomerular filtration rate (GFR). This is considered to wash any intrapelvic blood to the bladder and diminish the chance of clot colic, although proof is lacking.

Pulse and blood-pressure are recorded every 15 min for 2 hours, every 30 min for 2 hours and less frequently thereafter. The patient often sleeps for much of this period. He/she is allowed out of bed the following day, after the abdomen has been examined for a perirenal haematoma. A manual worker should perhaps take 2 days off before he/she returns to work; similarly, competitive sport should be avoided by all for a few days.

Complications

Considering the vascularity of the kidney, a complication of consequence is very infrequent. Given equal expertise, experience and post-procedure observation, renal biopsy is safer than liver biopsy. A death attributable to renal biopsy is very rare but not so rare following liver biopsy.

There is one major complication: haemorrhage. The majority of patients bleed initially – perirenal haematomata have been demonstrated by routine postprocedural computerized tomography (CT) scan or ultrasound. Microscopic haematuria occurs in all, macroscopic haematuria in about 10% and bleeding of clinical importance in less than 0.1%.

Case 1

A 20-year-old Afro-Caribbean woman with known lupus glomerulonephritis had defaulted from follow-up 2 years previously. She re-presented with fever, uraemic symptoms, pericarditis and arthropathy; she had a blood-pressure of 180/125 and a urine volume of less than 500 ml daily. The bipolar length of each kidney was 10 cm. Serum creatinine was 798 μmol/L.

Blood-pressure was controlled and plans were made for haemodialysis. Clinically it was not clear whether the patient had active systemic lupus erythematosus (SLE) or uncomplicated chronic renal failure. Because serological assessment of lupus takes some weeks, while the results of renal biopsy can be available a few hours after the procedure, the latter investigation was chosen. The biopsy was straightforward; two passes of a Tru-Cut produced two cores of very pale tissue. Advanced destruction of glomeruli was present, with tubular and interstitial fibrosis, together with prominent changes of accelerated-phase hypertension.

The following day urine became increasingly bloody, pulse-rate rose and blood-pressure fell. An arteriogram performed the same morning showed an arteriovenous fistula (Fig. 9.1). Attempts at embolization of the artery supplying the fistula were unsuccessful. A right nephrectomy was performed in the afternoon. The patient died 9 months later of uncontrollable SLE.

This case history illustrates three points. First, the morbidity of the procedure is increased in chronic renal failure. Secondly, it is unwise to perform renal biopsies unless expert help (in this case radiological and urological) is available should a complication arise. Finally, this is a rare complication: three in a personal series of over 1000 renal biopsies.

The following are other complications of renal biopsy:

1 Local discomfort lasting a few days. This is due to a perirenal haematoma. Explanation, analgesia, bed-rest and fluids suffice.

2 Perirenal infection has been reported: this is usually found at post-mortem. It is essential that aseptic technique be maintained.

3 The wrong organ may be biopsied. For the experienced and those who are guided by ultrasound this should never occur. Accidental biopsy of the spleen has been most commonly reported.

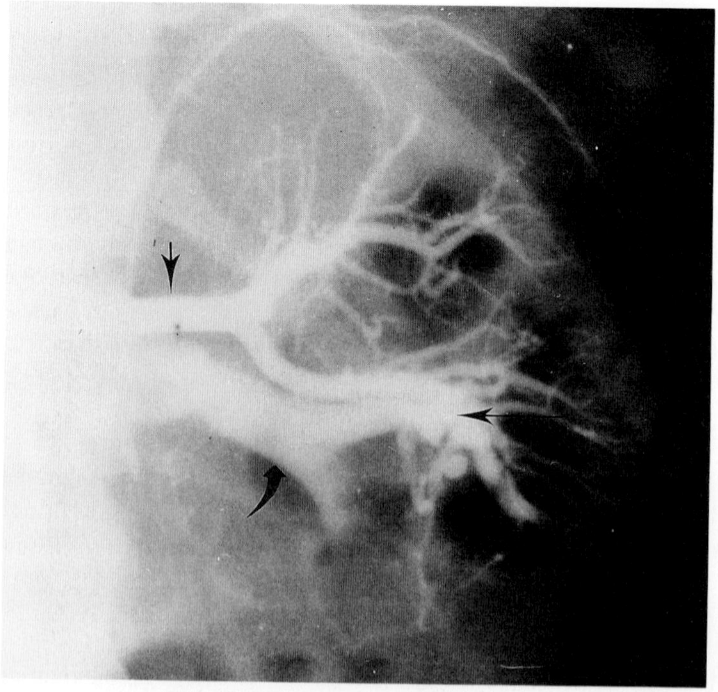

Fig. 9.1 A traumatic arteriovenous aneurysm between any interlobular artery and vein: a complication of renal biopsy. Contrast in the renal artery (vertical arrow) is seen draining (horizontal arrow) directly into the venous system and hence renal vein (broad arrow). Note also substantial pruning of the arterial tree, as found in chronic renal failure.

4 Distortion of a subsequent arteriogram. If arteriography is required, it should be performed before biopsy. In an unknown number of people, a small intrarenal arteriovenous aneurysm results.

Case 2

A woman aged 63 years was referred for biopsy because of hypertension, possibly secondary to nephritis. The histology was of secondary hypertension alone. Nine months later, because of increasingly severe hypertension, an arteriogram was performed to exclude atheromatous renal artery stenosis. The arteriogram was difficult to interpret until it was recalled that biopsy had been performed previously (see caption to Fig. 9.2).

Who should perform renal biopsies?

There are three groups of doctors who are appropriate to perform this procedure: renal physicians, general physicians with special interest in renal medicine and those training in the discipline. Renal biopsy, unlike liver biopsy, is not a technique that every registrar in medicine should master. These are the reasons:

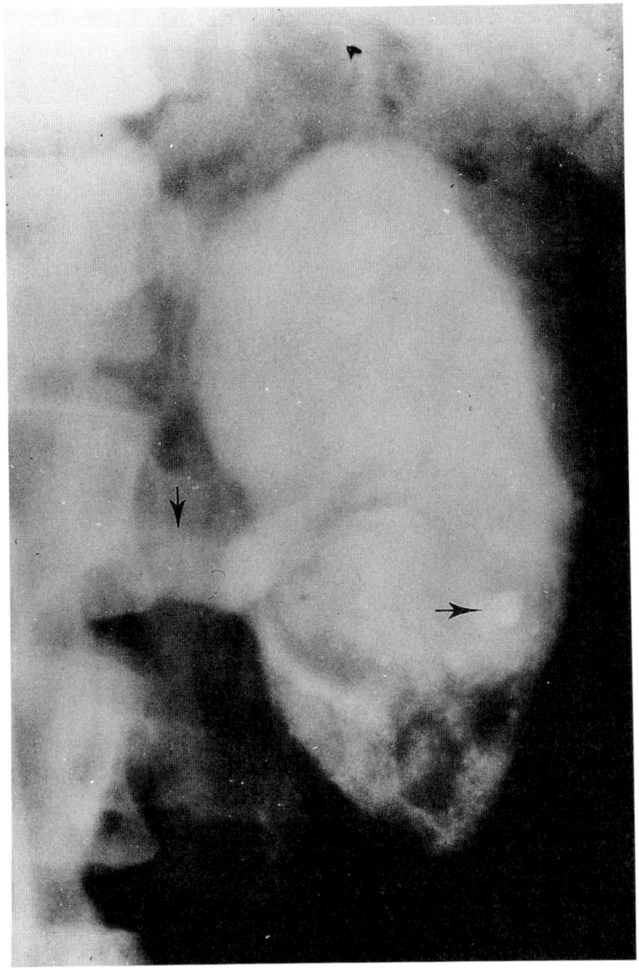

Fig. 9.2 Nephrogram immediately after intrarenal artery bolus injection of contrast (vertical arrow). A denser area is seen (horizontal arrow) in which contrast forms a so-called 'venous lake'. At this site there is an immediate connection between a small artery and its attendant vein. This was a consequence of a renal biopsy performed 9 months previously.

1 Only a small proportion of general medical patients require a renal biopsy: thus it would be impossible to train all registrars. At least 50 biopsies must be performed before a practitioner begins to become proficient.
2 It is not reasonable to subject patients to a potentially dangerous investigation unless the operator is trained or supervised.
3 To maintain familiarity with the technique two to three biopsies should be performed monthly.
4 Only a minority of histopathologists have training adequately to report upon renal biopsy tissue. In addition, technical staff must be skilled in the techniques of preparing small cores of tissue for light, immunoperoxidase and electron microscopy. Thus, to send renal biopsy tissue to a routine

department of morbid anatomy is inappropriate. The histopathologist, like his/her technical staff and the clinician, requires a minimum of 20 to 30 biopsies annually to maintain expertise.

Information required by the histopathologist

It is essential to inform the pathologist of the following:

1 The patient's current and past drug treatment.

2 The blood-pressure.

3 Current and previous creatinine clearances or some measures of GFR.

4 If the urine is infected.

5 The presence of systemic disease such as fever, SLE, polyarteritis or subacute bacterial endocarditis.

6 Urine protein excretion.

7 Plasma glucose concentration.

8 Serological variables: complement profile, double-stranded deoxyribonucleic acid (dsDNA) binding, ASOT, serum immunoglobulin concentrations and the current antineutrophil-cytoplasmic antibody (ANCA) titre.

This information allows the pathologist fully to interpret morphology. Often a precise diagnosis is made but at times discussion with a pathologist may be required to refine a differential diagnosis. In most renal centres regular meetings are held to discuss current biopsies: such gatherings are informative.

Summary

Renal biopsy is required to make the diagnosis of renal parenchymal disease. The major indications are unexplained renal impairment, proteinuria, recurrent haematuria and renal involvement in systemic disease. Coagulation disorders, uncontrolled hypertension and urinary obstruction are principal contraindications. Correct preparation is essential; the procedure should only be performed by renal physicians and those training in the discipline. The major complication is haemorrhage – one of the reasons why the procedure should be restricted to renal wards. It is important to supply the histopathologist who will report upon the biopsy with detailed clinical and laboratory information.

Further reading

1 Bearman, M. (1989) How to perform a renal biopsy. *Br. J. Hosp. Med.* **41**, 158–60.

2 Burstein, D.M. (1991) Percutaneous renal biopsy with use of real-time ultrasound. *Am. J. Nephrol.* **11**, 195–200.

3 Corwin, H.L., Schwartz, M.M. & Lewis, E.J. (1988) The importance of sample size in the interpretation of the renal biopsy. *Am. J. Nephrol.* **8**, 85–9.

4 de Caestecker, M.P., Hall, C.L., Basterfield, P.T. & Smith, J.G. (1989) Localisation of haematuria by red cell analysers and phase contrast microscopy. *Nephron* **52**, 170–3.

5 Gault, M.H. & Muehrcke, R.C. (1983) Renal biopsy: current views and controversies. *Nephron* **34**, 1–34.
6 Sinclair, R.A., Burns, J. & Dunhill, M.S. (1981) Immunoperoxidase staining of formalin fixed, paraffin embedded human renal biopsies with a comparison of the peroxidase–antiperoxidase (PAP) and indirect methods. *J. Clin. Pathol.* **34**, 859–65.
7 Striker, G.E. (1982) The role of renal biopsy in renal medicine. *Am. J. Kidney Dis.* **1**, 241–3.
8 Sutton, J.M. (1990) Evaluation of haematuria in adults. *JAMA* **263**, 2475–80.

Chapter 10
The Investigation and Management of the Glomerulonephritides

Roger Gabriel

This chapter will primarily discuss the clinical management of the glomerulonephritides, which may present with proteinuria, haematuria, proteinuria with haematuria, hypertension or, occasionally, progressive oliguria. These conditions are usually asymptomatic and are often found by chance. It is usually impossible to date the onset of disease. Population studies have shown that only about 2–5% of subjects have proteinuria, while proteinuria is common in hospital in-patients.

It is worth while to attempt from the history to date the onset of the proteinuria – oedema or frothing of the urine – so that with histology a composite picture of clinical events can be viewed. This helps the clinician to give a more accurate prognosis.

Initial assessment

A general approach to any patient with possible renal parenchymal disease includes the following:

1 Confirmation of urinary abnormalities – proteinuria, crenated red blood cells, granular casts.

2 Take a full history, including onset of oedema, if any, frothing of urine (proteinuria), whether haematuria has been noted, if the patient is diabetic, what drugs the patient has been taking (see Table 16.3, p. 228), any family history of renal disease or deafness (Alport's syndrome), and if any of these clinical events had occurred previously. If haemoptysis is mentioned, polyarteritis nodosa and anti-glomerular basement membrane (GBM) disease need rapid exclusion. Nasal or pharyngeal symptoms with urinary abnormalities raise the possibility of Wegener's granulomatosis. If there have been recent asthmatic symptoms, consider the Churg–Strauss syndrome.

3 A full clinical examination, with particular attention to blood-pressure, rashes (lupus, vasculitides, Henoch–Schönlein purpura (HSP)), the face (partial lypodystrophy is occasionally associated with mesangiocapillary glomerulonephritis (MCGN), the facies of scleroderma), joints (systemic lupus erythematosus (SLE) or rheumatoid arthritis), nails (white bands develop in chronic hypoalbuminaemia) and the presence and extent of oedema (ascites in childhood). If a patient who is over 55 years old presents as a nephrotic, the clinical examination should include a search for a malignancy – solid or haematological.

4 Measurement of serum creatinine – if possible two separate assays quite close in time so as to be sure that renal function is stable and not deteriorating rapidly. If the creatinine concentration has risen by, say, 100 μmol/L or more at the second assay, the patient may have rapidly progressive renal failure and must be referred to a renal physician that day (see p. 6).

5 The proteinuria is quantitated by asking the patient to collect urine for a 24-hour period. When this is returned, blood should be sampled for creatinine so that a clearance can be calculated. It is also useful to check on the completeness of the collection by using the formula quoted on p. 42. If there is a discrepancy of more than 5–10 ml/min, either the collection is incomplete or it may contain more than a 24-hour volume of urine.

6 It is wise in all patients, and especially Afro-Caribbean women, to have an assay for double-stranded deoxyribronucleic acid binding (dsDNAB) (p. 52) performed. Systemic lupus may present as a nephritis with no extrarenal symptoms or signs. A vasculitic lesion should prompt an assay for antineutrophil-cytoplasmic antibodies (ANCA) (p. 52). Haemoptysis should be investigated with assays for ANCA and anti-GBM antibodies.

7 An ultrasound study of the renal tract is necessary to learn the size and position of the kidneys and to verify the presence of two kidneys.

The kidneys in patients who are nephrotic are usually 2–3 cm longer than normal, provided renal function is normal. Patients with non-nephrotic-range proteinuria usually have normal-length kidneys (11–12 cm). Should the bipolar length of the kidneys be less than 10 cm, a substantial loss of glomerular filtration rate (GFR) has occurred.

8 Treatment of oedema is commenced as an out-patient. This is discussed later in this chapter.

9 Hypertension, if present, should be treated. Angiotensin-converting enzyme inhibitors or calcium channel-blocking drugs are very suitable.

10 Many patients in this category require a renal biopsy, the technique of which is described in Chapter 9, p. 127. A common exception is the presence of diabetic nephropathy, but occasionally a biopsy is required. This is discussed on p. 194.

11 The patient is reviewed in out-patients with the biopsy result. Specific therapy may be indicated. This is detailed in this chapter.

12 If the patient is likely to become a chronic nephrotic – membranous or mesangiocapillary nephropathies – dietary advice will be required for control of the attendant chronic hyperlipidaemia (see p. 142 and Chapter 20, p. 303).

Clinical types of proteinuria

Proteinuria of clinical importance is usually persistent and is of glomerular, non-glomerular, tubular or overflow type (see Fig. 4.1, p. 49). Glomerular proteinuria is the most common. Nephrotic-range proteinuria is the daily loss of 3.5 g or more. Proteinuric nephritic patients usually have daily urine protein losses of 5–7 g. Relatively infrequently is more than 10 g lost daily and only rarely is 30 g per day found. However, in younger patients there may be a sustained proteinuria of 20 g daily without hypoalbuminaemia, and hence peripheral oedema, developing. It follows, therefore, that the label 'nephrotic syndrome' is only of importance in therapeutic terms and, in adults, does not of itself carry any diagnostic or prognostic information.

When assessing a patient with proteinuria, the amount excreted is of general value to give an idea whether a glomerular lesion is or is not present. Generally, a daily excretion of 4–5 g or more is likely to be due to a glomerulonephritis. Smaller quantities of proteinuria are associated with a wider range of diseases.

If sequential 24-hour urines are assayed for their protein concentration, a daily variation of 2–3 g may well be found and is of no diagnostic or clinical importance.

Clinical management of proteinuria

Of patients with proteinuria perhaps only a quarter have peripheral oedema. Frequently, oedema is of concern because it is visible and inconvenient, impairs walking and shoe fitting and is cosmetically unattractive. Patients require reassurance that, of itself, oedema is not important and can be successfully treated in virtually all cases.

Treatment of peripheral oedema

This is usually straightforward and rarely requires admission.

Diuretic treatment

Bumetanide and frusemide are the main drugs used. The dose required to initiate a diuresis varies considerably. Before a treatment is commenced, the patient's weight should be recorded; this can be compared with later measurements to assess the success of therapy.

A small dose of bumetanide (1 mg) or frusemide (40 mg) is prescribed at first. The patient is advised of the time of onset, the duration and the possible ferocity of the diuresis. A morning diuresis is convenient for many; some prefer to take their diuretic at 4–6 p.m.

Diuretic treatment of nephrotic syndrome (Fig. 10.1)

Initial therapy is as above; it may be difficult to initiate and maintain a diuresis. Loop diuretics are the backbone of therapy and alone may prove adequate. Nevertheless, in a nephrotic avidly retaining sodium and despite a normal creatinine clearance, 500 mg of frusemide daily or an equivalent dose of bumetanide may be surprisingly ineffective. Generally, little is achieved by further increasing the dose of loop diuretic – in this circumstance there appears to be a flat dose–response curve.

The following additional strategies have to be tried:

1 The patient should weigh him/herself under standard conditions daily and record the weight, which is then used as an assessment of treatment.

2 The addition of 2.5–5 mg of metolazone to 500 mg frusemide may produce an impressive diuresis – perhaps leading to 1 kg weight loss daily. If such a diuresis is achieved, it may then be possible to control peripheral oedema with a reduced dose of frusemide and without metolazone (see p. 322).

3 In some diuretic-resistant nephrotics a short course of prednisolone (40–50 mg daily for 2–3 weeks) will induce a diuresis without diuretics. The following history illustrates this.

A 34-year-old man was referred because of nephrotic syndrome – weight 85 kg; serum albumin 25 g/L; proteinuria 24 g/L; estimated clearance 110 ml/min; renal biopsy: IgM-associated diffuse mesangial proliferative glomerulonephritis. This morphology does not, of itself, require prednisolone; accordingly the patient was treated with frusemide 80 mg daily. After 9 days of treatment he weighed 96 kg – proteinuria 36 g/L. Frusemide was withdrawn and prednisolone (50 mg daily) begun. Eight days later a diuresis began and, when seen 2 weeks

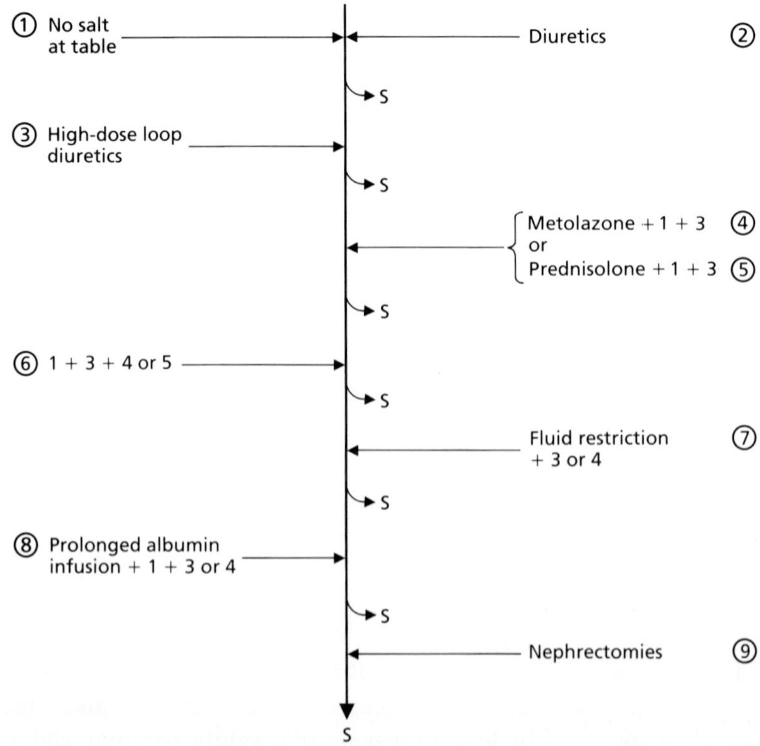

Fig. 10.1 A flow chart of the diuretic treatment of nephrotic syndrome. Rarely is strategy 8 required; strategy 9 is exceptional. For details see text. S, Success.

after beginning prednisolone, he weighed 76 kg and there was neither oedema nor proteinuria. Over 4 years of follow-up he has required no therapy, the estimated clearance remains normal and there is no proteinuria.

Types of glomerulonephritides that respond to a short course of prednisolone include the minimal-change lesion (although a long course is often required to prevent prompt relapse) and patients with various mesangial proliferative lesions. This strategy is not successful in lupus, mesangiocapillary or membranous nephrotics.

4 Prednisolone with loop diuretics. Some patients require long-term low-dose prednisolone in combination with a moderate dose of a loop diuretic to control peripheral oedema. Often one 5 mg dose of prednisolone alternate days with 40 mg of frusemide daily suffices. Without prednisolone this small group of patients become nephrotic and may not respond to even 500 mg doses of frusemide.

It is not known why these patients respond so differently from those described in number 3 above, especially as they share common morphologies of modest glomerular proliferative lesions.

Treatment of severe nephrotics

In the majority of nephrotics adequate control of peripheral oedema is obtained without difficulty, as described above. The term 'severe' in this context refers to difficulties in initiating and maintaining diuresis. The severity of sodium and water retention are only recognized as preliminary treatments fail.

During management much attention is paid to:

1 reducing the patient's salt intake; and
2 establishing a negative sodium balance with diuretics.

There are considerable difficulties in modifying a patient's sodium intake because such diets are unpalatable and impracticable. To maintain a patient's co-operation it is best to advise:

1 moderation with high-salt-containing foods; and
2 no additional salt at table.

Frusemide is probably the most widely used and is very safe provided that intravenous rapid-bolus doses are not given (ototoxicity) and that the daily dose does not lead to hypovolaemia. Bumetanide is a satisfactory alternative except for the myalgic symptoms which occur in some patients receiving large doses.

Dose of loop diuretics

It is prudent to begin therapy with 40–80 mg of frusemide or 1–2 mg of bumetanide daily, explaining the duration of action and allowing the patient to reduce the dose if a diuresis commences. After a week, assuming no diuresis and no decrease in weight, the dose is increased to 250 mg of frusemide or 5 mg of bumetanide. Again assuming no diuresis, the dose of either diuretic is doubled. At this level, little extra diuretic effect is gained from further doubling of dose, although a few nephrotics require about 750 mg frusemide or 15 mg bumetanide to gain control of peripheral oedema.

Loop diuretic resistance

If a nephrotic fails to achieve a diuresis when taking daily 500 mg of frusemide or the bumetanide equivalent, one of two possible strategies is employed:

1 the addition of metolazone, 2.5–5 mg daily; or
2 a course of prednisolone, provided the patient has a nephritis likely to respond, with a natriuresis, to steroid.

The strategies have been described above. It should be emphasized that prednisolone in this context is introduced for a few weeks only, to permit diuretics to function, and not on a long-term basis attempting to modify glomerular inflammation.

Occasionally, the addition of both metolazone and prednisolone to a loop diuretic is necessary and successful. If they fail, there is a tendency to maintain therapeutic doses of prednisolone in the hope that some good will be achieved. Nevertheless, if there is no reasonable hope of suppression of inflammation, prednisolone should be withdrawn to avoid the undesirable metabolic effects.

Assessing success of therapy

In the majority of nephrotics a diuresis can be achieved by one or more of the above. Success is confirmed by noting a daily weight loss.

When a diuresis has been established, it is wise to reduce the dose of diuretic by perhaps 50% so as to avoid a urine flow of more that 3 L daily, hypokalaemia and the distinct risk of acute hypovolaemia. The loss of 1 kg daily is adequate and safe.

Maintenance therapy

If the patient has a persistent proteinuria, maintenance diuretics will be required, usually at a substantially lower dose than that required to induce diuresis. Some patients prefer the relatively brief, predictable response to frusemide or bumetanide, while others may be satisfactorily maintained on a thiazide. If a thiazide proves inadequate and the patient prefers to avoid high-potency diuretics, chlorthalidone 50–100 mg daily is often beneficial. Amiloride is required to conserve urine potassium losses during chronic diuretic therapy.

Drug-resistant nephrotics

A minority of nephrotics are very resistant to the therapies discussed above. They are usually of two groups:

1 Those with chronic renal failure in addition.

2 Those in whom serum albumin is persistently 15 g/L or less.

A simple measure which may benefit patients in both groups is fluid restriction. This is easy to recommend but compliance may be difficult, particularly in the warmer months. Insensible loss in an adult is usually greater than 1 L; thus if a fluid intake of 1 L is not exceeded there will be weight loss approximately equal to that of the urine volume.

If no benefit has been obtained after a few weeks of fluid restriction and diuretic therapy, there is little purpose in pursuing this approach further. Fluid can readily be removed by arteriovenous haemofiltration. Treatment periods last 1–2 hours during which 2–3 L of fluid are removed. A succession of daily treatments produces an impressive gain in well-being but patients may relapse. In some cases, for reasons which are not clear, haemofiltration may induce a spontaneous diuresis or permit diuretic sensitivity to develop.

Exceptional measures

In a very small minority of nephrotics it is not possible to relieve symptoms. Such patients have marked hypoalbuminaemia and anasarca,

Table 10.1 The major complications of long-standing nephrotic syndrome

Venous and arterial thromboses
Hyperlipidaemia: vascular disease
Subnutrition
Acute renal failure
Increased incidence of bacterial infections

usually feel unwell and miserable and are unable to move or rest in comfort. They are at risk of, or demonstrate complications of, nephrotic syndrome (Table 10.1). Urine protein excretion is of the order of 25 g daily or more. Three measures may be considered.

Albumin infusions

While apparently a very logical treatment albumin infusions are often practised inexpertly by infusing an occasional bottle of human albumin. Such low-dose therapy produces transient and perhaps unmeasurable effects. If parenteral therapy is planned, a line via a subclavian or internal jugular vein should be inserted with the intention of infusing 50 g albumin daily for weeks or perhaps longer. Full remission of the nephrotic state has been reported.

Immersion therapy

It has been clearly shown that severe nephrotics, if placed in a bath at 34 °C, experience an improvement in renal haemodynamics such that increase in GFR, together with a diuresis and natriuresis, occurs for the duration of the immersion. The pressure of the bath water increases external hydrostatic pressure on the limbs and diminishes secretion of arginine vasopressin, which increases sodium and chloride delivery to distal tubules for excretion with water. Unfortunately, this is an impracticable therapy but it indicates that antigravity suits may have a place in therapy of chronic severe oedema.

Bilateral nephrectomy

In patients with incapacitating proteinuria, the source of the protein loss can be excised and the patient taken on to a haemodialysis programme. The decision is more straightforward if the patient has developed chronic renal failure.

'Medical nephrectomy' – the purposeful destruction of kidneys by drugs (non-steroidal anti-inflammatory drugs) (NSAIDs), aminoglycosides) or by theraputic embolization – leads to very substantial fever and discomfort. Surgical removal of irrevocably diseased organs is preferred.

Lipids in nephrotic syndrome

Hypercholesterolaemia and hypertriglyceridaemia are constant features of nephrotic patients. Further, hypercholesterolaemia is a consequence of steroid and cyclosporin therapies. Patients with focal sclerosing, membranous or mesangiocapillary glomerulonephritis may remain nephrotic for 5 or more years, during which time persistent hyperlipidaemia may accelerate the deposition of atheroma. It is logical to control, as far as feasible, the lipid abnormalities. These patients should consult a dietitian so as to limit their fat intake to providing one-third of daily calorie intake, and the ratio of polyunsaturated to saturated fat in their diets should be approximately 1.5 : 1.

Cholestyramine may be used in conjunction with diet to lower cholesterol concentrations, but gastric or colonic intolerance may prevent optimum doses. Drugs belonging to the fibrate and statin groups are relatively toxic and probably best avoided.

Specific glomerulonephritides

Before discussing the treatment of glomerulonephritis, it is necessary to define the renal morphology by renal biopsy. It is also necessary to have a classification, as shown in Table 10.2. Without a histological diagnosis, specific therapies, as opposed to diuretic treatment, should not be undertaken.

Table 10.2 A simplified classification of the major glomerulonephritides

PRIMARY GLOMERULAR DISEASES
1 Minor glomerular abnormalities (minimal change)
2 Focal and segmental lesions
Diffuse glomerulonephritides
3 Membranous glomerulonephritis (nephropathy)
Proliferative glomerulonephritides
4 Mesangial proliferative
5 Berger's disease (IgA/C3 nephropathy)
6 Endocapillary (postinfectious)
7 Mesangiocapillary (membranoproliferative)
8 Crescentic (extracapillary)
GLOMERULONEPHRITIS OF SYSTEMIC DISEASES
1 Lupus nephritis
2 Nephritis of Henoch–Schönlein purpura
3 Glomerular lesions in systemic infections:
Infective endocarditis
Human immunodeficiency virus-associated nephropathy
4 Anti-GBM disease

Primary glomerular diseases

Minor glomerular abnormalities (minimal-lesion glomerulonephritis)

The typical clinical course of minimal-lesion glomerulonephritis, or minimal-change nephrotic syndrome (MCNS), is one of spontaneous relapse and remission, but the severity of the nephrotic state is usually only partially controllable with diuretics and requires corticosteroids.

Prednisolone

With prednisolone given as a single daily dose of 50 mg (in adults), a rapid diuresis and cessation of proteinuria can be expected in 10–20 days after beginning treatment. Diuretics are withdrawn. After response to treatment, prednisolone is withdrawn stepwise over the next 4–6 weeks, changing from daily to alternate daily administration after 1–2 weeks. The alternate-day schedule is used to reduce the incidence of steroid side-effects. It may appear unnecessary for a relatively short course of prednisolone but it is desirable for the following reasons:

1 About 70% of patients with MCNS experience at least one relapse after the first successful course of prednisolone.

2 A number of these relapsing patients may require more prolonged therapy in order to induce remission.

3 Perhaps as many as 50% of these patients either frequently relapse or become steroid-dependent. In these two groups, which can only be recognized as treatment proceeds, the consequences of prolonged steroid therapy may be severe.

4 A small number of patients with MCNS, initially steroid-responsive, become steroid-resistant after two or more subsequent relapses.

Cyclophosphamide

Cyclophosphamide is reserved for those patients who prove to be frequent relapsers, steroid-dependent or steroid-resistant. The dose is 2–2.5 mg/kg body-weight daily for no more than 2–3 months. Generally, cyclophosphamide is a more successful drug than prednisolone in that remission for 5 or more years can be expected in approximately 60% of patients.

Although MCNS is not common in adults, a good argument can be made for using cyclophosphamide as the drug of first choice provided the patient has completed his or her family. For younger patients, gonadal toxicity is thought to be dose-related, and testicular and ovarian toxicity are uncommon if the total dose is less than 200 mg/kg. There is also the risk of opportunistic infection during therapy and the possibility of the late development of a malignancy.

Cyclosporin

In future cyclosporin may be used in a number of different ways:
1 In cyclophosphamide-resistant cases.
2 As a steroid-sparing agent.
3 If prednisolone is relatively contraindicated.

It is known that cyclosporin will induce remission but the correct duration of therapy to avoid relapse is not yet determined. Cyclosporin dependency has been described in this nephritis. It is premature to recommend this therapy in any general manner.

Conclusion

The long-term prognosis of MCNS in adults is very favourable provided that the complications of nephrotic syndrome (Table 10.1, p. 141) do not develop and that side-effects of therapy are not severe. Treatment is necessary because of the severity of the nephrotic state, which can usually be only partially controlled with diuretics. Chronic renal failure is not a feature of this nephropathy. It is probable that in adults remission eventually occurs, or is achieved, in all.

Failure of a high-protein diet and success of prednisolone therapy in MCNS is shown in Fig. 20.2, p. 308.

Focal and segmental glomerulosclerosis

Focal and segmental glomerulosclerosis (FSGS) is a severe nephritis, in terms of both morbidity and mortality. Many of these patients are persistently nephrotic, only about 25% responding to the conventional therapy of prednisolone and cyclophosphamide; many of these become dependent on continuous treatment to control the nephrotic state. Despite treatment, repeat renal biopsy will show progression of the disease.

Histology

The glomeruli show segmental increase in mesangial cells and matrix, occurring first at the juxtamedullary glomeruli. The initially affected areas become hyalinized, expand and lead to focal sclerosis of the lobule and eventually the glomerulus. IgM and C3 and C1q may be found in the sclerosing areas. Mesangial deposits are not seen at electron microscopy.

In the idiopathic form of FSGS progressive reduction in GFR is likely, particularly so in those who are persistently nephrotic. The 10-year survival rate is about 45% for those patients who remain nephrotic. For those patients who respond to prednisolone and cyclophosphamide the 10-year survival free of dialysis is approximately 70–80%. Persistent loss of GFR is probable in all patients with FSGS.

It has been found that cyclosporin can abolish all clinical features of the disease in at least 20% of patients. The success of therapy is not predictable and is not confined to those who responded to conventional therapy (prednisolone and cyclophosphamide). It is unknown whether renal morphology continues to deteriorate while clinical manifestations are held at bay by cyclosporin. Which FSGS patient to treat and the duration of therapy are likewise undecided. Cyclosporin dependency in FSGS has been documented.

Because, in practised hands, cyclosporin is straightforward to use, it is becoming established practice that, after a period of diuretics and observation, new patients with FSGS are treated with cyclosporin alone. If successful treatment must be continued for an unknown period of time. If after 3 months of therapy proteinuria still persists, prednisolone 10 mg daily is added. Success with combined treatment has been reported. Other physicians hold that initial treatment should still comprise conventional therapy and cyclosporin should be reserved for those who fail to respond. It is too early for conclusions to be reached, although the quality of life for a minority of patients with FSGS has been substantially improved by the use of cyclosporin.

Idiopathic membranous glomerulonephritis (nephropathy)

Idiopathic membranous glomerulonephritis (IMGN) may follow one of several well-defined clinical courses, which cannot be predicted with confidence at the time of diagnosis. Ten to fifteen years after diagnosis, about half of a group of patients with IMGN will have developed chronic renal failure and the others will be in remission or have mild proteinuria. Nephrotic syndrome is present in 80% at diagnosis; this tends to remit with time, but if persistent it is a marker for the eventual development of chronic renal failure (CRF). Generally, those patients with asymptomatic proteinuria are much less likely to have reduced GFR and may remit spontaneously.

Membranous nephropathy is idiopathic in at least 85% of European patients; identical or very similar morphological changes occur following a wide variety of different exogenous or endogenous events (Table 10.3). Drug-related membranous glomerulonephritis (MGN) is usually straightforward to diagnose and may resolve upon withdrawing the drug. It is good practice to request some measure of lupus serology (pp. 51 and 135) in all patients. A hepatitis B virus (HBV)- or parasite-related membranous nephropathy should be considered if a patient originates from, or has visited, those large parts of the world where such infections are commonplace. The association between membranous nephropathy and malignancy is very rare, although well documented. Many different types of carcinoma and lymphoma may be related to a glomerulonephritis. Membranous nephropathy is the most common morphology found. The nephropathy may precede clinical diagnosis of malignancy, or vice versa. Generally, the two diagnoses are closely related in time and complete removal of the tumour leads to resolution of the nephrotic state.

Table 10.3 The major conditions associated with membranous glomerulonephritis, listed in approximate order of frequency

Drugs	Gold Penicillamine Captopril NSAIDs Mercury
Infections	Hepatitis B virus Schistosomiasis Leprosy Syphilis Malaria
Autoimmune disease	Systemic lupus erythematosus
Diabetes mellitus	
Malignancies	Any solid tumour or lymphoma

World-wide, HBV infection is the most frequent association.

Drug treatment of idiopathic membranous glomerulonephritis

It is very difficult to determine beneficial treatment of this nephropathy in the context of the very protracted clinical course mentioned above. At least 1 year of observation should precede therapy unless renal function declines rapidly (a rise in serum creatinine of 50 μmol/L or more in 6 months).

Prednisolone

Prospective controlled studies using alternate-day prednisolone show that treated patients tend to go into remission and have lower average serum creatinine concentrations at 3–5 years than do the untreated controls, but there is no statistical significance between the two groups.

Cytotoxic therapy

Azathioprine, chlorambucil and cyclophosphamide have been used, usually in combination with corticosteroids. Azathioprine has not been shown to improve the clinical course of IMGN. Most studies have shown improvement (less proteinuria, less rapid decline in GFR) in patients when either chlorambucil or cyclophosphamide was added to prednisolone in this nephropathy.

At present, a 6-month course of alternating methylprednisolone (0.5 mg/kg daily) for the first month and chlorambucil (0.2 mg/kg daily) for the second month is recommended. At the end of the second month steroid is recommenced. The 2-month cycle is repeated three times. Under trial conditions, treated patients fared better than controls. Side-effects are likely to be minimal but regular white cell counts are required to avoid marrow suppression. It is not known whether the beneficial effects of cytotoxic therapy are outweighed by the increased chance of infection and the expected higher incidence of late malignancies. The methylprednisolone–chlorambucil regimen is recommended for patients above the age of 60 years and perhaps for selected younger patients, but not for those planning to reproduce. Fortunately IMGN is a disease of the middle-aged or older. There is considerable need to conduct 10-year clinical trials in this nephropathy so as to learn the best therapy.

Mesangial proliferative glomerulonephritis

Mesangial proliferative glomerulonephritis (MPG) is a quite common morphology found in 10–20% of cases when renal biopsies are performed in the assessment of asymptomatic proteinuria, nephrotic syndrome or haematuria with proteinuria. The diagnosis is made by light microscopy and to a certain extent is subjective in terms of the degree of proliferation noted, although quantification is possible. Further, while MPG is a specific morphology, patients with resolving postinfectious nephritis, lupus nephritis and HSP may appear identical with MPG and differentiation has to be made by history, examination and lupus serology. In addition, the presence of mesangial IgA in glomeruli would categorize the patient as having Berger's disease (p. 148).

Histology

All glomeruli have diffuse increased cellularity of the mesangium with an increased mesangial matrix and normal capillary walls. Granular deposits of IgM are found predominantly in the mesangium.

Course and therapy

Proteinuria or haematuria, or both, may remit spontaneously; in others it is persistent or intermittent. The following are suggested:

1 All patients require long-term follow up with regular assessment of GFR.

2 For those with haematuria or non-nephrotic-range proteinuria, no therapy is attempted.

3 Those who are nephrotic will require treatment as outlined in Fig. 10.1 (p. 138). If strategy 3 in the scheme is unsuccessful, strategy 5 should be used: it is frequently successful and may also suppress proteinuria, perhaps permanently.

4 If GFR declines in patients in number 2 above, prednisolone in similar doses to those suggested for minimal-change glomerulonephritis (p. 143) may be used. The major aim of therapy is to prevent further reduction in GFR and to regain normal function if possible. Any patient in whom the serum creatinine concentration is above the upper limit of normal should be offered a 6–8-week trial of therapy. The second aim of therapy is the suppression of proteinuria, which may occur while pursuing the first goal.

Prognosis

Prognosis has not been clearly defined. There is a tendency to progression to renal failure, particularly in those patients who fail to respond to steroids. For this reason, it is necessary to be sure which patients have reduced GFR and then concentrate upon their treatment.

Berger's disease (IgA nephropathy, IgA/C3 nephropathy)

Since the original description of IgA nephropathy (IgAN) in 1968 by Berger in Paris, there has been an increasing and expanding interest in the immunobiology of IgA in this nephropathy. Some prefer not to use the word 'disease' or 'nephropathy' because of the systemic features of this condition and because there are some virtually identical immunopathological features with HSP (p. 156). Nevertheless, for the sake of simplicity this discussion will concentrate upon the renal aspects of IgAN.

The commonest presenting features are macroscopic haematuria at times with aching loin pain, microscopic haematuria with or without intermittent proteinuria of 1–3 g daily or proteinuria with microscopic haematuria. Urine contains red cells of glomerular origin and granular and red cell casts. Haematuria is usually intermittent and recurrent, typically occurring at the height of, or shortly after, an upper respiratory tract infection. About equal numbers of patients have either haematuria or proteinuria.

Histology

Mesangial proliferation is present; this may be focal, segmental or diffuse. There is no abnormality of the capillary wall. The hallmark of this nephropathy is the presence of IgA and C3 in the mesangium of all glomeruli, whether or not the glomeruli are normal by light microscopy.

Course and therapy

As is to be exptected, those patients with hypertension, persistent proteinuria, nephrotic syndrome or renal impairment have an unfavourable prognosis and show more prominent changes in renal histology. Conversely, the majority – about 80% of patients – have a normal life expectation. It is debated whether recurrent macroscopic haematuria is a bad prognostic sign.

There is no known specific treatment to reduce the loss of GFR in the 20% of patients who will fare badly. In the early phases of IgAN, there are no clinical markers for either a benign or progressive course.

Diffuse endocapillary glomerulonephritis (postinfectious glomerulonephritis)

Postinfectious glomerulonephritis (PIGN) used to be called poststreptococcal nephritis, but it has become apparent that identical clinical events and morphological changes occur in the absence of streptococcal infection. Nevertheless, poststreptococcal nephritis is quite common in tropical parts of the globe. Very occasionally, PIGN follows staphylococcal or pneumococcal infection.

Clinical features of PIGN are very well known. Usually, the abrupt nephritic onset and reduced activity of serum complement make the diagnosis straightforward. If hypocomplementaemia persists for more than 6 weeks, the alternative diagnoses of lupus or mesangiocapillary nephritis should be considered, the appropriate serology requested and renal biopsy performed.

Postinfectious glomerulonephritis may present as nephrotic syndrome or, in adults, as rapidly progressive glomerulonephritis (RPGN). Such events occur very infrequently. Indeed, PIGN in an adult is, in Western Europe, an uncommon diagnosis.

Histology

At the acute stage, glomeruli show an increase in mesangial and endothelial cells. Polymorphonuclear leucocyte infiltration is often prominent. Glomerular basement membranes are intact. The histology is characteristic.

Course and therapy

There is a mortality of about 0.7% in the acute phase of PIGN; adults are much more likely to succumb than children. The prognosis is particularly excellent in children in that all clinical, biochemical and histological features resolve and microscopic haematuria ceases by 12 months from onset. It is thought that 10 years after PIGN about 1% of a hospital group of patients will have developed renal failure.

Management of the acute phase is straightforward and includes the following:

1 Streptococcal infection of throat or elsewhere, if present, should be eradicated by a course of penicillin.

2 The acute nephritic component involves control of sodium and water retention. Frusemide will induce a diuresis and captopril is recommended for management of hypertension.

3 Perhaps 5% of adult patients with PIGN require more intensive therapy – those who become nephrotic or have considerable reduction in GFR.

Mesangiocapillary (membranoproliferative) glomerulonephritis

Mesangiocapillary glomerulonephritis is usually an idiopathic nephritis with characteristic morphologies. It presents in teenagers and young

Table 10.4 Associated conditions in which mesangiocapillary glomerulonephritis may develop

1 Systemic immune complex diseases:
SLE
Mixed cryoglobulinaemia
Hereditary deficiency of complement components
2 Infectious diseases:
Usually bacteraemias, including SBE, occasionally parasitic infestation
3 Chronic liver disease:
Chronic active hepatitis in the presence of HBV
Cirrhosis
α-1-Antitrypsin deficiency
4 Malignant disease:
Light-chain nephropathy (multiple myeloma)
Various lymphomas and leukaemias
Hodgkin's disease
5 Miscellaneous:
Partial lipodystrophy
Recurrent infections
Sickle-cell disease
Scleroderma

SBE, Subacute bacterial endocarditis.

adults as nephrotic syndrome, proteinuria, recurrent haematuria or occasionally as an acute nephritis. In Western Europe 90% of patients have the idiopathic form of MCGN: the others, which are related to associated disorders, are presented in Table 10.4. This account will be restricted to the idiopathic form of MCGN.

Histology

The essential features of MCGN are:

1 Endocapillary cellular proliferation.
2 Increase in mesangial cells and matrix.
3 Thickening of capillary walls due to mesangial cell interposition.
4 The presence of immune complexes in capillary walls and mesangium.

Mesangiocapillary glomerulonephritis is divided into type I and type II varieties on the basis of immunoperoxidase studies and electron microscopy. Type I is the more common.

Serology

Fifty per cent of patients with type I MCGN and the majority with type II have reduced activities of C3, and hence haemolytic complement (CH50). These changes tend to persist for the duration of the clinical course, particularly so in type II MCGN. Reduced activity of C3 is due to the presence of an IgG autoantibody called nephritic factor (C3NF), which is directed against the C3 convertase of the alternative pathway of the complement cascade; this, in a complex manner, leads to persistent breakdown of C3 and thus reduced C3 and CH50 activities.

Course and therapy

Type I MCGN presents as nephrotic syndrome or proteinuria and type II is more likely to present as recurrent macroscopic haematuria or acute nephritis. Type II may be more aggressive than type I.

This nephritis is slowly progressive, with about 50–60% survival in type I at 10 years and about 10% less survival in type II. A poor outcome can usually be predicted in both types of MCGN if there is hypertension, loss of GFR or persistent nephrotic syndrome or if epithelial crescents are found at renal biopsy. Persistent nephrotic syndrome doubles the mortality rate compared with those with asymptomatic proteinuria.

In children, alternate-day prednisolone may delay the rate of progression of MCGN but at the cost of predictable side-effects. In adults, only symptomatic therapy is used because there is no proved therapy. Sexually active women with MPGN should be told that there may be a substantial and persistent loss of GFR in the third trimester: pregnancy is best avoided.

Idiopathic crescentic glomerulonephritis (rapidly progressive glomerulonephritis)

Idiopathic crescentic glomerulonephritis is uncommon; only a few cases are seen annually in a busy renal unit. Nevertheless, it is most important to recognize the condition because prompt treatment will allow restitution of renal function and avoid chronic dialysis. Clinical features and management are given in Chapter 11, p. 179.

Glomerulonephritides of systemic disease

Lupus glomerulonephritis

Systemic lupus erythematosus is a particularly complex disorder in which endogenous or exogenous factors lead to polyclonal stimulation of B cells, which in turn induces a loss of self-tolerance and further expansion of B cells or T cells or both. The B cells produce pathogenic antigen-dependent autoantibodies which can cause disease at many different sites – for example, electron-dense deposits in glomeruli.

Classification of lupus nephropathy

In 1975 the World Health Organization produced a very useful classification of lupus glomerulonephritis (LGN) which includes light,

Table 10.5 A histological classification of lupus nephritis based upon World Health Organization criteria

I	Normal
II	Mesangial hypercellularity alone (mild to moderate)
III	Segmental and focal glomerulonephritis – active necrotizing, active sclerosing and sclerosing
IV	Diffuse proliferative glomerulonephritis – with and without segmental necrotizing lesions
V	Diffuse membranous glomerulonephritis, which may include lesions found in groups I, III and IV
VI	Advanced sclerosing glomerulonephritis

Setting aside classes I and VI (see text), mesangial and segmental lesions occur in 35% of patients, class IV lesions in 50% and membranous nephropathy in 15%.

immunoperoxidase and electron microscopic features (Table 10.5). In addition, severity and chronicity can be scored, although the predictive value of these scores is debatable. Activity scoring relates necrosis, proliferation, polymorphonuclear infiltration crescents and hyaline thrombi in glomeruli. Chronicity is graded according to the amount of glomerular sclerosis, tubular atrophy and interstitial scarring.

Class I LGN may not represent a disease entity: it is found in patients who have no evidence of renal disease and does not *per se* require therapy. Patients with class II LGN have mild to moderate renal disease and a good prognosis. The changes of class III LGN are relatively severe and the clinical course is more aggressive than class II. The natural history is similar to that of class IV patients: classes III and IV are perhaps not different classes of lupus nephritis but a continuation of the same lesion. Class IV LGN (about 50% of patients studied) involves a wide range of histological changes and a severe nephrotic clinical picture, and has the worst prognosis because many progress to renal failure. The diffuse membranous variant (class V) is histologically indistinguishable from the idiopathic variety and the prognosis is similar to that of IMGN (p. 145). Class VI is primarily the result of progression of class IV; the patient requires preparation for dialysis.

A difficulty with the histological classification of LGN is that one morphology may transform to another, usually more severe, form, as demonstrated by repeated renal biopsy.

Renal biopsy in systemic lupus

All patients with proteinuria, haematuria or renal impairment, singly or in combination, require a renal biopsy. If tissue is sampled from patients with SLE but without any of the above features, it is likely that class I or mild class II lesions will be found. Also, if tissue is taken from patients with CRF, class VI changes will be demonstrated. Immunosuppressive therapy is not required in class I or VI LGN and therefore renal biopsy is not routinely required in these patients.

Correlation of disease activity and laboratory variables

Reduced serum haemolytic complement activity (consumption) and elevation of anti-dsDNAB titres are closely associated with active disease; return of these variables to normal indicates response to treatment. Nevertheless, once normal, these variables are of limited value in guiding therapy. Relapse is diagnosed if complement consumption recurs or dsDNAB rises to a high titre, or both. If lupus serology dose not gradually return to normal, the prognosis is substantially worse. In most patients, the above variables become normal if uraemia supervenes. Lupus serology must be requested repeatedly during and after therapy.

Laboratory help in monitoring progress in LGN is limited and assessment is mainly clinical. Regular assay of serum creatinine concentrations are the best single laboratory aid to therapy.

Treatment of lupus glomerulonephritis

Treatment of LGN is approached from the histological classification, disease activity and initial serology. General features include amelioration of oedema, control of hypertension and explanation of the consequences of a chronic disease. If necessary, treatment is adjusted for each patient individually – women, in particular, are naturally concerned by steroid side-effects on their facial appearance. Classes III and IV LGN require urgent treatment; there is usually time for attention to general features in classes II and V (Table 10.5) before specific therapy.

Patients with LGN may or may not have active SLE and vary from having acute life-threatening illness to having asymptomatic proteinuria. Extrarenal aspects of SLE will not be discussed save to indicate that at times extrarenal components may dictate the pace and dimension of therapy.

Prednisolone is the major drug used and an alternate-day regimen is introduced as soon as feasible. Azathioprine is an immunosuppressant and has prednisolone-sparing properties. Many physicians combine it with corticosteroids from the outset. Oral cyclophosphamide is as effective as azathioprine but more toxic. Intravenous cyclophosphamide is very potent and is reserved for those with life-threatening disease.

While details of treatment vary considerably the following is a summary of contemporary opinion.

Mild to moderate LGN (class II lesions)

Prednisolone is begun at about 50 mg daily and tapered to a maintenance dose of 10–15 mg daily, if possible given as 20–30 mg on alternate days. If there is renal functional impairment at the onset, azathioprine at a dose of 2 mg/kg body-weight daily is added to the prednisolone. The cytotoxic drug is best given in divided dose because of a short half-life. The dose is adjusted according to white cell counts.

After 12 months of treatment, prednisolone is reduced to less than 10 mg daily if the patient's health is good, the serum creatinine is normal for age, sex and body-weight, the erythrocyte sedimentation rate (ESR) and serological variables are normal and remain normal 2 months after reduction in steroid. Proteinuria in patients with class II lesions usually subsides to 1 g daily or less after 3–6 months of therapy. Failure to do so may be an indication for a repeat renal biopsy.

Segmental and diffuse proliferative LGN (class III and IV lesions)

Patients with class III and IV lesions constitute the majority requiring treatment. Therapy is urgent and admission is usually required. Prednisolone 50 mg daily is begun, together with azathioprine as discussed above. Serum creatinine or clearance has to be measured twice weekly – if there is impairment in function, some would give three daily 0.5 g doses of intravenous methylprednisolone (reducing oral prednisolone temporarily at this stage), while other physicians would recommend 500 mg doses of intravenous cyclophosphamide monthly for 3 months. Evidence is available that cyclophosphamide is the better drug in this cricumstance, but its use in young women is difficult.

The above strategies are usually adequate to maintain and regain GFR but, if unsuccessful, plasmaphaeresis may have a role by removing mediators of immune inflammation, although this treatment is controversial and expensive and requires very highly trained nursing staff.

Prednisolone is maintained at 50 mg daily for 2 or more months, tapered slowly and eventually given on alternate days. Steroid side-effects are an inevitable consequence of the treatment of what may be a life-threatening illness. Azathioprine is maintained for the duration of steroid therapy.

Diffuse proliferative LGN with crescents

Patients with diffuse proliferative LGN with crescents are infrequent, even in large renal centres. The clinical picture is that of rapidly progressive glomerulonephritis and detailed management is discussed in Chapter 11, p. 176.

Diffuse membranous LGN (class V)

In the pure form, class V LGN is an adynamic nephritis: low-dose prednisolone alone for 24 months is sufficient in many, provided GFR is unimpaired. For those with impaired GFR or if mixed membranous and other LGN histologies are present, more potent therapy is required.

Advanced sclerosing LGN (class VI)

There is little hope of treatment improving renal function in patients with class VI LGN. Treatment is only required if there are extrarenal features of SLE. In many patients with lupus, serology often becomes negative without treatment as uraemia advances. An explanation is awaited.

Duration of therapy

The duration of therapy is controversial but in general terms it is proportional to the severity of the initial renal histology and the ease with which it has been possible to control immune inflammation and hence maintain GFR. Before therapy is withdrawn, urine sediment should be normal, proteinuria about or less than 0.5 g/L and lupus serology negative.

For a mild class II LGN, 2 years of treatment should suffice, provided that the above criteria are fulfilled. Treatment is gradually withdrawn over a 3-month period, during which time clinical observation and the ESR are the main indicators of inactive disease. After treatment has been stopped, long-term follow-up is required, closely for the first 2 years and then less frequently for the next 5 years. With this cautious approach, it should be possible to detect relapse early.

Patients with classes III and IV LGN require much more prolonged treatment – 3–5 years. Some renal physicians repeat the renal biopsy before discontinuing drugs. The approach to withdrawing treatment is the same as described above in terms of urine sediment and lupus serology, but there is likely to be a persistent proteinuria of 2–3 g/L (reflecting scarred glomeruli, not necessarily active disease), which may elevate an ESR and make it unreliable. If the renal biopsy shows healing and little or no active inflammation, this is useful evidence which is used to reduce or withdraw therapy. Unfortunately, in a varying proportion the second tissue sample appears as severe as the first; in this circumstance therapy has to be continued and perhaps augmented.

Membranous lupus nephritis (class V) is treated in a similar manner to that of a class II nephritis, and partial remission of the nephrotic state is usually achieved.

Pregnancy and lupus nephritis

The majority of patients with LGN are of child-bearing years and the majority have unimpaired fertility. About 50% of these women will require cytotoxic therapy and, because LGN may be exacerbated by pregnancy, each patient should be advised that cyesis should be avoided during the years of treatment. Pregnancy in SLE is discussed more fully on p. 274.

Prognosis of lupus nephritis

Discussion regarding the prognosis of lupus nephritis will be restricted to LGN and will make no reference to extrarenal lupus. Only general statements can be made: treatment is often adapted to be the least inconvenient for the specific woman, which makes systematic analysis very difficult; it is held that prognosis is continually improving; in addition, one morphology may transform to another (usually to a more severe variety).

As expected, heavy proteinuria, persistent complement consumption and florid glomerular inflammation, particularly if fibrinoid necrosis and crescents are present, indicate a greater likelihood for progression into renal failure, but exceptions occur.

For patients with class II changes, at least an 80% 5-year survival is to be expected. Those women with segmental and focal changes (class III) fare less well, having perhaps 60–70% 5-year survival. The majority of therapeutic failures require dialysis or die in renal failure. The remaining patients die of lupus cerebritis or as a consequence, direct or indirect, of steroid or cytotoxic therapy or both. The diffuse proliferative nephritides of LGN (class IV) have a 5-year survival of 50–60% and it appears that prognosis is related to correct management in the first 2 months of therapy. Hypertension, cerebritis, atherosclerosis and infection are common causes for death in this subgroup. Nevertheless, it is in these patients that prognosis appears to be improving – some groups have reported an 80% and 60% survival at 5 and 10 years, respectively. The clinical course of lupus membranous nephritis (class V) is similar to that of the idiopathic variety, with about an 80% 5-year survival, except for those who transform to class III or IV morphologies.

Nephritis of Henoch–Schönlein purpura

Nephritis of HSP is common in childhood but is an unusual adult nephritis. Children develop skin and joint involvement, some with abdominal pain and a much small number with nephritis. Adults may present in the manner typical of children but the majority do not develop a rash or joint or abdominal features. Haematuria, gross or microscopic, proteinuria and, in some, progressive renal failure are the major events. There is a characteristic histological appearance in HSP. Where IgA deposition is present, a number of other conditions should be considered, as shown in Table 10.6. Usually the differential diagnosis is straightforward.

Table 10.6 A brief classification of nephropathies associated with IgA

Primary
IgA nephropathy (Berger's disease)
Secondary
Henoch–Schönlein purpura
Alcoholic liver disease
Coeliac disease
Dermatitis herpetiformis
Ankylosing spondylitis

Histology

The mesangium is chiefly involved, with varying degrees of hypercellularity, similar to IgAN. In adults, there is a greater chance of capillary thromboses or crescents, or both, developing than in children. Immunoperoxidase studies demonstrate widespread mesangial IgA deposition and, to a lesser extent, IgG or IgM.

Course and therapy

No adequate series of HSP in adults has been published. Further, because the course is indolent and insidiously progressive, the long-term benefit of treatment will be difficult to establish.

Probably the majority of adults with HSP will receive prednisolone and perhaps cytotoxic drugs, despite lack of evidence by which to gauge therapy. Treatment should be withheld if there is no loss of GFR. Conversely, loss of renal function and persistent nephrotic state are the principal indications for therapy, the correct nature and duration of which are unknown.

Nephritis of subacute bacterial endocarditis

Although classical subacute bacterial endocarditis (SBE) arising upon a rheumatic valve is now most uncommon, endocarditis or bacterial colonization of prosthetic inserts is not infrequent in the following circumstances:

1 Infection of valves previously distorted by earlier disease.

2 Infection of prosthetic valves.

3 Subacute bacterial endocarditis upon the tricuspid valve in intravenous drug addicts.

4 Infected ventriculoatrial shunts.

5 Infected intra-arterial or intravenous lines.

6 Visceral infections.

In each case, bacteria replicate within the bloodstream and hence bacterial antigen is available to make immune complexes. The varying ages of the above group of patients, the detailed clinical features and the differing bacteriology will not be discussed.

It is not clear what percentage of SBE or comparably infected patients develop renal involvement but this nephritis appears to develop in those who:

1 present late for treatment or are inadequately treated;
2 have fastidious or antibiotic-resistant bacteria.

Presentation is in the following ways:

1 As SBE but with haematuria, proteinuria or renal impairment.
2 As an unexplained systemic illness with renal involvement.

In any patient who is being treated for systemic infection, if renal function declines or does not improve, he/she should be considered to have SBE nephritis.

Laboratory findings

Anaemia is common, usually there is no leucocytosis, the ESR is raised and often the rheumatoid factor is elevated for the duration of the nephritis. A mixed cryoglobulinaemia has been reported in both SBE and 'shunt' nephritides. Complement is activated by the classical pathway in about 80% of patients; thus CH50, C4 and C3 are all reduced in activity. In practice, only an assay for C3 need be requested: if reduced, sequential measurement may be used for monitoring immune activity.

Histology

A diffuse cellular proliferation is the most common change; this includes polymorphs, macrophages and foci of necrosis. Crescents may form. IgG, IgM and C3 are to be expected. Less commonly, focal changes in a minority of glomeruli may be found. There is much overlap between the renal histology of SBE and that of acute bacterial endocarditis.

Course and therapy

It is usually possible to gain control and subsequently to eradicate both infection and nephritis by antibiotic therapy, but not always. Urinary abnormalities and reduced GFR may persist for months or more after successful antimicrobial treatment and thus are not necessarily measures of adequate therapy. Signs of a healing SBE nephritis during the course of antibiotics are a fall, if initially elevated, in the concentration of serum creatinine, and a rise in C3 activity. Rheumatoid factor, if present initially, usually becomes undetectable in serum, although this may be delayed until after hypocomplementaemia has departed.

It is usually straightforward to be sure of clinical success on the basis of clinical and laboratory observations. If a prosthesis has become infected, infection may be ineradicable until it has been replaced. Thus, valve or shunt replacement is not an uncommon procedure, once the bloodstream has been made sterile. Likewise, native heart valves may need to be replaced if they cannot be sterilized or if they are haemodynamically inefficient. After any of the above complex procedures are performed, there is usually a considerable improvement in health and GFR.

Human immunodeficiency virus-associated nephropathy (acquired immune deficiency syndrome nephropathy)

The most common morphology in human immunodeficiency virus (HIV)-associated nephropathy is an FSGS, although other immune-complex nephritides have been described. The nephropathy is most frequently seen in New York and Miami, is rare in San Francisco and is almost unknown in Britain.

In Africa a wide range of different glomerular morphologies occur in HIV-positive patients. This is briefly discussed in Chapter 22, p. 333.

Histology

There are three features leading to a fairly characteristic morphology:

1 Focal and segmental glomerulosclerosis lesions at all stages of evolution.

2 Mild tubular necrosis with mitotic figures indicating regenerating tubular epithelium.

3 Pale-staining tubular casts, which may be present in all segments of the nephron.

IgM, C3 and C1q are present in the sclerotic glomerular lesions (as in idiopathic FSGS).

Glomerular lesions observed in post-mortem material show progression from those in material obtained at renal biopsy a few weeks previously.

Course

Patients with HIV-associated nephropathy rapidly deteriorate to irreversible uraemia over a 4–16 week period. There is no treatment.

Anti-glomerular basement membrane nephritis/disease

The three essential features of anti-GBM nephritis – very rare but widely quoted systemic condition – are:

1 Pulmonary haemorrhage.

2 Nephritis.

3 Raised titres of circulating anti-GBM antibody.

The first two vary in severity; the third is diagnostic.

Lung haemorrhage and renal abnormalities *per se* coexist in a

Table 10.7 Conditions in which lung haemorrhage co-exists with renal features, including haematuria

Congestive heart failure with renal failure
SLE
Systemic vasculitis
Wegener's granulomatosis
Legionnaire's disease
Renal vein thrombosis with pulmonary embolism
Henoch–Schönlein purpura
Scleroderma
Anti-GBM disease

Some conditions are common, others infrequent. Anti-GBM nephritis is the least common.

number of conditions, as shown in Table 10.7. Some are straightforward diagnoses; others cannot be differentiated from each other without serology and renal biopsy.

Anti-GBM nephritis is most likely to be confused with a systemic vasculitis affecting kidney and lungs or with an RPGN (p. 172) because in all three there may be rapid reduction in GFR, recurrent macroscopic haematuria and recurrent haemoptysis or more prominent haemorrhage from the lungs. In anti-GBM nephritis, loss of GFR may be dramatically rapid: irreversible renal failure has been described 10 days after the first haemoptysis. Because very satisfactory treatment is available and because of the dynamic features of the nephritis, if anti-GBM disease is considered a diagnostic possibility, serum should be sent urgently to a regional centre for assay for anti-GBM antibody.

Histology

Light microscopy is not diagnostic: there is a crescentic glomerulonephritis, as in many patients with rapidly progressive glomerular lesions. Immunoperoxidase or immunofluorescence studies make the histological diagnosis because there is a continuous linear deposit of IgG on glomerular capillary walls.

Course and therapy

Once a raised titre of anti-GBM antibodies is found, the patient must be urgently referred to a renal unit. There, plasmaphaeresis and immunosuppression will be performed until the titre of anti-GBM antibodies falls.

Prognosis

The prognosis is directly related to the institution of therapy. If patients are referred late and oliguria has developed, the chance is

Table 10.8 Possible associations of primary glomerulonephritides and other conditions

Nephritis	Possible association
Minor glomerular abnormalities	Hodgkin's disease, lymphoma
Focal and segmental GN	Reflux nephropathy, heroin abuse
Membranous GN	Gold, penicillamine, NSAIDs, SLE, HBV infection, distant tumours, diabetes mellitus, syphilis
IgA nephropathy	Cirrhosis, HSP
Mesangiocapillary GN	Chronic bacterial infection, SLE, C3NF, complement component deficiency, partal lipodeficiency
Crescenteric GN	Chronic infection, polyarteritis nodosa, accelerated-phase hypertension

GN, Glomerulonephritis; HSP, Henoch–Schönlein purpura; C3NF, nephritic factor.

much reduced of a life independent of dialysis. Conversely, in those who receive treatment while still passing normal volumes of urine the outlook is favourable: life expectation is little reduced.

Conclusion

Many of the glomerulonephritides are primary conditions; other organs are involved in a secondary manner. Nevertheless, there are associations with other diseases, infections and drugs. Some of these have been mentioned in this chapter but Table 10.8 is a short summary of these associations.

Further reading

1 Adu, D., Howie, A.J., Scott, D.G.I. *et al.* (1987) Polyarteritis nodosa and the kidney. *Quart. J. Med.* **62**, 221–38.
2 Cameron, J.S. (1992) Membranous nephropathy – still a treatment dilemma. *N. Engl. J. Med.* **327**, 638–9.
3 Churg, J. (1991) Nomenclature of vasculitic syndromes. *Am. J. Kidney Dis.* **18**, 148–53.
4 Correia, P., Cameron, J.S., Lilian, J.D. & Hicks, D. (1985) Why do patients with lupus nephritis die? *Br. Med. J.* **290**, 126–31.
5 D'Amico, G. & Ferrario, F. (1992) Mesangiocapillary glomerulonephritis. *J. Am. Soc. Nephrol.* **2**, S159–S166.
6 Davidson, A.M., Cameron, J.S. & Kerr, D.N.S. (1984) Natural history of renal function in untreated idiopathic membranous glomerulonephritis in adults. *Clin. Nephrol.* **22**, 61–7.
7 D'Cruz, D. & Hughes, G. (1992) Systemic vasculitis. *Br. Med. J.* **304**, 269–70.
8 Donadio, J.V. & Glassock, R.T. (1993) Immunosuppressive drug therapy in lupus nephritis. *Am. J. Kidney Dis.* **21**, 239–50.
9 Glassock, R.J., Adler, S.G., Ward, H.J. & Cohen, A.H. (1991) Primary glomerular

diseases. In Brenner, B.M. & Rector, F.C. (eds), *The Kidney*, 4th edn. W.B. Saunders, Philadelphia, pp. 1182–279.

10 Glassock, R.J., Cohen, A.H., Adler, S.G. & Ward, H.J. (1991) Secondary glomerular diseases. In Brenner, B.M. & Rector, F.C. (eds), *The Kidney*, 4th edn. W.B. Saunders, Philadelphia, pp. 1280–368.

11 Goldstein, A.R., White, R.H., Akuse, R. & Chantler, C. (1992) Long-term follow-up of childhood Henoch–Schönlein nephritis. *Lancet* **339**, 280–2.

12 Jennette, J.C. & Falk, R.J. (1991) Diagnostic classification of anti-neutrophil autoantibody-associated vasculitides. *Am. J. Kidney Dis.* **18**, 184–7.

13 Kayson, G.A. (1992) Nutritional management of nephrotic syndrome. *J. Renal Nutrition* **2**, 50–8.

14 Keane, W.F. & Kasiske, B.L. (1990) Hyperlipidaemia in the nephrotic syndrome. *N. Engl. J. Med.* **323**, 603–4.

15 Kobet, S.M. & Schwartz, M.M. (1992) HIV infection and the nephrotic syndrome. *Am. J. Kidney Dis.* **20**, 97–103.

16 Lockshin, M.D. (1991) Therapy for systemic lupus erythematosus. *N. Engl. J. Med.* **324**, 189–91.

17 Meyrier, A. (1990) Treatment of glomerular disease with cyclosporin. *Nephrol. Dial. Transplant.* **4**, 923–31.

18 Olivero, J.J., Frommer, J.P. & Gonzalez, J.M. (1993) Medical nephrectomy: the last resort for intractable complications of the nephrotic syndrome. *Am. J. Kidney Dis.* **21**, 260–3.

19 Pettersson, E. & Heigl, Z. (1992) Antineutrophil cytoplasmic antibody (cANCA and pANCA) titres in relation to disease activity in patients with necrotizing vasculitis: a longitudinal study. *Clin. Nephrol.* **37**, 219–28.

20 Popović-Rolović, M., Kostic, M., Antic-Peco, A., Jovanovic, O. & Popovic, D. (1991) Medium and longterm follow up of patients with acute post-streptococcal glomerulonephritis. *Nephron* **58**, 393–9.

21 Raine, A.E.G. (1991) Renal biopsy and the prognosis of lupus nephritis. *Quart. J. Med.* **81**, 879–82.

Chapter 11
Rapidly Progressive Renal Failure

Guy Neild

Rapidly progressive renal failure (RPRF) is an emergency. The diagnosis should be made within 24 hours of presentation. Immediate treatment of a crescentic glomerulonephritis may mean the difference between recovery of adequate renal function, chronic dialysis and death.

Rapidly progressive renal failure develops over days or weeks, rather than months, in previously normal kidneys. In a patient with renal insufficiency, with no relevant past history, it must first be established whether there is acute renal failure (ARF), chronic renal failure (CRF) or acute-on-chronic renal failure. There is a distinction between ARF due to a sudden insult and kidney diseases of short duration leading to RPRF. The onset, presentation and management of RPRF are quite different from those of ARF. Commonly, RPRF is misdiagnosed as CRF and the tempo of the illness, together with the therapeutic implications, is not appreciated by the unwary. For the above reasons, RPRF is discussed separately from ARF because the differences between the two conditions are greater than the similarities.

Causes of renal failure may be divided into three pathophysiological groups:

1 Vascular or 'prerenal'.
2 Urinary obstruction.
3 Parenchymal injury.

Presenting symptoms, signs and biochemical investigations of ARF are described in Chapter 16, p. 230. Obstructive nephropathy is discussed on pp. 17 and 116. This chapter will concentrate on inflammatory parenchymal renal injury.

Diagnosis of acute renal parenchymal injury

In renal failure, if renal perfusion is adequate and urine flow not obstructed, there is parenchymal disease affecting either glomeruli, tubules, interstitium or blood-vessels. When the patient presents for the first time, a diagnosis of ARF, CRF or acute-on-chronic renal failure must be made. If the kidneys are of normal size, the condition is probably acute.

Initial approach to rapidly progressive renal failure

There is no uniform clinical picture of patients presenting with RPRF, as will be appreciated by reading the lists of causes in Tables 11.1–11.4. The conditions are not common, so few physicians have experience in diagnosis of RPRF. A general approach to a patient suspected of having RFRF includes:

1 Not accepting a single raised blood urea or creatinine concentration as being indicative of CRF. At presentation, patients with RPRF almost invariably have some degree of renal failure.
2 Taking a careful drug history (see Table 11.3).
3 Measuring the blood-pressure and assessing the patient for atheroma (see Table 11.2).
4 Examining the skin: the butterfly rash of lupus, the vasculitic lesions of fingers and nails, the facies of scleroderma.
5 Microscopy of urine: an abnormal sediment will invariably be present.
6 A blood film should be scanned for fragmented erythrocytes: a major clue in the diagnosis of haemolytic uraemic syndrome (HUS) and thrombotic thrombocytopenic purpura (TTP).
7 An urgent ultrasound assessment of the renal tract: in most cases the

Table 11.1 Common causes of rapidly progressive renal failure

Non-glomerulonephritic
Haemolytic uraemic syndrome
Acute interstitial nephritis
Accelerated-phase hypertension
Primary glomerulonephritic
Idiopathic crescenteric glomerulonephritis
Secondary glomerulonephritides
Microscopic polyarteritis nodosa
Lupus nephritis

kidneys will be of normal size or enlarged. In addition, this investigation will exclude an obstructive uropathy.

8 The patient should be admitted to hospital without delay. It is not unusual for the creatinine concentration to have risen by 50–100 μmol/L over 24–48 hours. If this is found, it is essential that the patient be referred to a renal unit that day (see Fig. 1.2, p. 6).

The commonest causes of RPRF are listed in Table 11.1.

Clinical signs and symptoms of rapidly progressive renal failure

Pain

Constant renal or loin pain is an unusual renal symptom. It may occur when the kidney is acutely swollen – usually with acute pyelonephritis or acute interstitial nephritis, much less commonly with acute tubular necrosis (ATN) or acute glomerulonephritis. It may also occur when segmental infarction of the kidney extends to involve the renal capsule.

Urine volume

Anuria strongly suggests obstruction. Nevertheless, it may very rarely occur with severe glomerular disease such as anti-glomerular basement membrane (GBM) antibody-mediated nephritis. Oliguria is not diagnostic in RPRF, but normal or increased volumes of urine in the presence of severe renal dysfunction (serum creatinine >1000 μmol/L) suggest tubular rather than glomerular disease. A history of nocturia may give a guide as to the duration of renal dysfunction.

Haematuria

Macroscopic haematuria in RPRF suggests pathology of the outflow tract but may occur with glomerulonephritis. Often, in severe crescentic glomerulonephritis there is sufficient haematuria to discolour the urine but it is not recognized as blood by the patient. Descriptions such as smoky, rusty, cold tea or even blackcurrant juice may be used.

Oedema

Peripheral oedema may be due to salt and water retention or to hypoalbuminaemia. The former will be associated with signs and symptoms of fluid overload, such as pulmonary oedema, raised central venous pressure and added heart sounds. Oedema occurring as a prominent early feature of RPRF suggests glomerular pathology.

Acute nephritis or acute nephritic syndrome was common and seen typically in children with poststreptococcal glomerulonephritis. This condition is now very uncommon in Western Europe.

Laboratory diagnosis

Particular features of individual causes of RPRF are described in the relevant sections. General features are discussed first.

It must be emphasized that careful examination of the urine is important. Urine should be microscoped and cultured and its osmolality and concentration of sodium measured.

Microscopy

Prominent microscopic haematuria (many red cells per high-power field in unspun urine) is always found in acute crescentic glomerulonephritis. Red cell casts confirm glomerular bleeding. With phase-contrast microscopy, red cell morphology can be examined and dysmorphic red cells of glomerular origin may be seen. Red cells all of normal morphology indicate bleeding in the collecting system.

Prominent, sterile leucocyturia (more than 100 cells per mm^3 of unspun urine) suggests an interstitial nephritis.

Proteinuria

Proteinuria greater than 3 g/L usually indicates glomerular pathology. However, proteinuria of 10 g/day may occur with acute allergic interstital nephritis. Proteinuria less than 1 g/day together with absence of cells in the urine suggests outflow obstruction.

Urea and electrolytes

In ARF simultaneous measurement of urea and sodium concentrations in urine may help to distinguish between prerenal and established renal failure. Urinary sodium concentrations are difficult to interpret following diuretic therapy. Biochemical investigation of urine in early ARF is discussed on p. 237.

Vascular causes of rapidly progressive renal failure

Pathological conditions leading to obstruction of the major vessels of the kidney are shown in Table 11.2. Renal failure is often acute and the extrarenal symptoms dramatic. Clinical examination and routine investigations normally indicate the diagnosis. Sometimes the onset of renal failure may be more insidious.

Atheromatous or cholesterol emboli

Cholesterol embolization is a rare complication of severe atheromatous involvement of the aorta, typically affecting men over 60 years of age. It usually follows a surgical procedure, trauma or catheterization, but may occur spontaneously. There may be evidence of systemic

Table 11.2 Vascular causes of rapidly progressive renal failure

Renal artery and large intrarenal branches
Aortic dissection
Atheroma
Stenosis
Thrombosis
Embolus
Cholesterol
Atheroma
Thrombus
Arteritis
Polyarteritis nodosa
Giant-cell arteritis
Takayasu's arteritis
Small arteries and arterioles
Accelerated hypertension
Arteritis
Scleroderma
Haemolytic uraemic syndrome

embolization with skin infarcts, livedo reticularis, retinal artery emboli and central nervous system (CNS) involvement. Eosinophilia and hypocomplementaemia are said to be common. Anticoagulants do not help: it has been suggested that they may precipitate the condition.

Renal artery stenosis

Severe bilateral renal artery stenosis leads to a slow decline in renal function. Sudden deterioration may be due to complete occlusion of an artery. When the blood-supply is precarious, the kidney is particularly vulnerable to other nephrotoxic or ischaemic insults, and renal function may decline when blood-pressure is reduced, diuretics are increased (accentuating prerenal failure) or angiotensin-converting enzyme inhibitors are used.

Accelerated (malignant) hypertension

Diastolic pressures of 120 mmHg or higher may sometimes be tolerated for several years without symptoms. Transformation to an accelerated phase leads rapidly to renal failure. Diastolic blood-pressures of 130 mmHg or higher are associated with retinal haemorrhages and exudates or papilloedema. Untreated, mortality is 80% at 1 year.

Accelerated hypertension is commonest in the fourth decade. It is both more frequent and occurs earlier in Blacks. There is usually a preceding history of hypertension. As well as rapidly deteriorating renal function, there is microscopic haematuria with proteinuria, usually less than 5 g/day. The reason for the rapid rise in blood-pressure is unknown.

In man and experimental models, severe hypertension is often associated with a natriuresis leading to salt depletion and weight loss. In some patients, hypertensive encephalopathy or cardiac failure occurs. Microangiopathic haemolytic anaemia and thrombocytopenia may develop.

Long-term management requires complete control of blood-pressure but the pressure should not be reduced abruptly. Steady control over the first 48 hours can usually be obtained by gradual introduction of β-blockers and calcium antagonists. Subsequently, more potent agents may be necessary. This important therapeutic area is fully discussed on p. 222.

Arteritis

Vasculitis of the smaller branches and glomeruli is discussed below. Acute polyarteritis nodosa may affect the main renal arteries as part of a life-threatening, systemic arteritis, also affecting other splanchnic organs.

Giant-cell arteritis, associated with cranial arteritis, very rarely involves main renal arteries.

Aortitis, such as Takayasu's arteritis, may involve the renal arteries, leading to a subacute or chronic renal artery stenosis.

Scleroderma

Renal failure is a major cause of death in systemic sclerosis. Proteinuria and hypertension are common. The classical type of renal involvement in systemic sclerosis is characterized by the abrupt onset of severe hypertension with RPRF or ARF, which may be associated with cardiac failure and convulsions. Thrombocytopenia and haemolytic anaemia with fragmented red cells (microangiopathic haemolytic anaemia) are common.

Although most patients have a history of systemic sclerosis, renal failure may be the presenting feature and may occur in the absence of detectable skin changes. This presentation may be indistinguishable from HUS.

There is no specific treatment. Hypertension should be controlled. There is increasing evidence that angiotensin-converting enzyme inhibitors may be the drug of choice and that they may even reduce renal injury. If thrombocytopenia and haemolysis are prominent, treatment as for HUS may be tried (see below).

Haemolytic uraemic syndrome and thrombotic thrombocytopenic purpura

Haemolytic uraemic syndrome is not a single disease entity. It is characterized by:

1 Sudden onset of renal failure.

2 Thrombocytopenia.
3 Microangiopathic haemolytic anaemia.

Typically it occurs as an acute and often epidemic illness, with a diarrhoeal prodrome in infants and young children. This has recently been shown to be frequently associated with gut infection by *Escherichia coli*, which produce verotoxin. In this form, there is acute renal failure, glomerular thrombosis and severe endothelial damage. The natural history is one of spontaneous 'recovery', but anuria or the absence of diarrhoea or both are adverse features.

A sporadic form of HUS may affect older children and adults, developing insidiously following a respiratory or other viral infection. The sporadic form in children may follow a relapsing course and is sometimes familial.

Clinical presentation is varied and the diagnosis is often not suspected until thrombocytopenia or anaemia with fragmented red cells is noted. Frequently, patients present relatively late in the disease with oliguria and severe or accelerated-phase hypertension. By this time, there is irreversible vascular pathology. In adults, renal biopsy is often necessary to establish the diagnosis and to determine the potential degree of reversibility.

Thrombocytopenia is only detected in 50% of patients. Anaemia may be mild and fragmented red cells may be few and mistaken for the burr cells of uraemia. Associated with red cell haemolysis, serum lactate dehydrogenase concentrations are raised and haptoglobin may be reduced. With severe haemolysis, bilirubin is raised. Coombs' test is negative. The prothrombin and kaolin clotting times are normal although the thrombin time may be slightly prolonged.

In the closely related syndrome of TTP, similar vascular injury occurs simultaneously in many organs, and associated haematological findings are correspondingly more severe. Thrombotic thrombocytopenic purpura is a multisystem disease characterized by fever, fluctuating CNS abnormalities, renal failure, microangiopathic haemolytic anaemia and thrombocytopenia. Bacterial sepsis should always be suspected as the primary diagnosis when thrombocytopenia occurs with prolongation of clotting times. Fragmented red cells may also occur, with septicaemia.

Treatment

In addition to the standard management of severe anaemia and renal failure, several treatments may be tried to inhibit the vascular injury. Fresh frozen plasma (FFP) has been given with considerable success. Plasma exchange may not have any special advantages, except that in oliguric patients it may be the only way of infusing sufficient FFP without fluid overload. Intravenous prostacyclin may produce vasodilatation in the renal vasculature.

Failure to respond to prostacyclin may represent vascular injury too advanced to expect recovery. 'Antiplatelet' drugs have not been shown to be of benefit, but this may reflect timing of treatment. Dipyridamole may potentiate the action of prostacyclin and could be used in combination. Anticoagulants have not been shown to be of benefit.

Urinary obstruction causes of rapidly progressive renal failure

Anuria strongly suggests the presence of obstruction but obstruction does not necessarily cause anuria or oliguria. It is ill appreciated that kidneys may be incompletely obstructed, causing severe renal insufficiency with polyuria. Obstruction can never be excluded until a definitive examination, such as ultrasound, has been performed (see p. 69).

Complete obstruction to one ureter and irreversible loss of that kidney may occur insidiously and painlessly.

Insidious obstruction leading to bilateral hydronephrosis and renal failure is usually due to bladder outflow obstruction, tumour involvement of ureteric orifices or retroperitoneal disease causing extrinsic compression of ureters. These topics are discussed in Chapter 2, p. 12.

Renal parenchymal causes of rapidly progressive renal failure

Tubulointerstitial disease

Recognized causes of ARF due to tubular injury are shown in Table 11.3. Not infrequently, the cause of ATN is never found.

Acute interstitial nephritis may present as RPRF or ARF.

Acute pyelonephritis

Acute interstitial nephritis, with severe diffuse infiltration with neutrophils and microabscesses, is caused by septicaemic spread and occasionally by ascending urinary tract infection. Pyuria and proteinuria (2–3 g/L) occur. There may be widespread and irreversible parenchymal destruction.

Acute allergic interstitial nephritis

Acute allergic interstitial nephritis appears 2 days to 5 weeks (mean 15 days) after administration of the 'causal' drug. A large number of drugs have been incriminated but the most common are the penicillins, rifampicin and nonsteroidal anti-inflammatory agents. Fever (39–40 °C) occurs in most cases and is accompanied by a maculopapular rash in 25% of patients. Arthralgia is less common. Loin pain may be severe and unilateral. Oliguria occurs in 20–50% and some degree of renal insufficiency in 60%.

There is a sterile pyuria, rarely with an eosinophiluria. Haematuria is

Table 11.3 Tubulointerstitial conditions which may present with severe renal insufficiency and normal-sized kidneys

TUBULAR TOXINS	
Chemicals	Paraquat Organic solvents, e.g. carbon tetrachloride Glycols, e.g. ethylene glycol Haemolytic agents, e.g. sodium chlorate
Drugs	Tetracycline Aminoglycosides
Elements	Calcium Heavy metals, e.g. mercury
Foodstuffs	*Cortinarius* mushrooms
TUBULAR OBSTRUCTION	
Casts	Myeloma
Crystals	Urate, sulphonamides
TUBULOINTERSTITIAL DISEASE	
Acute	
Allergic interstitial nephritis	Ampicillin, NSAIDs
Infections	Pyelonephritis Legionnaire's disease Leptospirosis Viral haemorrhagic fevers
Autoimmune interstitial nephritis	
Chronic	
Infections	Malacoplakia Tuberculosis
Infiltrates	Lymphoma Leukaemia

common and may be macroscopic. Proteinuria up to 3 g/L is present in 75%; rarely proteinuria is greater and leads to nephrotic syndrome. A transient eosinophilia occurs in 80%. IgE concentration is raised in half the cases. Ultrasound examination demonstrates two normal or large kidneys. Urinary electrolytes are usually those typical of ATN (see also p. 237).

Acute interstitial nephritis and systemic infections

When an interstitial nephritis is secondary to systemic disease, the symptoms of the underlying disease predominate. Legionnaire's disease may be associated with acute renal dysfunction and should always be suspected when ARF complicates pneumonia. Leptospirosis should be suspected when there is hepatitis with jaundice.

A number of 'tropical' viruses cause a syndrome of a febrile illness with shock, haemorrhage and renal failure. The Hantaan virus is a major cause of this syndrome in Asia (Korean haemorrhagic fever). An attenuated form of this virus is now prevalent in Western Europe and causes ARF.

Acute idiopathic interstitial nephritis

In acute idiopathic interstitial nephritis, there is typically a 2-week prodrome with myalgia, anorexia and malaise. It may be associated with uveitis and granulomata in bone marrow and lymph nodes.

Treatment and outcome

Following withdrawal of the initiating drug or resolution of the precipitating infection, recovery can be expected in the majority. Poor outcome has been associated with older age at onset, the severity of interstitial infiltrate and duration of oliguria for more than 3 weeks.

Although there have been no controlled studies, early use of high-dose oral steroids appears to be associated with more rapid and total recovery than that in untreated patients. When the damage, judged histologically, appears acute and reversible, it would be apropriate to treat aggressively with a short, tapering course of oral prednisolone, starting at 60 mg/day, lasting 6–8 weeks.

Chronic interstitial nephritis

Chronic interstitial nephritis may, rarely, present as an acute illness. The kidneys may be of normal size, or irregular and enlarged when chronic infection occurs with renal stones and obstruction. In this setting, the rare conditions of xanthogranulomatous pyelonephritis or malacoplakia may be found.

Glomerular disease

Rapidly progressive glomerulonephritis including renal vasculitis

Rapidly progressive renal failure due to glomerular disease is a very important condition. Delay in diagnosis and treatment has serious consequences. The term rapidly progressive glomerulonephritis has been used to describe a rare syndrome characterized:

1 clinically by an acute nephritic syndrome with the rapid development of renal failure; and

2 pathologically by a severe glomerulonephritis with crescents ('extracapillary proliferation').

Glomerulonephritis with crescents may occur with many forms of primary glomerulonephritis and is also associated with various systemic diseases (Table 11.4). The most important of these is polyarteritis.

Table 11.4 Causes of rapidly progressive glomerulonephritis with crescents

PRIMARY GLOMERULONEPHRITIS (NG)
Common forms of proliferative glomerulonephritis
Diffuse endocapillary GN
Mesangiocapillary GN (MCGN)
Idiopathic proliferative GN
Anti-glomerular basement membrane antibody GN
Rare forms of proliferative glomerulonephritis
Membranous GN
Mesangial IgA GN
Non-proliferative glomerulonephritis
Idiopathic necrotizing GN
SECONDARY GLOMERULONEPHRITIS
Systemic lupus erythematosus
Henoch–Schönlein purpura
Cryoglobulinaemia
Polyarteritis
Microscopic polyarteritis
Polyarteritis nodosa
Wegener's granulomatosis
Churg–Strauss arteritis

Vasculitis

Polyarteritis nodosa is a rare and severe disease, affecting predominantly the larger muscular arteries of splanchnic organs. At autopsy, vessel involvement may be visible with the naked eye. Systemic vasculitis, affecting smaller branches, is, in comparison, relatively common. The term 'microscopic' polyarteritis is used to describe an arteritis that is only detectable by light microscopy. When the kidneys are involved, there is typically a segmental inflammatory necrosis of the glomerulus (necrotizing glomerulonephritis) with crescents. An arteritis will only be seen in about 20% of biopsies. Immune deposits in glomeruli are not found. Many patients with rapidly progressive glomerulonephritis have a clinical illness suggestive of a vasculitis. In spite of these prodromal symptoms, necrotizing glomerulonephritis with crescents may be the sole histopathological manifestation of a microscopic polyarteritis.

Glomerulonephritis

Rapidly progressive renal failure may sometimes be due to severe, acute proliferative glomerulonephritis with few or no crescents, which may occur following infection, such as streptococcal infection, or with mesangiocapillary glomerulonephritis (MCGN) or systemic lupus erythematosus (SLE).

Irrespective of the precise diagnosis, patients can be broadly divided into two groups based on the morphology of the glomerular lesion:

1 Those with glomerular proliferation (capillary and mesangial cell proliferation showing diffuse deposits of immunoglobulins and complement).

2 Those with segmental glomerular necrosis (necrotizing glomerulonephritis) but without diffuse proliferation, immunoglobulins or complement – this is associated with systemic polyarteritis.

Clinical features

Patients with proliferative glomerulonephritis (Table 11.4) typically present with acute nephritis, usually preceded by mild flu-like symptoms. Macroscopic or heavy microscopic haematuria occurs with nephrotic syndrome in about half the cases.

In contrast, patients with necrotizing glomerulonephritis often have vague multisystem symptoms present for several weeks or months, suggestive of a systemic vasculitis. The renal disease often has a more insidious onset. Macroscopic haematuria is less common and nephrotic syndrome is very rare.

Complete accounts of the different forms of glomerulonephritis are given in Chapter 10, p. 134, but particular features related to RPRF are commented on below.

Diffuse endocapillary glomerulonephritis (postinfectious nephritis)

Classically acute nephritis follows a streptococcal infection. The glomerular lesion is a diffuse endocapillary proliferation with polymorph exudation into the glomerular tuft. Electron microscopy shows characteristic large subepithelial deposits called 'humps'; these contain IgG and C3. Acute nephritis following a streptococcal sore throat is now very rare in Britain. Poststreptococcal nephritis is seen in the Third World, sometimes associated with streptococcal skin infection.

Endocapillary nephritis may follow a pneumococcal or staphylococcal infection, but often the preceding pathogen is not identified. It may occur in association with bacterial endocarditis.

During the acute illness there is a transient fall in C4 and C3 activity. Recovery is spontaneous, even when there is oliguria with or without crescents.

Mesangiocapillary glomerulonephritis (mesangioproliferative glomerulonephritis)

Mesangiocapillary glomerulonephritis may be seen with certain systemic diseases, such as SLE, bacterial endocarditis, cryoglobulinaemia, visceral infections or shunt-nephritis. It is more usually idiopathic.

Occasionally, typical primary MCGN will present as acute nephritis, with or without crescents, leading to RPRF. More commonly, the diagnosis is known and acute deterioration in renal function follows an intercurrent illness.

Unlike other forms of proliferative glomerulonephritis with crescents, primary MCGN responds poorly or not at all to aggressive treatment.

Idiopathic glomerulonephritis

Not infrequently with crescentic nephritis, there is a diffuse proliferative glomerulonephritis which cannot be classified as one of the primary forms and for which no cause can be found. Often, at electron microscopy a mixture of subepithelial and subendothelial deposits is seen, or occasionally deposits may be absent. Complement activity may be transiently reduced. Immune complex disease appears to be the cause. This form of nephritis usually responds well to aggressive therapy, although cases may improve spontaneously.

Anti-glomerular basement membrane antibody disease

Anti-GBM antibody disease, which is associated with lung haemorrhage, was called Goodpasture's syndrome. This form of glomerulonephritis is becoming more common. It should be suspected when a previously fit person notices bloody or discoloured urine followed by severe oliguria or even anuria. In patients with severe oliguria, a biopsy will often show 100% infarction of glomeruli. When the diagnosis is suspected, serum should be sent immediately to the local reference laboratory for measurement of anti-GBM antibodies.

The glomeruli characteristically show linear IgG on the GBM but there may be such extensive glomerular damage that it is not seen. If the patient is already oliguric, treatment is unsuccessful and renal function does not recover. Treatment should be reserved for those with remaining renal function or with lung haemorrhage, particularly as, in elderly patients, treatment with plasmaphaeresis, cytotoxic drugs and steroids is potentially dangerous.

Lung haemorrhage should always be suspected if the haemoglobin is disproportionately low (less than 8 g/dl). In the absence of haemoptysis and radiological signs of alveolar haemorrhage, the partial pressure of oxygen ($P\text{O}_2$) and the carbon monoxide diffusion constant ($K\text{CO}$) should be measured serially.

Secondary forms of glomerulonephritis

Systemic lupus erythematosus

Rapidly progressive renal failure due to severe lupus nephritis is part of a severe systemic illness; the diagnosis is usually straightforward. Treatment (detailed below) should precede a renal biopsy so as to gain rapid control of the immune inflammation. Nevertheless, a renal biopsy is essential to assess the activity of the inflammation and to guide later stages of therapy.

The management of lupus nephritis is much more difficult when acute-on-chronic deterioration in function occurs, particularly in the absence of systemic disease activity. A biopsy is essential to assess the degree of activity and reversibility.

Occasionally other explanations may be found for deteriorating function, such as renal vein thrombosis or progression of disease to a frank polyarteritis.

Henoch–Schönlein purpura

Henoch–Schönlein purpura (HSP) may occasionally present as, or relapse into, an RPRF. Henoch–Schönlein purpura with crescents usually responds poorly to aggressive treatment, although treatment should be tried if the histology appears reversible. In an adult, HSP must always be assumed to be microscopic polyarteritis until proved otherwise. The presence of mesangial deposits with IgA favour the diagnosis of HSP.

Treatment and management of rapidly progressive glomerulonephritis

Rapidly progressive glomerulonephritis is a serious disease. Prompt and adequate treatment is essential. Few kidneys with necrotizing glomerulonephritis recover function once they become oliguric. Recovery is relatively common if the underlying lesion is a proliferative glomerulonephritis.

The aggressiveness of the treatment directed at the kidneys should match the histological severity of the disease. For severe crescentic disease, both steroids and an immunosuppressive drug are necessary. High-dose oral prednisolone should be given in an initial dose of about 60 mg/day (35 mg/m^2/day), together with either azathioprine or cyclophosphamide in a dose of 2–2.5 mg/kg/day. Azathioprine has the merit of being relatively safe in both the short and long term, with marrow suppression and other side-effects being unusual at this dose. Cyclophosphamide may be more efficacious in Wegener's granulomatosis.

Sometimes, this disease is not controlled by azathioprine but responds to cyclophosphamide. Cyclophosphamide is more toxic than azathioprine and may cause marrow suppression, alopecia and haemorrhagic cystitis. After 3 months, there is an increasing incidence of gonadal failure, and change to azathioprine is appropriate. During the acute phase of the disease, high-dose intravenous 'pulses' of methylprednisolone may be beneficial. It is likely that its action is principally anti-inflammatory. Usually 0.5–1 g is given on 3 consecutive days. If the disease is not controlled by these measures, plasmaphaeresis has been advocated. It is of particular value if the patient is already oliguric.

Without plasmaphaeresis, very few such patients have recovered renal function.

If oliguric patients show no sign of recovery after 3–4 weeks, immunosuppressive treatment should only be used for controlling extrarenal vasculitis. Combined immunosuppression and plasmaphaeresis are associated with mortality from infection. The prednisolone dose can usually be tapered over 2–3 months to 20 mg/day (12 mg/m^2/day). Over the next 2–3 months the does should be tapered more slowly to a maintenance dose of 10–15 mg/day. Side-effects, such as a cushingoid appearance or myopathy, may be reduced if the drug is given on alternate days. After 2 years of disease inactivity, an attempt can be made to wean the patient off the steroids and immunosuppressive drugs. If the disease is in complete remission, an earlier tapering or withdrawal of prednisolone can be tried.

Assessment of activity can be difficult, particularly when the kidneys are the prime or only site of disease. Measures of renal activity are changes in urine sediment proteinuria, in haematuria and in renal function. Glomerular filtration rate (GFR) must be monitored closely and accurately. Otherwise, apart from overt clinical signs of activity in other organs, sequential measurements of haemoglobin, erythrocyte sedimentation rate (ESR) and C-reactive protein are made, together with antinuclear factor (ANF), complement, antineutrophil-cytoplasmic antibodies (ANCA) and anti-GBM antibody, as appropriate. Some patients have a once-only disease and will remain in remission off treatment. Others will relapse and require further treatment, and a third group have a continuing disease which is controlled by immunosuppression.

Summary

Many of the conditions discussed in this chapter are uncommon but, if correctly diagnosed and treated, long-term dialysis may be avoided. It is most important, when assessing any new patient apparently with CRF but without an appropriate history, to consider whether he may have RPRF. Frequently these patients are misdiagnosed as CRF and the opportunity of treatment is lost. The concentration of serum creatinine or plasma urea is much less important than the rate of change in concentration.

Correct management involves early diagnosis, a renal biopsy, dialysis or haemofiltration if required, removal of any 'causal' drug and immunoregulatory therapy in many. It follows, therefore, that a patient with RPRF needs urgent referral to a physician with the necessary experience, equipment and nursing staff.

Further reading

1 Bennett, W.M., Elzinga, L.W. & Porter, G.A. (1991) Tubulointerstitial diseases. In Brenner, B.M. & Rector, F.C. (eds), *The Kidney*, 4th edn. W.B. Saunders, Philadelphia, pp. 1430–86.

2 Cameron, J.S. (1985) Glomerulonephritis. In Marsh, F.P. (ed.), *Postgraduate Nephrology*. Heinemann, London, pp. 237–95.
3 Cassidy, M.J., Gaskin, G., Savill, J., Pusey, C.D. & Rees, A.J. (1990) Towards a more rapid diagnosis of rapidly progressive glomerulonephritis. *Br. Med. J.* **301**, 329–31.
4 Glassock, R.J., Adler, S.G., Ward, H.J. & Cohen, A.H. (1991) Primary glomerular diseases (ch. 26) and secondary glomerular diseases (ch. 27). In Brenner, B.M. & Rector, F.C. (eds), *The Kidney*, 4th edn. W.B. Saunders, Philadelphia, pp. 1182–279 and 1280–368.
5 Ives, H.E. & Daniel, T.O. Vascular diseases of the kidney. In Brenner, B.M. & Rector, F.C. (eds), *The Kidney*, 4th edn. W.B. Saunders, Philadelphia, pp. 1497–550.
6 Neild, G.H. (1985) Renal vasculitis: a review. *J. Roy. Soc. Med.* **78**, 667–71.
7 Neild, G.H. & Williams, D.G. (1987) Polyarteritis and related syndromes. In Weatherall, D.J., Ledingham, J.G.G. & Warrell, D.A. (eds), *Oxford Textbook of Medicine*, 2nd edn. Oxford University Press, Oxford, p. 16.28.

Chapter 12
The Kidney in Systemic Diseases

Roger Gabriel

The kidney is susceptible to damage in the presence of many systemic diseases which are not renal conditions *per se*. In addition, renal involvement in myeloma and amyloid is not uncommon. The toxic nephropathies represent a renal response to a heterogeneous and wide range of drugs and chemicals. Examples of the above conditions are not infrequently seen in medical and surgical wards. This chapter outlines the main examples, except for renal involvement in diabetes mellitus, which is discussed in the next chapter, p. 190.

Acute interstitial nephritis

There are two main varieties of acute interstitial nephritis which present as acute renal failure (ARF) or subacute renal failure: acute allergic interstitial nephritis (often drug-related) and acute infective interstitial nephritis. The differentiation is important because treatment is quite different. The topics are discussed in Chapter 11, p. 163, tabulated in Table 11.3 (p. 171), and are also mentioned in Chapter 16, pp. 226 and 228.

Chronic tubulointerstitial nephritides

Chronic tubulointerstitial nephritides (CTIN) present as asymptomatic proteinuria or chronic renal failure (CRF), or both.

The major causes are shown in Table 12.1; the list is not exhaustive. At presentation, proteinuria of 1–3 g daily is found, with renal failure proportional to the degree of histological damage.

Table 12.1 Conditions which may cause chronic tubulointerstitial nephritis listed in approximate order of frequency of occurrence

1	Ischaemia secondary to long-standing hypertension
2	Lithium
3	Myeloma
4	Gout
5	Reflux nephropathy
6	Analgesic nephropathy
7	Sarcoid
8	Tuberculosis
9	Sickle-cell disease
10	Lymphoma or leukaemia
11	Medullary cystic disease
12	Sjögren's syndrome
13	Radiation nephritis

Biochemical investigations are straightforward, mainly involving measurements of clearance and proteinuria. Because renal tubules are involved, tubular dysfunction occurs in an undefined number of these patients. Where distal tubules or medulla or both are involved, apart from impairment in the ability to concentrate urine, sodium reabsorption may be less than adequate, which occasionally is of clinical importance. The resulting postural hypotension responds to oral sodium chloride replacement. Nevertheless, sodium-wasting states are infrequently met.

Histology

A wide range of changes may be found. There is an increase in volume due to interstitial fibrosis, which is accompanied by varying degrees of infiltration with chronic inflammatory cells. Associated tubular atrophy and degeneration is invariable. The lesions are patchy. Glomerular sclerosis, periglomerular fibrosis and atrophy may be found at presentation or develop as the lesions progress. Eventually, an end-stage kidney histology occurs which is indistinguishable from that of end-stage kidney disease due to other causes.

Occasionally, the cell infiltrate may be diagnostic or highly suggestive: the best examples are sarcoid, mycobacterial infection and, very occasionally, leukaemias or lymphomas. Nevertheless, in the majority of patients the cellular infiltrate is non-specific.

Intracellular crystals are seen in hyperuricaemia and cystinosis.

Tissue diagnosis

Many of the conditions listed in Table 12.1 can only be diagnosed by renal biopsy, but sampling of tissue is only essential if myeloma, sarcoid, tuberculous infection or infiltration by malignant tissue is suspected. Conversely, such diagnoses may only be considered in the light of the renal histology when investigating a patient with asymptomatic proteinuria or persistent renal impairment.

Specific investigations

Once a tissue diagnosis has been made, obvious investigations and the rate at which they need to be performed come to mind.

Lithium nephropathy presents with polyuria and polydipsia. A renal biopsy is not essential but histological confirmation is often of psychological benefit. Distinguishing organic symptoms due to the renal disorder from those of the primary psychiatric condition may be difficult. The working diagnosis is made not from measurement of clearance or serum lithium concentrations but by demonstrating that urine passed at 6.00 a.m. has a very similar osmolality to that passed at any other time of day – isosthenuria. Indeed, if psychiatrists regularly measured the osmolality of early-morning urine in patients taking lithium carbonate, it might be possible to avoid this nephropathy entirely by reducing the dosage of lithium when early loss of concentrating overnight urine first occurs.

Course and therapy

Because the CTIN (Table 12.1) represent a very heterogeneous group of conditions, generalizations regarding course and therapy are impossible, except that there is a strong possibility of progression to terminal renal failure and that hypertension occurs only when the disease process is advanced, in contrast to glomerular disease, where hypertension usually develops early.

The clinical course reflects the primary cause and the dimension and duration of the initiating event. From Table 12.1 it is clear that there is a wide range of rates of loss of renal function. Myeloma may cause terminal renal failure within months; conversely, lithium nephropathy may evolve over many years.

There is no restorative treatment available for patients with sickle-cell or medullary cystic disease or radiation nephritis. It is debatable whether long-standing hypertensive ischaemic renal damage can be ameliorated. Leukaemic infiltration of kidneys may perhaps respond to chemotherapy. Renal involvement in myeloma may be very refractory to treatment: this is discussed later (p. 184).

The other conditions related to CTIN are amenable to intervention. Analgesic and lithium nephropathies may respond well to withdrawing the causal agents and finding satisfactory substitutes. Chronic damage resulting from years of ingestion of non-steroidal anti-inflammatory drugs (NSAIDs) or mixtures of analgesics occurs in only a small minority of such people. Lesions are less likely to develop if a continuous water diuresis is maintained, presumably by washing out drug and metabolites from medulla and papillae.

Chronic tubulointerstitial nephritis develops in an unknown proportion of people with chronic hyperuricaemia. It is probable that long-term use of allopurinol will reduce the incidence of interstitial disease. Presumably, those with hyperuricaemia but with decreased urinary uric acid excretion who develop CTIN are those with persistent hyperacidity of their urine. Uric acid is substantially less soluble in acidic urine, which facilitates precipitation in the distal nephron. Crystals of urate excite a giant-cell reaction which is the beginning of the CTIN. Traditionally, a nocturnal dose of sodium bicarbonate has been used, but the efficacy is unproved.

Interstitial granulomas are infrequently found. It is held that they may be present in the kidneys in 30% of patients with sarcoid and very occasionally may be the only manifestation of this condition. In an unknown proportion, sarcoid granulomas may cause renal failure which responds to prednisolone therapy. The granulomas related to mycobacterial infection may be eradicated by antituberculous treatment but may leave residual fibrosis.

Renal amyloid

Renal amyloid is found in 5–10% of renal biopsies undertaken annually in a renal unit, the usual indications in these patients being asymptomatic proteinuria or nephrotic syndrome.

Amyloidosis represents a series of chronic infiltrative disorders characterized by extracellular deposits of insoluble fibrillar proteins. It was usual to classify amyloid into primary (heart, tongue, gut, peripheral nerves and skin deposition) and secondary varieties but these patterns are known to be inconsistent. Amyloid is now classified according to the type of fibril deposited, as judged by immunochemical staining. Such a classification is presented in Table 12.2. Only the AL and AA types are deposited in kidneys. About 80% of patients with amyloid have renal involvement and the AA variety comprises about 88% of all cases.

There are many conditions which may be complicated by AA amyloid: Table 12.3 is a list of the major associations.

Table 12.2 A classification of amyloid according to constituents

Original terminology	Current terminology
1 Primary amyloid, myeloma-associated	AL
2 Secondary types, FMF-related	AA
3 Hereditary amyloid, polyneuropathy	AF
4 Senile – brain or heart	AS
5 Endocrine-associated	AE

FMF, Familial Mediterranean fever.

Table 12.3 Conditions which may be complicated by secondary amyloidosis

Chronic inflammatory disorders
Rheumatoid arthritis
Juvenile rheumatoid arthritis
Ankylosing spondylitis
Psoriatic arthritis
Reiter's syndrome
Inflammatory bowel disease
Chronic infectious diseases
Paraplegia (neurogenic bladder with recurrent infection)
Tuberculosis
Osteomyelitis
Bronchiectasis
Multiple skin abscesses (heroin abuse)
Leprosy
Neoplastic diseases
Multiple myeloma (but AL amyloid)
Renal cell carcinoma
Hodgkin's disease

Clinical features

The 'initiating' condition (Table 12.3) may be very obvious and the development of proteinuria may therefore be not surprising. Nevertheless, it is not uncommon to diagnose AA amyloid by renal biopsy and not to detect any precipitating cause, even after prolonged follow-up. In any patient older than 60 years, the development of progressive renal failure should prompt a search for myeloma. AL amyloid may be present, together with other renal changes of myeloma.

Generally, the onset of proteinuria in patients with amyloid is gradual; asymptomatic proteinuria may precede nephrotic syndrome by years. While there is an overall correlation between proteinuria, renal failure and glomerular amyloid, surprising variations are at times found. If AA amyloid is deposited predominantly on vascular and tubulointerstitial sites, little or no proteinuria develops. Heavy proteinuria is more common in AA than in AL amyloid; this is due to glomerular deposition. Hypertension is not a common feature in renal involvement in amyloid.

Course and therapy

Almost invariably, progressive renal failure develops. Spontaneous remissions occasionally occur but are rare. Remissions usually result after eradication of chronic infection, the most usual example being the successful treatment of tuberculosis.

Nephrotic syndrome reduces survival to about 10% at 3 years. Azotaemia has a similar or worse prognosis. About 50% of patients with familial Mediterranean fever become nephrotic, with a rapid decline in glomerular filtration rate (GFR). Myocardial involvement in AA amyloid is not common but is prognostically ominous.

There is no known treatment for renal or systemic amyloid: the insoluble fibrils continue to be deposited. If organs other than the kidney are not involved, dialysis and transplantation are entirely appropriate, although amyloid may well be deposited in the graft.

Renal involvement in myeloma

Multiple myeloma causes a number of renal abnormalities and leads to death secondary to infection or to renal or cardiovascular failure. The characteristic feature is an unbalanced proliferation of a clone of B-lymphocyte-derived cells which normally synthesize immunoglobulins. The abnormal proliferation leads to a paraproteinaemia in serum or urine, or both, a proliferation of marrow plasma cells and suppression of normal immunoglobulin production. An excess of the light-chain portions of immunoglobulins is made, such that the normal urinary concentrations (κ: 2.4 mg/day; λ: 1.8 mg/day) are much exceeded. More than 12 g daily may be recovered (relating to tumour mass). Light chains circulate as monomers (κ chains; MW 22 kDa), which are freely filtered by glomeruli, and as dimers (λ chains; MW 44 kDa), of which only about 10% are recoverable in urine. Light chains constitute Bence-Jones proteinuria (BJP) and are found in variable percentages in patients

Table 12.4 An immunochemical classification of multiple myeloma together with approximate percentage frequency of Bence-Jones proteinuria and chance of renal failure

Immunoglobulin class	Frequency of myeloma class (%)	Light-chain proteinuria (%)	Renal failure (%)
IgG	55–60	50–70	50
IgA	20–25	50–70	60
Light-chain disease	15–20	100	90
IgD	1	90	90
IgM	1	?	?

Ig, Immunoglobulin.

Table 12.5 Causes of Bence-Jones proteinuria

1 Benign gammopathy	
2 Multiple myeloma	
3 Waldenström's macroglobulinaemia	
4 Systemic amyloid	
5 Heavy-chain (μ) disease	rare
6 Chronic lymphoproliferative disorders	rare

with myeloma (Table 12.4). It should be noted that BJP is not invariable in myeloma but the absence of urinary light chains does not exclude this plasma cell dyscrasia. Likewise, BJP is not diagnostic of myeloma; the other causes are shown in Table 12.5.

From Table 12.4 it is clear that there is a relationship between BJP and the development of renal failure. The most likely exaplanation is that light chains directly interfere with the metabolic activity of renal tubular cells.

Histology

There are three groups of morphological changes that may be found on renal biopsy: overlap occurs between these.

1 Myeloma cast nephropathy (myeloma kidney). Here, some collecting tubules are filled with 'hard' BJP casts. Multinucleate giant cells develop in relation to these casts.

2 Deposition of light chains as:

(a) amyloid deposits on tubular basement membrane, blood-vessel walls and interstitium and, less commonly, in glomeruli;

(b) κ light chains on glomerular loops, which leads to tuft lobulation not dissimilar from mesangiocapillary glomerulonephritis.

3 Lesions secondary to infection, hypercalcaemia or hyperuricaemia.

Indications for renal biopsy

Renal biopsy is required in patients with multiple myeloma:

1 if light-chain deposition is suspected;

2 when symptoms are unexplained by the degree of renal failure;

3 if ARF occurs.

Clinical features

There are many possible renal manifestations in multiple myeloma, as shown in Table 12.6. Renal failure is often the presenting feature of multiple myeloma and it should always be considered in the middle-

Table 12.6 Morphological, fluid and electrolyte changes in multiple myeloma

Myeloma cast nephropathy	Bence-Jones proteinuria
Light-chain nephropathy	Hypercalcaemia
Hypercalcaemic nephropathy	Dehydration
AL amyloid	Hyperviscosity
Pyelonephritis	Hyperuricaemia
Chronic renal failure	Hyperkalaemia
Uric acid nephropathy	Metabolic acidosis
Acute renal failure	Pseudohyponatraemia
Tubular dysfunction	

aged and elderly if there is unexplained, fairly rapidly advancing CRF. Additional features that suggest this malignancy include recurrent infections, hypercalcaemia (which occurs in 30–50%; it is usually less than 3.3 mmol/L and is not associated with raised serum concentrations of alkaline phosphatase), light chains in serum or urine or both, an abnormal bleeding tendency, hyperviscosity or the chance finding of cryoglobulins or AL amyloid deposition.

The most common tubular disorder in multiple myeloma is the adult Fanconi syndrome, diagnosed by the clustering of glycosuria and increased quantities of urinary bicarbonate, uric acid, phosphate and amino acids, together with a tubular proteinuria and possible osteomalacia and pseudofractures.

Course and therapy

General features of management include:

1 Maintenance of adequate hydration.
2 Avoiding dehydration.
3 Avoiding nephrotoxic drugs and X-ray contrast.
4 Prompt treatment of hypercalcaemia and hyperuricaemia.

Drug therapy involves allopurinol together with melphalan or cyclophosphamide and prednisolone. The cytotoxic agents have to be reduced in dose proportional to renal function. Plasmaphaeresis is occasionally necessary for hyperviscosity or if there is a high serum concentration of light chains.

Acute renal failure occurs in approximately 10% of these patients; it should be treated aggressively because there are a number of reports of successful therapy of this complication. Chronic renal failure occurs in up to 50% of patients: there is a fairly close relationship to BJP and progressive renal failure. As in ARF, in myeloma dialysis is indicated if extrarenal involvement is not severe and chemotherapy is planned. Acute renal failure and CRF may be irreversible: in this circumstance, chronic haemodialysis or peritoneal dialysis is appropriate. Nevertheless, these patients do not fare well: the 1-year survival on dialysis is about 50%.

Toxic nephropathies

The toxic nephropathies are a heterogeneous group of disorders, caused by a very wide range of drugs and chemicals (Table 12.7), which cause combinations of proteinuria, nephrotic syndrome, haematuria, ARF or CRF and tubular dysfunction. Glomeruli, tubules, interstitium or blood-vessels, variously, may bear the brunt of injury. Presumably the kidney is vulnerable because of the high blood supply, the large vascular endothelial surface area and the concentrating mechanisms of the medulla, all of which lead to a higher concentration of initiating agent per unit volume of kidney than that in any other organ.

Table 12.7 A classification of the toxic nephropathies

ACUTE RENAL FAILURE
Prerenal – prostaglandin synthesis inhibitors
NSAIDs
Renal – toxic tubule cell injury
Antibiotics: aminoglycosides, cephalosporins, tetracyclines, others
Heavy metals: mercury, arsenic
X-ray contrast (iodine)
Chemotherapeutic agents: cisplatin, methotrexate, streptozotocin, others
Acute allergic tubulointerstitial nephritis: antibiotics, diuretics, analgesics, others
Obstructive: uric acid sludge, oxalate, sulphonamides
CHRONIC RENAL FAILURE
Tubulointerstitial nephritis
Analgesic nephropathy
Heavy metals: lead, cadmium, lithium
Glomerular lesions
Organic solvents
Heroin addiction
Nephrotic syndrome or proteinuria
Heavy metals: gold, mercury, bismuth
Drugs with sulphydril groups: D-penicillamine, captopril
NSAIDs
Lupus-like syndrome: hydralazine, anticonvulsants
Hydrocarbon exposure
Rifampicin

See also Tables 8.2, p. 110, and 16.3, p. 228.

A number of the toxic nephropathies are immunologically induced and therefore entirely different from the above structural and functional features. Evidence suggesting an immune origin of a drug-induced nephropathy involves the following:

1 The event is not dose-related.

2 Remission usually occurs after the drug has been withdrawn.

3 Frequently there are extrarenal manifestations: fever, rash, arthropathy.

4 Laboratory features, including eosinophilia, eosinophiluria, raised serum concentrations of IgE, anti-drug antibodies and deposition of complement and immunoglobulins in glomeruli.

5 Patients with the DR3 antigen are at higher risk of gold-induced proteinuria than comparable individuals bearing other DR antigens.

Clinical course

From Table 12.7 it is clear that widely different renal syndromes occur as a result of a toxic nephropathy. The acute dynamic aspects of ARF are discussed in Chapter 16, p. 224; acute renal parenchymal injury is described on pp. 170–177. Initial management of CRF is covered in Chapter 14, p. 198. The various strategies will not be reiterated.

Table 12.8 The risk factors of radiocontrast-induced renal damage ranked in order of importance

Pre-existing renal failure
Diabetic nephropathy
Ischaemic kidney
Dehydration
Multiple myeloma
Previous contrast-induced nephrotoxicity
High-dose contrast
Advanced age

Renal failure worsened by the administration of intravenous iodinated contrast is worthy of specific mention because it remains common and is avoidable. The risk factors are shown in Table 12.8. Studies have shown that, after the majority of intravenous urograms (IVUs) in routine clinical practice, serum creatinine is up to 50% higher than before the investigation and particularly so in patients with pre-existing impairment of renal function. The dangers of an IVU in patients with plasma cell dyscrasias have perhaps been overemphasized; nevertheless, if intravenous or intra-arterial contrast has to be given to a patient with myeloma, a diuresis (> 2 ml/min) should be initiated before the procedure and maintained for 2–3 hours after (see also p. 260). Currently, with the use of ultrasound and dimercaptosuccinic acid (DMSA) renal scans (p. 78) the need for contrast studies is less than formerly.

The possibility of a drug-related glomerulonephritis should be considered in all patients with proteinuria more than 1 g daily. In particular, demonstration of a membranous glomerulonephritis should lead one to consider whether it is secondary to a drug – see Table 10.3, p. 146. After withdrawal of gold or penicillamine, proteinuria and haematuria usually cease by 12–18 months. Likewise, the nephrotic state and subsequently the proteinuria usually recede entirely and renal function returns to normal after a causal NSAID is withdrawn. If the association is not made, CRF probably ensues.

Further reading

1 Bluestone, R., Waisman, J. & Klinenberg, J.R. (1977) The gouty kidney. *Semin. Arthritis Rheum.* **7**, 97–113.
2 Brezis, M. & Epstein, F.H. (1989) A close look at radiocontrast-induced nephropathy. *N. Engl. J. Med.* **320**, 179–81.
3 Donohoe, J.F. (1992) Scleroderma and the kidney. *Kidney Int.* **41**, 462–77.
4 Duffy, T.P. (1992) The many pitfalls in the diagnosis of myeloma. *N. Engl. J. Med.* **326**, 394–6.
5 Hall, C.L. (1988) Gold nephropathy. *Nephron* **50**, 765–72.
6 Hawkins, P.N. (1988) Amyloidosis. *Blood Rev.* **2**, 270–80.
7 Iggo, N. & Parsons, V. (1990) Renal disease in multiple myeloma: current perspectives. *Nephron* **56**, 229–33.
8 Porile, J.L., Barks, G.L. & Garella, S. (1990) Acute interstitial nephritis with

glomerulopathy due to NSAIDs: a review of the clinical spectrum and effects of steroid therapy. *J. Clin. Pharmacol.* **30**, 468–75.
9 Roy, A.T., Brautbar, N. & Lee, D.B. (1991) Hydrocarbons and renal failure. *Nephron* **58**, 385–92.

Chapter 13
Diabetic Nephropathy

Roger Gabriel

Diabetic renal failure is the second commonest cause of chronic renal failure (CRF) in Europe. Such patients are of both the insulin-dependent variety (type I) and the non-insulin-dependent diabetics (type II). There is much interest in the topic of diabetic renal failure in the hope that the frequency of renal failure in diabetics can be reduced. If proteinuria (more than 0.5 g) daily develops in a diabetic, there is about a 70% chance of developing terminal renal failure over the next 5–10 years.

Pathogenesis of diabetic nephropathy

The aetiology of type I and type II diabetics is different. Nevertheless, patients with either form of diabetes have an increased risk of microvascular, macrovascular and neurological complications when compared with non-diabetic controls. Much attention has been paid to serum concentrations of glycosylated haemoglobin as a measure of glycaemic control. Unfortunately, in the majority of patients glycosylated haemoglobin concentrations are usually elevated above the upper limit of normal. The glycosylated material, over a period of decades, becomes chemically bonded with collagen, producing what is termed advanced glycosylated end-products (AGEs). It is thought that AGEs lead to irrevocable tissue damage which is eventually clinically recognized as a diabetic complication. These events lead, for example, to the increase of thickness of the glomerular basement membrane – the earliest diabetic change detectable in the kidney. It is of interest that after transplantation serum concentrations of AGEs fall, implying that the kidney has an important role in the clearance of AGEs. There are, in addition, multiple other hormonal and structural alterations in the diabetic patient; an outline of the renally important ones is given in Fig. 13.1.

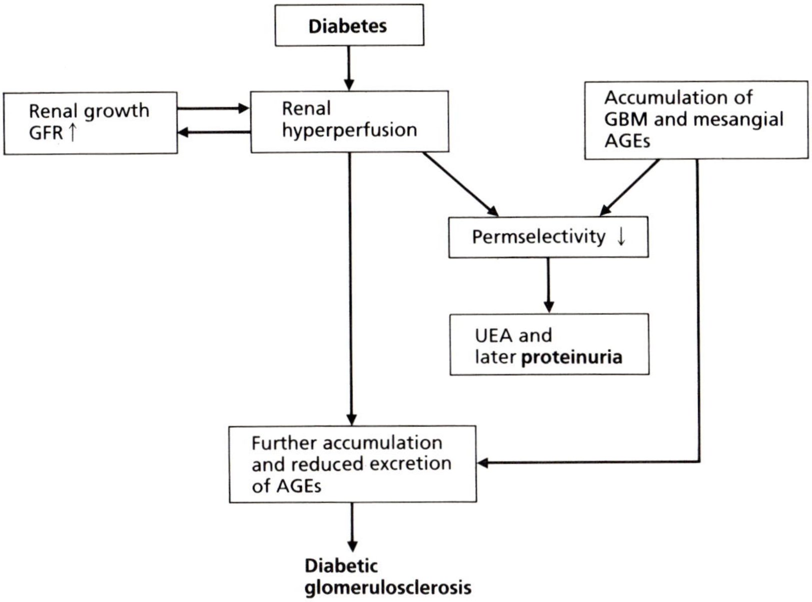

Fig. 13.1 A possible explanation of the development of diabetic glomerulosclerosis. The renal growth and increased glomerular filtration rate (GFR) are present at onset of type I diabetes; the GFR subsequently declines after 1–2 years. Permselectivity is a measure of glomerular capillary wall discrimination between molecules of different size, charge and configuration. A fall in permselectivity implies GBM (glomerular basement membrane) damage. AGEs, Advanced glycosylated end-products; UEA, urinary excretion of albumin.

Stages of diabetic nephropathy

A clear idea of renal events which may occur in a patient who has insulin-dependent diabetes is of value so that a clinician is able to interpret the stages of nephropathy and offer appropriate advice. Renal involvement in diabetes mellitus is now expressed in five stages, as shown in Table 13.1. While the table is correct in general terms, there are wide variations in progression from patient to patient. It is not possible to predict for a specific patient who, at stage II, will progress to stage III. Likewise patients at stage III do not necessarily progress to stage IV, but all at stage IV develop CRF (stage V).

Stages I and II

Stages I and II (Table 13.1) are clinically silent and do not routinely require analysis. Many patients after 15 years of insulin dependence have a normal glomerular filtration rate (GFR) and urinary albumin excretion (UAE). Nevertheless, in some, UAE may be elevated at 10 years or even sooner. It is not possible to predict which patients will deteriorate so quickly.

Table 13.1 The stages of diabetic nephropathy

Stages	Clinical and laboratory events	Time course
I	Renal hypertrophy and hyperfunction	Present at diagnosis
II	Clinically silent. Normal UAE. Thickening of GBM begins which persists but does not necessarily deteriorate	After 2 or more years
III	Renal function normal. No proteinuria on routine testing but UAE may be present and increase	After >7 years, usually 10–15 years
IV	Clinical nephropathy with hypertension and proteinuria	After 15–20 years
V	CRF secondary to diabetic sclerosis and hypertensive renal damage	*c.*25 years

UAE, Urinary albumin excretion (microalbuminuria); GBM, glomerular basement membrane. There is no automatic progression from stage to stage for every patient.

Stage III

Stage III is the high-risk phase for development of diabetic nephropathy. Longitudinal and cross-sectional studies continue to be analysed. At present, it appears that UAE increases while GFR remains normal. There is a tendency towards hypertension which is aggravated by exercise. Angiotensin-converting enzyme inhibitors (ACEI) should be used early to control even minor sustained elevation in blood-pressure. At stage III renal involvement in diabetics, raised UAE predicts poor prognosis but the microalbuminuria may be returned to normal concentrations ($<20\,\mu g/min$) by adequate hypotensive treatment. It is not yet clear whether control of UAE at stage III can be maintained indefinitely and thus prevent development of progressive renal damage.

Modest protein restriction (*c.* 50 g daily) is appropriate to reduce or ameliorate intraglomerular pressure and diminish stimuli to increasing glomerular mesangial sclerosis (see p. 119).

Stage IV

Unfortunately, at present about 40% of insulin-dependent diabetics develop diabetic nephropathy 15–25 years after presentation. Renal histology shows the classical structural abnormalities – thickening of glomerular basement membrane, especially of the lamina densa, together with mesangial expansion and sclerosis.

At this stage UAE has progressed into clinical proteinuria of >0.5 g daily. Hypertension will be established and the GFR will fall progressively. Decline in renal function can be reduced by careful blood-pressure control and perhaps by additional dietary protein restriction, as described on p. 300.

Stage V

Gradually, without any clear demarcation, all stage IV patients deteriorate to stage V – CRF. Glomeruli become obsolescent, tubules atrophy and kidneys shrink. Unless severe vascular damage elsewhere precludes selection, continuous ambulatory peritoneal dialysis (CAPD) is commenced before creatinine clearance falls below 5 ml/min. Because diabetes is a common disease, approximately 25% of dialysis patients are diabetic with end-stage diabetic glomerular sclerosis.

Microalbuminuria – urinary albumin excretion

The measurement of microalbuminuria has considerable academic interest but its routine clinical value remains to be fully evaluated. A specific immunochemical assay is required to detect this minor proteinuria measured in micrograms per minute. Urinary albumin excretion is not measured by routine assays of urinary protein or by dipstick testing of urine for protein. Normal UAE is $< 20\,\mu g/min$; it is best measured in overnight urine but 24-hour samples are also used.

Microalbuminuria is present when UAE is $> 20\,\mu g/min$ and $\leq 200\,ng/min$. The GFR tends to fall when UAE is persistently greater than 70 ng/min. This albuminuria is abnormal but the concentration is too low to be detected by dipstick urine testing. When UAE exceeds 200 ng/min on two or three consecutive urine samples, the patient has clinical nephropathy. At this stage, routine (dipstick) testing of urine will demonstrate a proteinuria.

Management of diabetic nephropathy

Ideally, patients with stage IV diabetic nephropathy are seen jointly by a diabetologist and a renal physician, but this is not possible for the majority of patients: 1–2% of the British population are diabetic.

The following are suggested:

1 Regular screening for proteinuria, preferably biannually. Screening for microalbuminuria twice annually if the assay is locally available.

2 Regular measurement of lying and standing blood-pressure. A pressure taken with the patient sitting or lying will miss the postural fall of an autonomic neuropathy.

3 Urine culture at each visit. It is not known whether diabetics have an increased incidence of urinary infection, but antibiotic eradication of bacteria, if present, is sensible.

4 Regular measurement of the serum creatinine concentrations if proteinuria is present – 6-monthly until the concentration reaches 150 μmol/L and then every 3 months until the serum creatinine is above 200 μmol/L and subsequently every 1–2 months.

5 Strict control of hypertension, using ACEI, having satisfied oneself that atheromatous renal artery stenosis is not present (see p. 216).

6 Tight glycaemic control if possible.
7 Regular attention to vascular disease in the feet.
8 Annual ophthalmic assessment or more frequently if a retinopathy develops. Retinopathy and nephropathy often coexist.
9 Referral to a renal physician when serum creatinine is greater than 250 μmol/L.
10 Protein restriction to 0.5 g/kg body-weight/day when serum creatinine reaches 500 μmol/L and carbohydrate increased to supply sufficient calories.

Until the mid-1980s many diabetics were not referred for dialysis because it was thought that the generalized atheroma and other diabetic complications were contraindications to treatment. Continuous ambulatory peritoneal dialysis is suitable for many such patients and, when used with intraperitoneal insulin, glycaemic control may be very good. Results of renal transplantation in younger diabetics are similar to those with other causes of renal failure.

General physicians tend not to refer diabetic patients because of a misapprehension that renal units are invariable over-subscribed. A patient should be referred with diabetic nephropathy (24-hour urine protein 0.5 g or more) early because loss of GFR may be very rapid and also unpredictable. Hypertension appears to accelerate loss of renal function.

Protein restriction is used in an attempt to break the cycle of glomerular hyperfiltration and glomerular sclerosis but it is not clear if this dietary approach is beneficial because multiple other variables make precise analysis difficult. Protein restriction does control anorexia.

Glycaemic therapy in uraemic diabetics

1 Insulin requirements often fall as uraemia increases. The doses of insulin have to be judged from blood glucose concentrations. Testing the urine for glucose is valueless because, with progressive nephron loss, there may be no glycosuria in the presence of hyperglycaemia.
2 In type II uraemic diabetics, biguanides are contraindicated because of their propensity to precipitate lactic acidosis.
3 Chlorpropamide is potentially dangerous because of the long half-life of about 33 hours.
4 Tolbutamide, which has a half-life of 6 hours, is the oral hypoglycaemic of choice in uraemia.

Indications for renal biopsy in diabetic patients

It is not often necessary to perform a renal biopsy in diabetics with or without diabetic nephropathy. The main indications are:
1 An unexpected nephrotic syndrome, suggesting renal pathology other than diabetic glomerulosclerosis.
2 Glomerular haematuria, reflecting an immune-complex nephritis.

3 A disproportionate loss of GFR according to the stage of the patient (see Table 13.1).

Some studies have suggested that the diabetic kidney may develop nephritides more than would be expected by chance; the issue has yet to be clarified.

Treatment of hypertension in patients with diabetes mellitus and renal impairment

Until recently it was not thought to matter which hypotensive drug was used in patients with diabetic nephropathy and renal impairment (DMRI), provided that the blood-pressure was satisfactorily controlled and side-effects were acceptable. It now appears that ACEI are the drugs of choice.

The kidney contains all components of the renin–angiotensin system. The actions of angiotensin II include regulation and redistribution of renal blood flow, differential vasoconstrictor effects on glomerular efferent and afferent arterioles, contraction of the mesangium and suppression of renin synthesis and release. It is not surprising that ACEI have major effects on renal function; these may be divided into two groups, one harmful and the other beneficial:

1 *Harmful effects on renal function.* Patients with low, fixed, renal blood flow, particularly those who are sodium- and volume-depleted by diuretic therapy, are at risk of increased renal impairment if ACEI are given. If bilateral tight renal artery stenosis is present, acute renal failure occurs following ACEI. This is because, in this condition, glomerular blood flow and hence GFR are directly dependent upon efferent glomerular vasoconstriction – maintained by angiotensin II. Loss of postglomerular angiotensin II activity immediately leads to a sharp sustained fall in glomerular perfusion, with decrease in an already reduced GFR and acutely worsening uraemia. The effects are less dramatic in patients with unilateral renal artery stenosis (see p. 216) because the contralateral kidney is able to compensate for the loss of function in the affected kidney.

2 *Beneficial effects on renal function.* It is now held that ACEI maintain GFR, reduce proteinuria and possibly retard development of diabetic glomerulosclerosis. It has also been shown that ACEI therapy reduces microalbuminuria and this effect appears to be unique to ACEI. Angiotensin-converting enzyme inhibitors may therefore have effects that prevent or retard the development of diabetic glomerulosclerosis in both normotensive and hypertensive patients.

There are also endogenous renin–angiotensin systems in many tissues (brain, heart, vascular tree, gonads and gastrointestinal tract) which serve autocrine or paracrine functions, or both. The clinical advantages of tissue renin–angiotensin system inhibition with ACEI include:

1 Increased arterial wall compliance.

2 Improved left ventricular function.

3 Longer survival in heart failure.

4 Regression of vascular and left ventricular hypertrophy.
5 Delay in the progression of DMRI.

Angiotensin-converting enzyme inhibitors do not have first-order kinetics. The plasma, drug or metabolite concentration–time profile is a function of linear elimination kinetics, together with saturable drug-binding to tissue and circulating ACEI. Tissue rather than circulating ACEI correlate better. The varying degrees of tissue-binding of different ACEIs account for the different dosage schedules.

At present no one ACEI appears to have any clinical advantage over another except that some patients find a single daily dose more convenient than a twice-daily regimen. In patients without renal insufficiency, treatment is straightforward. If the concentration of serum creatinine is 250 μmol/L or more, care is needed in both diabetics and non-diabetics.

Potassium excretion in urine is influenced by aldosterone, which is dependent upon angiotensin II. Thus, with continuous reduction in angiotensin II activity, fractional potassium excretion decreases, plasma potassium concentrations may rise and hyperkalaemia may occur. The higher the serum creatinine concentration, the more likely is serious potassium retention to develop. In addition, entirely separate from a renal arterial stenosis, a minor reduction in renal function occurs in uraemic patients when receiving ACEI therapy. This is accentuated if over-large doses of loop diuretics are given. Other side-effects of ACEI are described, the most frequent of which appears to be a chronic dry cough, which resolves if the drug is stopped. The incidence of cough is thought to be the same in DMRI patients, both in non-diabetic CRF and in subjects with normal renal function.

Summary

Diabetic nephropathy is important because in those patients with type I disease who have developed proteinuria during the second decade of their disease have a 100-fold greater risk of dying than those without proteinuria. They also have the same chance of death from cardiovascular disease. Management is lifelong and the best hope for longevity is strict glycaemic control and rigid control of hypertension with ACEI.

The outlook for patients with type II diabetes is less depressing but neither CRF nor death from macrovascular disease is uncommon.

Further reading

1 Bank, N. (1991) Mechanisms of diabetic hyperfiltration. *Kidney Int.* **40**, 792–807.
2 Borch-Johnsen, K., Norgaard, K., Hommel, K. *et al.* (1992) Is diabetic nephropathy an inherited complication? *Kidney Int.* **41**, 719–22.
3 Catalano, C. & Marshall, S.M. (1992) Epidemiology of end-stage renal disease in patients with diabetes mellitus. *Nephrol. Dial. Transplant.* **7**, 181–90.
4 Epstein, M. (1991) Calcium antagonists and diabetic nephropathy. *Arch. Intern. Med.* **151**, 2361–4.

5 Manske, C.L., Sprafka, J.M., Strong, J.T. & Wang, Y. (1990) Contrast nephropathy in azotaemic diabetes undergoing contrast arteriography. *Am. J. Med.* **89**, 615–20.
6 Morgensen, C.E. & Christensen, C.K. (1984) Predicting diabetic nephropathy in insulin dependent patients. *N. Engl. J. Med.* **311**, 89–93.
7 Morgensen, C.E. (1992) Angiotensin converting enzyme inhibitors and diabetes mellitus. *Br. Med. J.* **304**, 327–8.
8 Narins, G. & Kirshma, G.G. (1988) Diabetic nephropathy: the basis for dietary and converting enzyme therapy. *Am. J. Hypertension* **1**, 215–20.
9 Payton, C.D. & Boulton-Jones, J.M. (1989) Treatment of renal failure in diabetic patients. *Hosp. Update* **15**, 249–60.
10 Ritz, E., Nowack, R., Fliser, D., Koch, M. & Tschope, W. (1991) Type II diabetes mellitus: is the renal risk adequately appreciated? *Nephrol. Dial. Transplant.* **6**, 679–82.
11 Sirmon, M.D. & Kirkpatrick, W.G. (1991) Diabetic nephropathy: new directions in management. *Renal Failure* **15**, 51–60.
12 Steffes, M.W. & Mauer, S.M. (1991) Towards a basic understanding of diabetic complications. *N. Engl. J. Med.* **325**, 883–4.
13 Valentino, V.A., Wilson, M.D., Weart, W. & Bakris, G.L. (1991) A perspective on converting enzyme inhibitors and calcium channel antagonists in diabetic renal disease. *Arch. Intern. Med.* **151**, 2367–72.
14 Viberti, G.C. (1989) Interventions based on microalbuminuria screening and low protein diet in the treatment of kidney disease of diabetes mellitus. *Am. J. Kidney Dis.* **13**, 1341–4.
15 Watkins, P.J. (1990) Diabetic nephropathy. *Quart. J. Med.* **76**, 767–9.
16 Zeller, K., Whittaker, E., Sullivan, L., Rankin, P. & Jacobson, H.R. (1991) Effect of restricting dietary protein on the progression of renal failure in patients with insulin dependent diabetes mellitus. *N. Engl. J. Med.* **324**, 78–84.

Chapter 14
Initial Management of Chronic Renal Failure

David Carmichael

Chronic renal failure (CRF) is the gradual, progressive and irreversible loss of renal function and may be caused by almost any renal disease. The conditions which are most frequently seen are:

1 Chronic glomerulonephritis.
2 Diabetes mellitus.
3 Severe hypertension.
4 Obstructive uropathy – usually of the bladder neck but also bilateral ureteric and urethral.
5 Adult polycystic disease.
6 Interstitial nephritides – with and without obstruction or reflux, including analgesic abuse.

It is often impossible to find a definite cause when patients present in advanced uraemia. Chronic renal failure is not the same as end-stage or terminal renal failure, when there is virtually no residual renal function and no prospect of reversibility. The term CRF is often used to indicate that the creatinine clearance has fallen below 50 ml/min.

Although the rate of deterioration of patients with CRF varies from disease to disease, there seems to be a more important variation from patient to patient. The rate of decline in renal function can be estimated by using a plot of the reciprocal of serum creatinine against time (see Fig. 17.1, p. 253). This has been employed to assess the effects of diet, treatment of hypertension and other measures used to ameliorate decline in renal function, but variation from patient to patient makes evaluation of a particular treatment difficult.

It is essential that the early management of CRF includes diagnosis and treatment of any reversible component (Table 14.1). Once this has been done, treatment is directed at minimizing the effects of CRF and slowing its progression to end-stage disease.

Pathophysiology

The kidney has a large functional reserve which allows compensation in homoeostatic, excretory and endocrine functions, even when there is considerable loss of glomerular filtration rate (GFR). It is possible that large numbers of nephrons fail simultaneously, particularly in diseases primarily affecting the medulla. The more likely final common pathway to declining renal function is described by the 'intact nephron hypothesis'. Remaining nephrons adapt to maintain renal function by hypertrophy (as can be seen on histological sections) to enable adequate filtration to take place. Sustained hyperfiltration is detrimental to the structure of the glomerulus as it produces mesangial cell damage, cellular proliferation and mesangial matrix over-production, all of

Table 14.1 Reversible and treatable features in chronic renal failure listed in approximate order of frequency

Reversible factors in chronic renal failure
1 Hypertension
2 Urinary infection
  Primary
  Secondary to obstruction
3 Analgesic nephropathy
4 Recent obstruction
5 Tuberculosis
6 Glomerulonephritis secondary to infection

Disorders aggravating chronic renal failure
1 Infection
2 Drugs
3 Salt and water depletion
4 Hyperphosphataemia
5 Hypercalcaemia
6 Hyperuricaemia
7 Renal vein thrombosis

Treatable types of renal parenchymatous disease
1 Pyelonephritis
2 Lupus nephritis
3 Analgesic nephropathy
4 Acute hypertension nephropathy
5 Multiple myeloma
6 Hypercalcaemic nephropathy
7 Haemolytic uraemic syndrome
8 Rapidly progressive glomerulonephritis
9 Renal vein thrombosis
10 Sarcoid infiltration

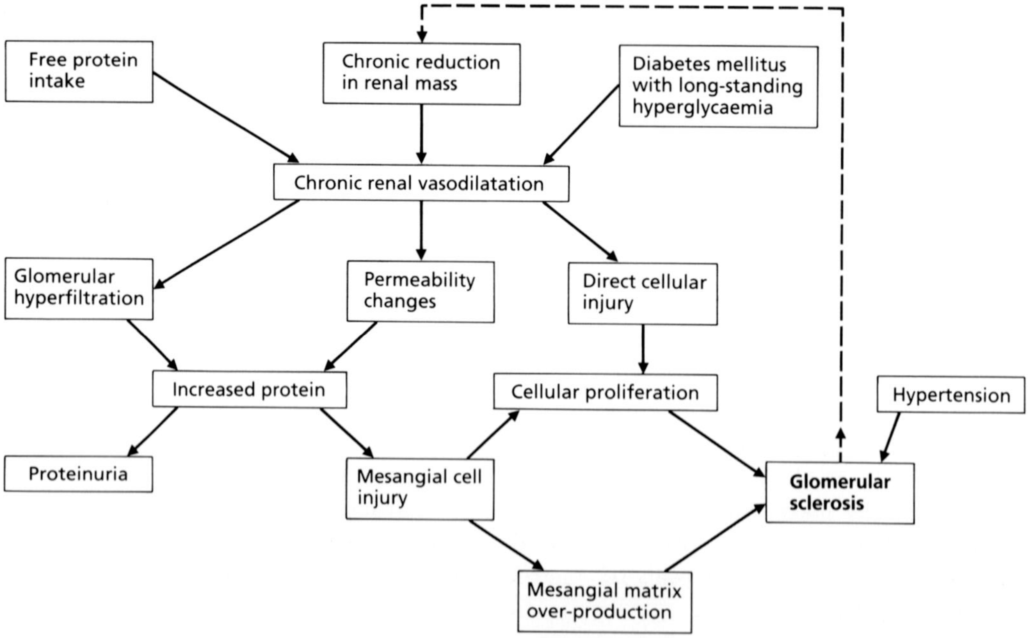

Fig. 14.1 The consequences of glomerular hyperfiltration and hypertension upon glomerular structure and function.

which may lead to glomerulosclerosis (Fig. 14.1). As more nephrons are destroyed, the remainder take on more work themselves, becoming sclerosed until ultimately insufficient are left.

Mechanisms producing hyperfiltration include chronic renal vasodilatation, which occurs in response to a reduced renal mass, a large protein intake (as protein or peptide fragments) and hyperglycaemia in diabetic nephropathy. For these reasons, attention is being paid to the use of diets to halt or slow decline in renal function and to ensure adequate blood sugar control, together with restricted protein intake, in diabetics early in the course of renal disease. Other mechanisms that may influence decline in renal function are presented in Fig. 14.2 but will not be discussed.

In CRF, secondary hyperparathyroidism occurs, with phosphate retention. This causes a fall in the concentration of serum ionized calcium. In addition, the kidney is unable to metabolize 25-hydroxycholecalciferol into the active component 1,25-$(OH)_2$-cholecalciferol (see Fig. 14.2).

Parathyroid hormone

As GFR declines and assuming a constant dietary phosphate intake, phosphate retention occurs, leading to increase in serum phosphate concentrations. Such retention is closely related to the development of secondary hyperparathyroidism.

Persistent phosphate retention reduces the renal production of cal-

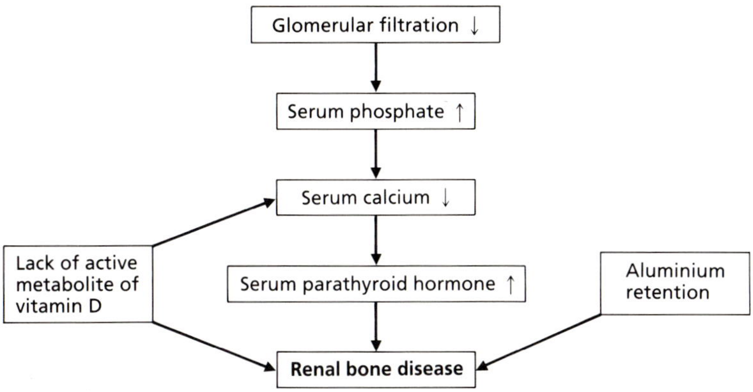

Fig. 14.2 Sequence of metabolic events in causing renal bone disease. Osteomalacia is less common than osteitis fibrosa cystica.

citriol (1,25-$(OH)_2$-cholecalciferol, the most active form of vitamin D_3). Secondary hyperparathyroidism ensues because the concentration of plasma ionized calcium falls and because of the inhibitory effect of calcitriol upon parathyroid hormone (PTH) secretion. Such an increase in PTH production is initially appropriate because it tends to return the concentrations of ionized calcium and serum phosphate to normal. In the long term (advancing CRF), chronic over-secretion of PTH leads to renal osteodystrophy. When the GFR is persistently below 30 ml/min, PTH is unable to increase renal phosphate secretion further and the net effect of the hormone is to enhance bone phosphate release.

Relatively recently, an assay for the intact PTH molecule has become available. Regular assay of the hormone, in combination with serum concentrations of calcium, phosphate and alkaline phosphatase, is of considerable value in judging the correct long-term dose of calcium carbonate and 1-α-Hydroxycholecalciferol (1-α-HCC) (see p. 206). Additionally, with good metabolic care, the concentration of PTH can be lowered towards normal, which reduces the development of osteodystrophy and the later need for parathyroidectomy and prevention of tertiary hyperparathyroidism.

Intact-molecule PTH should be measured relatively frequently in the first months of CRF and thereafter twice annually.

Initial management

A general approach to any patient with possible CRF includes:

1 Confirmation of CRF.

2 Diagnosis of the cause with particular reference to reversibility.

3 Detection of aggravating factors.

4 Assessment of the severity, chronicity and presence of sequelae of renal failure.

5 Assessment of complications of uraemic syndrome.

6 Treatment of reversible and aggravating factors.

7 Treatment of the consequences of CRF.
8 Renal replacement therapy.

A full history, physical examination and appropriate investigations can be applied within this framework.

Clinical presentation

Patients present in a variety of ways and at different stages of renal impairment (Table 14.2). A chance finding of an elevated blood urea (although not always caused by renal failure) may be the first indication of renal disease. Symptoms are unlikely to be due to renal failure alone until creatinine clearance has fallen below 20 ml/min. A careful clinical history may suggest the aetiology and important reversible factors. As renal function declines, symptoms of uraemia supervene.

History and examination

The following topics need to be covered when taking a history:
1 *Family history*. Renal disease, particularly polycystic disease, hypertension, gout or deafness (hereditary nephritis).
2 *Past medical history*. Previous blood-pressure readings and urine tests (details may be available in previous hospital notes), enuresis and obstetric history.
3 *Drug history*. Analgesics, diuretics, antibiotics, non-steroidal anti-inflammatory agents, heavy-metal exposure and radiographic contrast material (hospital notes may be helpful).
4 *Presenting complaint*:
(a) Symptoms suggesting chronicity: poor health for months, thirst, polyuria, polydipsia or nocturia.
(b) Symptoms suggesting the cause: urinary difficulties (of which the patient may be unaware), rashes and joint pains.
(c) Symptoms suggesting consequences of hypertension: underlying systemic diesease or uraemia.

The history may provide some assessment of the duration of the renal failure, particularly with symptoms of uraemia. In patients with advanced renal failure, it may be difficult to obtain a clear history and it is worth while obtaining information from notes of any previous medical consultations.

Examination may provide further evidence of chronicity and occasionally provide information on aetiology. The major features to be considered are:
1 Signs of chronic uraemia: skin excoriation (may be due to hypercalcaemia), brown arcs on nails, pigmentation, anaemia, neuropathy and pericardial friction rub.
2 Cardiovascular system, including examination of forearm veins with regard to fistula formation prior to haemodialysis.
3 Hypertension.

Table 14.2 Symptoms, signs and associated features of chronic renal failure

Early (creatinine clearance > 20 ml/min)
Chance finding
Hypertension
Urinary symptoms
Proteinuria
Haematuria
Intermediate (creatinine clearance 10–20 ml/min)
Anorexia
Nausea and vomiting
Tiredness
Anaemia
Bone disease
Amenorrhoea
Impotence
Growth failure
Late (creatinine clearance < 10 ml/min)
Drowsiness
Fits
Neuropathy
Fluid overload
Pulmonary oedema
Pericarditis
Hyperkalaemia
Acidosis

4 Fluid status.
5 Abdomen, with emphasis on previous surgery and hernias, in anticipation of acute or chronic peritoneal dialysis.
6 Palpable kidneys.
7 Urinary obstruction, including rectal and pelvic examination.
8 Rashes.

Searching for these specific features in each patient ensures a competent examination.

Investigations

The presentation and initial clinical assessment will indicate which investigations are most immediately relevant. A solitary serum creatinine concentration of, say, 200 μmol/L should not necessarily be interpreted as indicating CRF. Rapidly progressive renal failure is easy to overlook (see Chapter 11, p. 163). Thus, in every patient in the early stages of diagnosis, blood should be reassayed for creatinine concentration less than a week from the first sample to assess the tempo of decline.

There are many possible investigations in patients with CRF; they are listed in Table 14.3. Much of the skill in investigating these patients lies in the order and frequency with which these investigations are

Table 14.3 The major investigations necessary in patients with chronic renal failure

1 Urine	Protein, blood, casts, bacteria
2 Blood	Serum creatinine, plasma urea, sodium, potassium glucose, serum calcium, phosphate, alkaline phosphatase, urate, immunoglobulins, HBV, PTH
3 Urine biochemistry	Clearance, proteinuria, sodium, potassium, Bence-Jones proteinuria
4 ECG and chest X-ray	
5 Radiological	Ultrasound, skeletal survey
6 Renal biopsy	For diagnosis of parenchymal disease
7 Renal arteriogram	Exclusion of renal artery stenosis

HBV, Hepatitis B virus.

requested and repeated. These topics have been discussed in Chapters 4–7 and 9 (pp. 38, 58, 67, 90 and 125).

Medical treatment in early chronic renal failure

Dietary measures

Protein

Protein restriction is used for two reasons:
1 To alleviate symptoms of advanced uraemia.
2 To slow the rate of decline in renal function.

As GFR falls below 10 ml/min, uraemic symptoms begin to develop. Protein restriction at this stage may reduced anorexia, nausea, vomiting and pruritis and slow the development of neuropathy, pericarditis and anaemia. Very severe protein restriction (20 g daily) leads to increased muscle breakdown and malnutrition and is undesirable. Most patients are managed on approximately 0.6 g of protein/kg body-weight/day. The main protein sources are meat, fish, eggs and milk. The calorie intake should be kept at approximately 2500 calories/day (10 000–12 000 kJ/day), with carbohydrate in a greater proportion than fat. As GFR falls, anorexic patients may need supplements, such as Hycal (glucose 1000 kJ/100 ml) or Caloreen (glucose 17 kJ/g), to maintain calorie intake.

Protein restriction to influence the rate of decline in renal function should be started early (creatinine clearance 30 ml/min or even higher) but its benefits are perhaps controversial (see p. 300).

Lipids

Hyperlipidaemia is common in CRF and should be corrected by dietary measures because vascular disease is a major cause of morbidity and mortality. Reduction in intake of saturated fatty acids is advisable but there is no evidence that reducing concentrations of triglycerides below normal confers any benefit.

Potassium

Hyperkalaemia does not occur until the clearance falls below 10 ml/min and then often because of injudicious intake of high potassium-containing foods or administration of potassium-sparing diuretics. Acidosis and infection often induce hyperkalaemia. Foods rich in potassium include:

Soya flour	Chocolate
All Bran	Coffee (instant > ground)
Fruit (dried > fresh)	Nuts
Meat	Marmite
Cooked vegetables	Treacle

Sodium

Patients tend to retain sodium as the clearance falls below 10 ml/min. Those who retain sodium and therefore fluid will develop hypertension and peripheral or pulmonary oedema or both. Sodium intake should be restricted by avoiding processed food and by not adding salt in cooking or at table. This will lower the intake to approximately 100 mmol/day. Many are unable to comply and need regular loop diuretics to produce a naturiesis and diuresis.

Some have salt-losing states (see p. 111) up to, and sometimes after, starting dialysis. It is essential to maintain an adequate sodium intake in these patients because they are at risk of developing fluid depletion, which may further compromise their renal function.

Water

Until terminal renal failure most patients need to maintain a high fluid intake because they will have an osmotic diuresis from raised concentrations of plasma urea. It is unusual to need to restrict the fluid intake until dialysis is required but it may be necessary in those with heart failure or nephrotic syndrome. Restriction of fluid is much easier to follow in conjunction with sodium restriction.

Phosphate

There is experimental evidence that phosphate restriction may slow the decline in renal function. Phosphate-reduced diets are unpalatable.

Oral agents are used to reduce serum phosphate function by binding phosphate in the gut so that less is absorbed. Calcium carbonate is the preferred agent. It is prescribed with meals when serum phosphate is persistently above 2 mmol/L or if the calcium × phosphate product is greater than 6 (or 70 if mass concentrations are used). The dose is 500 mg to 2 g daily, judged by concentrations of serum phosphate and calcium and increased slowly because there is a risk of inducing hypercalcaemia. The aim of treatment is to reduce serum phosphate to about 1.5 mmol/L and the calcium × phosphate product to about 3.5–4.0.

Preparations containing aluminium hydroxide are infrequently used because some aluminium is absorbed and, in the presence of renal failure, is not excreted into the urine. It is deposited in brain and bone, producing fatal dialysis encephalopathy or fracturing renal osteodystrophy, which is complicated to treat. Aluminum preparations are only used if calcium or mixed calcium and magnesium salts induce hypercalcaemia.

Calcium

The hypocalcaemia of advanced renal failure is partially corrected by calcium carbonate, used to bind gut phosphate by producing insoluble calcium compounds.

Closely related to the hypocalcaemia, hyperphosphataemia and acidosis of CRF is osteodystrophy. A large majority of patients with terminal renal failure have renal osteodystrophy if they have not been correctly managed. At this degree of renal failure (GFR < 5 ml/min), the serum calcium tends to be below 2 mmol/L and requires treatment. Calcium carbonate alone does not correct this hypocalcaemia: the synthetic analogue of vitamin D, 1-α-HCC, increases gut calcium absorption. It has a short half-life and hence adjustments in dose are straightforward. Frequent measurement of serum calcium and phosphate and calculation of the calcium × phosphate product are essential to diminish the risk of metastatic calcification. 1-α-Hyroxycholecalciferol is begun at a dose of 0.25 μg daily and increased at 2-weekly intervals. More than 1.0 μg daily is needed rarely. If 1-α-HCC and calcium carbonate are prescribed together, great care is needed to avoid dangerous iatrogenic hypercalcaemia. With good control of serum calcium and phosphate, the concentration of PTH will fall towards normal.

Vitamins

In the absence of specific deficiencies, routine vitamin supplements are unnecessary.

Anaemia

When creatinine clearance falls below 30 ml/min, the normochromic, normocytic anaemia of CRF gradually develops. There is a slight bleeding tendency in uraemia and minor blood loss in the gut occurs. In CRF absorption of iron is poor.

The anaemia of CRF usually does not usually produce troublesome symptoms until clearance is below 10 ml/min and the haemoglobulin concentration has fallen to about 8–10 g/dl. There is considerable variation in the above two values from patient to patient. Blood transfusion is contraindicated if renal transplantation is planned. The anaemia of CRF responds to erythropoietin but this hormone is expensive. Few funds exist for the treatment of patients before they begin dialysis.

Hypertension

Rapid reduction in blood-pressure, particularly in the presence of volume depletion, may be deleterious to renal function. Satisfactory control of blood-pressure may reduce the rate of reduction of GFR caused by glomerulosclerosis. This appears to be the case in diabetic nephropathy. Causes and treatment of hypertension in CRF are dealt with in Chapter 15 (p. 214).

Infection

The topic of infection has been discussed in Chapters 7 and 8, pp. 90 and 108.

The toxicity of tetracyclines is important and is illustrated in the following case history.

Case 1

Chronic renal failure was diagnosed in a 67-year-old woman in 1981. An intravenous urogram (IVU) showed small unobstructed kidneys. Renal function gradually deteriorated and she was referred for dialysis in March 1984. The serum creatinine was 829 μmol/L, creatinine clearance 5 ml/min and plasma urea 29 mmol/L (Table 14.4). After 3 months of continuous ambulatory peritoneal dialysis (CAPD) her renal function had improved: serum creatinine 650 μmol/L, urea 20 mmol/L. The CAPD catheter was removed. Her renal function remained stable until March 1985, when she developed anorexia, malaise and severe dehydration. Renal function had deteriorated (see Table 14.4). The patient had developed an upper respiratory tract infection, which had been treated with oxytetracycline 250 mg four times daily for the 7 days before presentation. Rehydration produced an improvement in renal function: serum creatinine 794 μmol/L and blood urea 29.9 mmol/L. Her health remained satisfactory for a further year but when dialysis became necessary again she decided against this treatment and died peacefully.

This case history shows that not only the hospital doctor following a patient but any other doctor who may prescribe for a patient with CRF must be aware of the diagnosis.

Table 14.4 Biochemical data, treatment and comments regarding the woman described in Case 1

Date	Serum creatinine (μmol/L)	Blood urea (mmol/L)	Serum calcium (mmol/L)	Serum phosphate (mmol/L)	Alkaline phosphatase (U/L)	Comments
10/1981	385	16.5	1.94	1.57	230	
1/1982	400	16.7	1.91	1.40	250	
5/1983	450	19.2	1.62	1.48	224	1-α-HCC 0.25 μg/day started
9/1983	526	21.9	2.1	1.58	187	Aluminium hydroxide 10 ml twice daily
2/1984	715	30.1	2.58	1.92	152	1-α-HCC discontinued
3/1984	829	28.6	2.45	2.1	134	1-α-HCC 0.25 μg/day restarted; referred for dialysis
4/1984						Commenced CAPD but this was never established
7/1984	650	20.0	1.96	1.99	60	Spontaneous recovery in renal function
12/1984	693	25.2	1.93	2.23	62	Aluminium hydroxide 10 ml three times daily
2/1985	981	50.0	1.87	3.18	76	Dehydrated and uraemic after tetracycline
4/1985	794	29.9	1.98	2.3	69	
7/1985	830	30.0	1.93	2.23	58	
2/1986	915	32.0	1.90	2.25	84	Remained well

Diabetic renal failure

Diabetic renal failure is the second commonest indication for dialysis in Western Europe. The topic is discussed in detail is Chapter 13, p. 190.

Obstruction

Obstruction can usually be relieved and therefore is one of the most important potentially reversible causes of CRF. It may also contribute to a decline in function in renal failure from other causes. Recovery of function after relief will depend upon the duration of the obstruction and whether there has been infection (see p. 116). The site of obstruction may be obvious from the history and examination. This is not always so and ultrasound examination of the urinary tract in every patient with renal failure is essential. An ultrasound evaluation provides information about the upper renal tract, pelves and bladder regardless of renal function. Intravenous urography with tomography has become obsolete.

Lower tract obstruction should be relieved by catheterization and upper tract obstruction by percutaneous nephrostomy tubes. They can also be used for antegrade contrast studies (see p. 75).

Bladder decompression should be slow, because rapid release of urine may lead to haemorrhage. If there is a large diuresis and natriuresis, fluid depletion may occur and acute-on-chronic renal failure may supervene – see p. 323. Definitive management of obstructive uropathy is the province of a urologist.

Follow-up and referral

Patients with CRF may present to any branch of medicine and it is important that doctors are able to make a proper initial assessment. Maintenance dialysis will not be needed in all patients. Although some patients may not be taken on to a renal replacement programme because of age, ischaemic heart disease, decrepitude and social circumstances, the main reason why patients do not receive treatment is that they are never referred to a renal physician.

Late referral or inadequate preliminary assessment may mean that renal function has deteriorated past the point of recovery in those patients with a reversible cause or component. Late referral of those patients who need renal replacement therapy imposes considerable difficulties as it not only adversely affects their prognosis but also disrupts day-to-day management of a dialysis unit when additional unforeseen patients are accepted. Inevitably, there are some patients who are seen for the first time in terminal renal failure for whom therapeutic plans have not been made. Thus the patient commences dialysis with inadequate preparation and is unlikely to be in optimum physical and mental condition. This is illustrated in the comparison of two patients accepted for dialysis, described on pp. 210–11.

Preparation for dialysis

The decision about the type of dialysis suitable for a particular patient will be taken in a renal unit. Nevertheless, the general physician should be aware of the different possibilities and foresee some of the difficulties. This may mean earlier referral of a patient.

Haemodialysis

Fewer patients are now trained for home dialysis because more peripheral, minimal care units have been, or are being, established. Hospital patients comprise:

1 Those awaiting a transplant (who in some units will therefore not train for home dialysis).

2 Those training to dialyse at home or at a minimal care unit.

3 Those who are too frail for or unsuited to minimal care dialysis.

When a patient is accepted for haemodialysis, the first priority is to plan vascular access. The preferred method is an arteriovenous (Cimino) fistula created in the non-dominant forearm. It is essential that all veins of, if possible, both arms are preserved and never used for routine venepuncture or insertion of intravenous cannulae. It takes approximately 4–6 weeks after fashioning for a fistula to be ready for insertion of dialysis needles. Women with small arms (particularly Asian women) are less likely to have suitable veins and other surgery may be needed such as transplantation of a portion of a saphenous vein into the arm. This requires more time and greater expertise than fashioning a fistula.

Continuous ambulatory peritoneal dialysis

Continuous ambulatory peritoneal dialysis and other forms of peritoneal dialysis were offered to older patients, those with ischaemic heart disease and diabetics with retinopathy. Chronic peritoneal dialysis may be tolerated better than haemodialysis by some patients in these categories. Patients without satisfactory vascular access are treated with CAPD and increasing numbers of young patients opt for this therapy. Patients can be transplanted from CAPD. Previous abdominal surgery, particularly if there was peritonitis, reduces available peritoneal surface area and may make this form of dialysis impracticable.

Examination of the abdominal wall for inguinal, femoral, umbilical or incisional hernias is important because the pressure exerted by the intraperitoneal fluid may make hernias worse and prevent satisfactory dialysis. Repair of such hernias is more easily carried out before CAPD is needed.

Transplantation

Patients are usually dialysed before transplantation even if there is the possibility of a living related donor. Discussion at an early stage with the patient and family can be useful as it may influence the decision about the type of dialysis used.

Psychological factors

Patients with progressive CRF leading to renal replacement therapy may find their condition difficult to accept. Early referral to a renal physician may help because the patient will then have the opportunity to learn about various forms of treatment by discussion with staff and patients.

Case 2

A male waiter aged 54 presented in 1978 with a blood-pressure of 140/100. His serum creatinine was 323 μmol/L, plasma urea 24.8 mmol/L and proteinuria 2.6 g/24 hours. There had been possible pyelonephritis 20 years before. The IVU showed small scarred kidneys and the renal arteriogram normal renal arteries. The diagnosis was CRF of unknown cause. Blood-pressure was controlled with atenolol 100 mg/day. He remained abroad for the next 5 years and was referred back to a general medical clinic with symptoms of tiredness and malaise. His serum creatinine was 744 μmol/L, creatinine clearance 8 ml/min, blood urea 40.6 mmol/L and haemoglobin 10.9 g/dl. He was immediately referred to a renal unit and accepted for long-term haemodialysis and probable transplantation. A forearm fistula was created in June 1983. There was slow deterioration over the next 2 years, with a considerable increase in symptoms from March 1985, when the serum creatinine was 856 μmol/L and plasma urea 48 mmol/L. The transition to haemodialysis was extremely smooth with easy needling of an excellent fistula. He has since received a cadaveric transplant.

Case 3

A male newsagent aged 43 was diagnosed as having gout in 1970. He immigrated to the United Kingdom in 1979, when allopurinol therapy was commenced. He presented to his local hospital with symptoms of CRF in July 1984. He denied analgesic abuse but there was a history of depression and excessive alcohol consumption. Investigations at that time showed haemoglobin 5.5 g/dl and creatinine clearance 5–9 ml/min. The ureters were not obstructed; the right kidney was small and irregular and the left of normal size. His symptoms improved but his renal function remained unchanged. A diagnosis of urate nephropathy and possible analgesic abuse was made. Plans were laid for out-patient referral to a renal physician. Comment was made about his ability to cope with his illness and he was encouraged to stop drinking alcohol.

He was readmitted 6 weeks later after two *grand mal* convulsions. A referral letter had not been written. His plasma urea had risen from 25 to 52 mmol/L and serum creatinine from 600 to 1600 μmol/L. He was transferred for treatment and was noted to be uraemic, twitching and dehydrated. Despite rehydration, his renal function deteriorated further and he was started on haemodialysis. A wide-bore dialysis catheter was inserted into the left subclavian vein and a forearm fistula fashioned a few days later. Twice-weekly hospital haemodialysis was commenced but in the interval before his fistula could be used the subclavian catheter had to be repositioned. He was depressed for a year after starting dialysis before he could adjust to diagnosis and treatment. He trained successfully for home dialysis and 18 months later received a transplant, which continues to function well.

The patient described in Case 3 spent over 2 months in hospital, suffering from the sudden need to acclimatize to dialysis, for which no mental preparation time had been given.

Summary

Patients with CRF present in any speciality. The minority are first seen in a renal unit. Those with advanced renal failure (serum creatinine >700 μmol/L) need urgent assessment to diagnose the cause of their renal failure and to find reversible or treatable elements. If a patient has a creatinine clearance of <10 ml/min (serum creatinine 400–700 μmol/L), referral to a renal unit is indicated; with a creatinine clearance between 30 and 20 ml/min (serum creatinine 250–400 μmol/L), referral is not urgent but is necessary so that dialysis plans may be made. The referring physician assists in this process. He should:

1 Search for reversible causes of CRF.
2 Diagnose the cause when possible and start any specific treatment.
3 Institute a reduced protein diet.
4 Continue regular follow-up and treatment to minimize the effects of CRF.
5 Refer to the regional renal unit when creatinine clearance falls below 20 ml/min (serum creatinine >500 μmol/L).
6 Refer diabetics when serum creatinine reaches approximately 250 μmol/L.

Further reading

1 Baker, L.R.I., Abrams, S.M.L., Roe, C.J. *et al.* (1989) 1,25(OH)$_2$D$_3$ administration in moderate renal failure: a prospective double-blind trial. *Kidney Int.* **35**, 661–9.
2 Barsotti, G., Giannoni, E., Morelli, E. *et al.* (1984) The decline of renal function slowed by very low phosphorus intake in chronic renal failure patients following a low nitrogen diet. *Clin. Nephrol.* **21**, 54–9.
3 Coburn, J.W. & Salusky, I.B. (1989) Control of serum phosphorus in uraemia. *N. Engl. J. Med.* **320**, 1140–2.
4 Cundy, T., Hand, D.J., Oliver, D.O. *et al.* (1985) Who gets renal bone disease before beginning dialysis? *Br. Med. J.* **290**, 271–5.
5 Editorial (1988) What causes diabetic renal failure? *Lancet* **i**, 1433–4.
6 Editorial (1989) Low dose vitamin D analogues for renal osteodystrophy. *Lancet* **i**, 1364–5.
7 El Nahas, A.M. & Coles, G.A. (1986) Dietary treatment of chronic renal failure: ten unanswered questions. *Lancet* **i**, 597–60.
8 Giovanetti, S. (1985) Dietary treatment of chronic renal failure: why is it not used more frequently? *Nephron* **40**, 1–12.
9 Mitch, W.E., Walser, M., Buffington, G.A. & Lemann, J. (1976) A simple method for estimating progression of chronic renal failure. *Lancet* **ii**, 1326–8.
10 Muirhead, N., Catto, G.R.D., Edward, N. *et al.* (1984) Suppression of secondary hyperparathyroidism. *Br. Med. J.* **288**, 177–9.
11 Nairns, R.G. & Kirskna, G.G. (1988) Diabetic nephropathy: basis for dietary and converting enzyme inhibitor therapy. *Am. J. Hypertension* **1**, 215–20.
12 Nath, K.A. (1992) Tubulointerstitial changes as a major determinant in the progression of renal damage. *Am. J. Kidney Dis.* **20**, 1–17.
13 Ratcliffe, P.J., Phillips, R.E. & Oliver, D.O. (1984) Late referral for maintenance dialysis. *Br. Med. J.* **288**, 441–3.
14 Rostand, S.G., Brunzell, J.D., Cannon, R.O. & Victor, R.G. (1991) Cardiovascular complications in renal failure. *Am. Soc. Nephrol.* **2**, 1053–62.
15 Sakhaee, K. (1992) Management of renal osteodystrophy. *Semin. Nephrol.* **12**, 101–8.

16 Slatopolsky, E., Weerts, C., Norwood, K. *et al.* (1989) Calcium carbonate as a phosphate binder in patients with chronic renal failure. *N. Engl. J. Med.* **315**, 157–61.

17 Watson, M.L. (1990) Adult polycystic kidney disease. *Br. Med. J.* **300**, 62–3.

Chapter 15
Combined Hypertension and Renal Failure

David Carmichael

Hypertension very commonly accompanies chronic renal failure (CRF). It is an important cause of vascular morbidity causing deterioration in renal function by producing glomerulosclerosis. A small minority of patients with CRF do not become hypertensive until glomerular filtration rate is almost zero.

The pathophysiology of hypertension in renal failure is probably multifactorial; possible explanations include sodium and water retention, increased activation of the renin–angiotensin system, essential hypertension causing renal failure, central and autonomic system activity, reduced renal prostaglandin production and increased cardiac output.

All patients with hypertension should be screened for renal disease. A careful history and physical examination, as outlined in Chapter 14, p. 198 are important. Clinical assessment must be directed at the effects of a raised blood-pressure upon the heart and circulation. Retinal examination is necessary because haemorrhages, exudates or papilloedema indicates the presence of accelerated-phase (malignant) hypertension.

Ninety per cent of the hypertensive population has essential hypertension, which causes mild renal impairment in some. In moderate hypertension, renal parenchymal disease is more common. In severe, particularly terminal, renal failure, sodium and water retention are likely to be responsible for sustained hypertension. The kidney may be 'causal' by different mechanisms. These include:

- renal parenchymal disease;
- essential hypertension;
- renoprival hypertension;
- accelerated-phase hypertension;

- renovascular hypertension;
- acute renal failure.

They may be interrelated. Proposed mechanisms of these conditions are discussed in reference texts of renal medicine.

Investigations

The minimum investigations of any hypertensive patient are listed in Table 15.1. Proteinuria may suggest a primary renal cause. In essential hypertension, proteinuria is unusual and indicates renal damage. Heavier proteinuria, seldom in the nephrotic range, may occur in accelerated-phase hypertension. Hypertension in renal parenchymal disease or renal vascular disease is invariably associated with proteinuria. The additional findings of haematuria or granular casts point to an underlying glomerular lesion. Plasma electrolytes may very rarely reveal secondary causes of hypertension, such as hyperaldosteronism or Cushing's syndrome, which may be accompanied by mild to moderate renal failure. Hyponatraemia may occur in accelerated-phase hypertension and hyperkalaemia is found in more advanced renal failure.

Serum creatinine rather than blood urea is a test of renal function in hypertensive patients. If preliminary investigation suggest renal failure or a possible renal cause, the patient should then be investigated as outlined in Chapter 14, p. 198, both to confirm the diagnosis and to search for reversible or ameliorating factors.

Clinical conditions

Acute renal failure

A glomerular lesion is more likely if the patient is hypertensive: raised systemic pressure is not a feature of uncomplicated acute tubular necrosis. Hypertension in acute glomerulonephritis is usually volume-dependent, although there may be activation of the renin–angiotensin system. This is most common in ischaemia or damage to the juxtaglomerular apparatus.

Accelerated-phase hypertension

The diagnosis of accelerated-phase hypertension is clinical, confirmed by finding haemorrhages, exudates and papilloedema, together with

Table 15.1 Major investigations of the hypertensive patient

Urine examination for proteinuira, haematuria and casts
Serum creatinine
Plasma electrolytes
Electrocardiography
Chest X-ray

hypertension and impairment in renal function. Fibrinoid necrosis of arterioles occurs when there is a sudden sustained increase in systemic pressure. In addition, there may be focal and proliferative glomerular lesions, which resolve if the blood-pressure has been treated adequately.

Renal parenchymal disease

Hypertension can occur with any renal parenchymal disease. Examples include:

- chronic glomerulonephritis;
- diabetic nephropathy;
- polycystic disease;
- chronic pyelonephritis;
- analgesic nephropathy;
- ureteric reflux;
- hydronephrosis.

Hypertension is more common in glomerular than in tubulointerstitial disease. Unilateral parenchymal disease does not usually produce renal impairment because of the reserve capacity of the contralateral healthy kidney. The renin–angiotensin system may be responsible in some circumstances for initiating hypertension. Excess renin is produced by an ischaemic kidney with suppression of renin from the contralateral organ, shown by bilateral renal vein renin sampling for measurement of plasma renin activity. Removal of a damaged kidney at an early stage may cure the hypertension, providing it was not sufficiently severe or prolonged to produce contralateral glomerulosclerosis.

It is important to assess what proportion of renal function the affected kidney is contributing, particularly if overall function is diminished. This is easily achieved using a dimercaptosuccinic acid (DMSA) isotope scan. The following conditions may, by surgical intervention, reverse the hypertension:

- unilateral pyelonephritis (resection);
- small atrophic kidney (resection);
- unilateral hydronephrosis (repair);
- pelviureteric junction malformation (repair);
- recent ureteric obstruction (relieve).

If there is no reversible cause for the renal lesion, control of hypertension by drugs may slow deterioration in renal function. When clearance falls below 10 ml/min, salt and water retention often becomes apparent; dietary protein restriction and loop diuretics will be needed.

Renovascular hypertension or renal artery stenosis

Renal artery stenosis may account for 5% of all patients with hypertension. Renal failure may occur under the following circumstances:

1 Bilateral parenchymal disease.

2 Unilateral disease in a single kidney or an only functioning kidney.

3 Renal artery stenosis in patient who already has intrinsic renal disease, including glomerulosclerosis secondary to long-standing hypertension.
4 Renal artery stenosis with prolonged or severe hypertension, leading to glomerulosclerosis in the contralateral kidney.

Revascularization by surgery or angioplasty at an early stage will cure the hypertension in the majority of patients. In long-standing disease, the response is less predictable and most patients still require drug treatment, albeit in reduced dose. It is likely that at this stage mechanisms other than over-production of renin, and hence angiotensin II, are operating to maintain the hypertension.

The aim in most cases of renal artery stenosis is to control the blood-pressure. The atheromatous type of the disease, which occurs in older patients, is progressive and may lead to occlusion of one or both renal arteries. Under these circumstances, renal failure occurs and treatment must also be directed at reversing this process. Fibromuscular hyperplasia occurs in younger patients and it is less usual for this form of the disease to cause renal failure unless the hypertension is severe and prolonged.

There are no pathognomonic features of uncomplicated renal artery stenosis but the following are suggestive in a hypertensive patient:
1 Age less than 35 years.
2 Presence of an epigastric bruit.
3 Difficulty in controlling hypertension.
4 Widespread disease with worsening renal failure.

Investigation

Various screening tests are available. They are:
1 Intravenous urogram.
2 Isotope renogram (with and without a small intravenous dose of captopril).
3 Peripheral plasma renin activity.
4 Effect of chronic administration of angiotensin-converting enzyme inhibitors (ACEIs) upon blood-pressure.
5 Bilateral renal vein renin assay.
6 Renal blood flow.

There is controversy about the value of these tests. If there is advanced renal impairment their usefulness is further diminished.

Once the decision has been made to investigate a patient, the first step is to define the anatomy of the renal arteries. Intravenous digital subtraction angiography is a newer technique than conventional arteriography but the quality of images is insufficient adequately to delineate ostial lesions. Aortography and selective catheterization of the renal arteries are necessary. Unfortunately, in atheromatous stenosis a catheter may cause dissection or thrombotic occlusion. Selective arteriography may detect branch vessel disease. Whilst still in the X-ray department, percutaneous transluminal angioplasty can be performed.

Divided renal vein renin studies have been used to predict the value of revascularization. The results are conflicting and this is more evident in patients with renal failure.

The decision to revascularize a kidney in combined renal failure and renal artery stenosis should be based on the following criteria:

1 Satisfactory general condition of the patient.
2 Need to control blood-pressure, preserve renal function or both.
3 The presence of viable renal tissue (as assessed by isotope scanning).
4 Surgery or angioplasty technically feasible. Some of the difficulties are emphasized in the case discussed below.

Case history

A male aged 62 years had presented at the age of 56 with a blood-pressure of 160/100 mmHg. Blood urea at that time was 8.6 mmol/L. Serum creatinine was not measured. Treatment began with methyldopa and a diuretic. Four years later, he pressure was 220/110 whilst taking atenolol 100 mg daily, cyclopenthiazide 0.25 mg daily, hydralazine 25 mg tds and a potassium supplement. Plasma urea was 11.2 mmol/L. A year later he presented with accelerated-phase hypertension. His blood-pressure was eventually controlled with labetalol 1200 mg daily, navidrex K and hydralazine 25 mg tds. The blood urea had risen to 22 mmol/L. Six months later he presented in pulmonary oedema, despite frusemide. He was treated with increasing doses of captopril (up to 100 mg tds) but rapid deterioration in renal function occurred (plasma urea 40 mmol/L, serum creatinine 500 μmol/L). The dose of captopril was reduced but renal function did not substantially improve.

He was referred for further investigation with fluid retention, papilloedema and a blood-pressure of 190/135. He was taking methyldopa 500 mg qds and frusemide 200 mg daily. Investigations showed plasma urea 38.5 mmol/L, serum creatinine 352 μmol/L, creatinine clearance 11 ml/min and severe left ventricular hypertrophy on electrocardiography; chest X-ray showed an enlarged heart and pulmonary oedema. Arteriography showed an occluded right renal artery and a tight stenosis of the left. Renal function deteriorated further after arteriography; haemodialysis became necessary. The right kidney was revascularized by endarterectomy and end-to-side vein graft, using the gastroduodenal artery. Dialysis was needed for 2 weeks postoperatively.

Four weeks later, he was discharged with a pressure of 160/100, taking hydralazine 50 mg daily and frusemide to control his heart failure. Serum creatinine was 215 μmol/L and clearance 25 ml/min. Renal function and blood-pressure remained stable but he died 3 months later of cardiac failure after a myocardial infarction.

This case illustrates several points:

1 Early investigation of this man would have led to a diagnosis and radiological or surgical correction.
2 Renal failure probably would not have occurred.

3 Adequate treatment of his blood-pressure alone probably would have avoided hypertensive heart failure.
4 Revascularization of a kidney helps in blood-pressure control and improvement in renal function.
5 Angiotensin-converting enzyme inhibitors cause deterioration in function in renal artery stenosis (see p. 195).
6 The clue which should have prompted investigation in the first years was the raised plasma urea disproportionate to the patient's blood-pressure.

Treatment of hypertension in patients with chronic renal failure

Reducing blood-pressure in patients with CRF must be achieved with the minimum of side-effects. Over-vigorous (particularly intravenous) treatment may cause reduced renal perfusion and deterioration in renal function, which may be irrecoverable. It is not possible to predict which patients will respond in this way but use of diuretics in those susceptible to excess urinary sodium loss is most likely to lead to difficulties. Blood-pressure control is more difficult in those with glomerular lesions, particularly glomerulosclerosis. Patients with accelerated-phase hypertension may give cause for concern as renal function may deteriorate rapidly when hypotensive therapy is begun. It is not clear if this is a consequence of the hypertension or of over-vigorous treatment. If blood-pressure cannot be controlled adequately with drugs, an underlying cause such as renal artery stenosis should be excluded. Other causes of secondary hypertension rarely cause severe renal failure but should be considered in mild to moderate renal impairment.

A stepwise approach to treatment is used, as in other patients with hypertension; drugs with differing actions in combination will ususally prove satisfactory.

Diuretics

Thiazides

Thiazides are useful in mild to moderate renal failure but are less effective when clearance falls below 20 ml/min. They act by increasing sodium and water excretion, with an additional direct effect on arterioles, producing vasodilatation. Metolazone, which is often classified as a thiazide but has a different structure, is effective when the clearance is below 20 ml/min.

Hyperuricaemia is common in renal failure and may be exacerbated with diuretics. Allopurinol is indicated if gout or uric acid stones occur. Treatment of asymptomatic hyperuricaemia is controversial because there is no clear evidence that it produces benefit. Side-effects of thiazides, such as impotence, hyperglycaemia or hypercalcaemia, may necessitate stopping the drug.

Loop diuretics

Frusemide and bumetanide are effective at very low levels of renal function. They are particularly useful in patients with fluid retention. Large intravenous doses (up to 500 mg of frusemide) may be needed, but deafness may occur if they are infused too rapidly. The use of loop diuretics in CRF is discussed further on p. 322.

Beta-blockers

Besides the usual precautions in using β-blockers, the effects on renal perfusion should be considered. Propranolol probably reduces perfusion; atenolol, metoprolol, acebutalol and pindolol have little effect and nadolol may improve renal blood flow. If renal function is monitored during treatment, all are safe, as any deterioration is reversible. Labetalol, an α- and β-blocker, can be used in renal failure. It is particularly useful in the emergency treatment of hypertension, when it can be given intravenously (initial dose 50 mg and repeated to 200 mg until desired effect is achieved) or by continuous infusion.

Vasodilators

Vasodilators are used in a similar fashion whatever the cause of hypertension and therefore primarily as second-line drugs, although prazosin is often used on its own. The vasodilators may enhance renal blood flow. There are no special precautions with regard to dose, which is titrated against the desired hypotensive effect.

Doxazosin

Doxazosin is a new α-blocker with fewer side-effects than prazosin. Tachyphylaxis does not occur. The starting dose is 1 mg daily increasing to a maximum of 16 mg daily. No dose adjustment is needed in renal failure.

Minoxidil

Minoxidil is the most powerful vasodilator: it acts on arterioles. It may be particularly useful in renal failure, as there are reports of a beneficial effect on renal function, presumably by an effect on increased renal perfusion. Reflex tachycardia and severe sodium retention occur; the drug should be combined with a loop diuretic and a β-blocker. Reversible hirsutism occurs, which may be unacceptable in women. Depilatory creams may be needed. The dose of minoxidil is 5 mg once a day, rising to a maximum of 50 mg daily.

Calcium antagonists

Nifedipine and verapamil can both be used, but experience with the former in hypertension is more extensive. They are used in all forms of hypertension, either as first-line therapy or in combination with other drugs. There appear to be no special precautions in renal failure. They act by producing vasodilatation. Slow-release nifedipine is well tolerated, although it can produce headaches, flushing, fluid retention or nocturia. It has no deleterious effects on renal perfusion. Nifedipine is sometimes given to lower blood-pressure acutely, either as a capsule swallowed whole or broken up and held sublingually, when absorption is more rapid. Here, the rate of fall of blood-pressure may be very prompt. The dose of the slow-release preparation is 10–40 mg twice daily. A single daily dose preparation of nifedipine has recently been marketed.

Angiotensin-converting enzyme inhibitors

High circulating concentrations of angiotensin II may be found in association with chronic renal disease: the rationale for the use of ACEI is clear. In renovascular hypertension, ACEIs have been used both as investigative tools and in treatment. Careful monitoring of renal function is needed in these patients because these drugs may produce a deterioration in renal function in patients with a solitary functioning kidney (including transplanted kidneys) and in bilateral renal artery stenosis. This is particularly important with the concomitant use of diuretics, as glomerular filtration is even more dependent upon intrarenal concentration of angiotensin II. It is necessary to measure renal function in all hypertensives receiving ACEI, because the diagnosis of renovascular hypertension may have been overlooked (see case history, p. 218).

Plasma potassium may rise with ACEI because of the lack of effect of angiotensin II on aldosterone release. Captopril and enalapril are well tolerated and lisinopril perhaps even better.

Proteinuria has been reported: it appears to be transitory, although nephrotic-range proteinuria has been seen with captopril, in association with membranous and interstitial nephritis.

The dose should be low to start with, and built up until the desired antihypertensive effect is achieved: captopril 6.25 mg bd rising to 50 mg tds; enalapril 2.5 mg to 25 mg daily; lisinopril 2.5 mg to 20 mg daily in a single dose. There are now many 'me-too' ACEIs on the market, but it is far from clear if they have advantages over the three mentioned above.

Choice of hypotensive agents

With the large number of effective compounds available, it is preferable to prescribe a relatively small number of hypotensive agents and thus become highly proficient in their use. Table 15.2 represents a personal choice of drugs which are effective at differing degrees of chronic renal

Table 15.2 Choice of hypotensive drugs for patients with hypertension and chronic renal failure. Loop diuretics are required as clearance falls

Blood-pressure	Drug
>160/95–105	Single agent: nifedipine ACEI β-blocker
If no response after dose increase	Add a thiazide
If diastolic still 105–120	Use two agents: nifedipine ACEI
If no response after dose increase	Add high-dose loop diuretic
If diastolic still >120	Use three drugs: minoxidil 5–50 mg atenolol 50 mg frusemide 250–500 mg

impairment. Dose reduction in the presence of renal failure is necessary for β-blockers and ACEIs. Conversely, the dose of bumetanide or frusemide should be substantially increased, which has the advantage of rendering the patient normokalaemic or slightly hypokalaemic.

Within renal medicine, calcium channel-blockers and ACEI are now used as first-line hypotensive drugs. Whether anti-angiotensin agents will prove effective in the hypertensive patient with renal failure has yet to be established. The use of ACEIs in diabetics with renal failure is discussed on pp. 195–6.

Summary

Hypertension is common in renal failure from whatever cause. Conversely, renal disease accounts for a small but important percentage of patients with hypertension. Recognition of such patients is necessary because there may be remediable causes such as renal artery stenosis or obstruction to the urinary tract. Early renal disease may be identified and correct management started.

Every hypertensive patient should, at presentation, have the urine examined for protein and blood and have serum creatinine and plasma electrolytes measured. This will demonstrate the majority of patients with renal parenchymal disease. The diagnosis of renal artery stenosis may be suspected from the history and presentation, but an arteriogram is the only method which definitely excludes the diagnosis.

Hypertension is an important cause of vascular morbidity in renal failure, and blood-pressure control is essential. A balance is needed between adequate control and renal perfusion. Hypotensive drugs should be prescribed as in other forms of hypertension. Loop diuretics rather than thiazides are needed when the glomerular filtration rate falls. Angiotensin-converting enzyme inhibitors or calcium channel-blocking drugs are particularly useful in the presence of renal failure.

Further reading

1 Brazy, P.C., Stead, W.W. & Fitzwilliam, J.F. (1989) Progression of renal insufficiency: role of blood pressure. *Kidney Int.* **35**, 661–9.
2 Brown, J.J., Davies, D.L., Morton, J.J. *et al.* (1976) Mechanisms of renal hypertension. *Lancet* **i**, 1219–21.
3 Carmichael, D.J.S., Mathias, C.J., Snell, M.E. & Peart, S. (1986) Detection and investigation of renal artery stenosis. *Lancet* **i**, 667–70.
4 Curtis, J.R. (1990) Interventions in chronic renal failure. *Br. Med. J.* **301**, 622–4.
5 Editorial (1991) Hypertensive emergencies. *Lancet* **338**, 220–1.
6 Fukuoha, K.A. *et al.* (eds) (1990) ACE inhibitors and the kidney. *Nephron* **55** (suppl. 1), 1–59.
7 Kelleher, C.C. (1990) ACE inhibitors in the prevention and therapy of diabetic nephropathy: what is their role? *Drugs* **39**, 639–45.
8 McKinney, T.D. & Stein, J.H. (1992) Management of hypertensive crises. *Hosp. Practice* **27**, 228–36.
9 Mathias, C.J., May, C.N. & Taylor, G.M. (1984) The renin–angiotensin system and hypertension – basic and clinical aspects. In Malcolm, A.D.B. (ed.), *Molecular Medicine.* IRL Press, Oxford, pp. 178–208.
10 McKinney, T.D. & Stein, J.H. (1992) Management of hypertensive crises. *Hosp. Practice* **27**, 228–36.
11 Peart, W.S. (1977) The kidney as an endocrine organ. *Lancet* **ii**, 543–8.
12 Ravine, D., Walker, R.G., Gibson, R.N. *et al.* (1991) Treatable complications in undiagnosed cases of autosomal dominant polycystic disease. *Lancet* **337**, 127–9.
13 Salusky, J.G., Foley, J., Nelson, P. & Goodman, W.G. (1991) Aluminium accumulation during treatment with aluminium hydroxide. *N. Engl. J. Med.* **324**, 527–31.
14 Schmitt, J. (1991) Selecting an appropriate phosphate binder. *J. Renal Nutrition* **1**, 38–40.
15 Scoble, J.E. & Hamilton, G. (1990) Atherosclerotic renovascular disease. *Br. Med. J.* **300**, 1670–1.
16 Siampolous, K., Sellars, L., Mishra, S.C. *et al.* (1983) Experience in the management of hypertension with unilateral chronic pyelonephritis: results of nephrectomy in selected cases. *Quart. J. Med.* **52**, 349–62.
17 Taverner, D., Bing, R.F., Heagerty, A. *et al.* (1983) Improvement of renal function during long-term treatment of severe hypertension with minoxidil. *Quart. J. Med.* **52**, 280–7.
18 Ying, C.Y., Tifft, C.P., Gavias, H. & Chobanian, A.V. (1984) Renal revascularization in the azoetemic hypertensive patient resistant to therapy. *N. Engl. J. Med.* **311**, 1070–5.

Chapter 16
Management of Acute Renal Failure

Ken Farrington

Acute renal failure (ARF) is often clinically dramatic at onset and has a very high mortality. Acute tubular necrosis (ATN) is the commonest histology in ARF. This will heal spontaneously if the patient can be kept alive and the cause of the ARF diagnosed and successfully treated. Infection is the major cause of ARF and unfortunately it is often impossible to eradicate the sepsis. This is the chief reason for the high mortality. This chapter reviews management of ARF, with particular emphasis on initial assessment, treatment of emergencies and other aspects which are important for a non-specialist.

Acute renal failure is a reversible syndrome characterized by an abrupt decline of previously normal renal function, causing retention of nitrogenous waste products. Potential reversibility is the main distinction between ARF and chronic renal failure. When an acute and potentially reversible deterioration of renal function occurs in a patient with pre-existing renal impairment, this is known as acute-on-chronic renal failure.

Aetiology of acute renal failure

Acute renal failure has many causes, which are seen in almost any branch of medicine. Causes are divided into three groups:

1 Prerenal – renal hypoperfusion.
2 Intrinsic renal – renal parenchymal damage or dysfunction.
3 Postrenal – acute obstruction to the flow of urine.

Prerenal causes

In health, autoregulatory mechanisms ensure stable renal blood flow and glomerular filtration rate (GFR) over a wide range of perfusion pressures. Prolonged hypoperfusion can overwhelm autoregulation, which results in a marked loss of GFR and retention of waste products. Prompt correction of hypoperfusion rapidly restores normal renal function, but if correction is too late, or inadequate, ARF develops. The chance of ARF developing may be increased by prior injection of non-steroidal anti-inflammatory drugs (NSAIDs) or angiotensin converting agents (ACEIs).

Intrinsic renal causes

There are a wide range of intrinsic renal causes, as shown in Table 16.1, with an accordingly broad range of clinical features. ATN is most commonly a result of medullary ischaemia or a nephrotoxin. Myoglobinuria due to skeletal muscle necrosis (rhabdomyolysis) is now detected relatively frequently in patients with ATN. The causes of rhabdomyolysis are shown in Table 16.2

Kidneys are susceptible to damage by drugs. There are a large number of drugs and poisons that may precipitate ARF (Table 16.3). The most common nephrotoxins include NSAIDs, gentamicin, paracetamol in overdose and radiographic contrast. Acute drug-related interstitial nephritis may present as ARF: the diagnosis is made by renal biopsy.

It is important to diagnose the primary parenchymal disorders early because treatment is different. This has been discussed in Chapter 11, p. 172.

Postrenal causes

An accurate diagnosis is essential because often specific surgical treatment is required, which may be curative. Obstruction to the urinary tract typically produces anuria if the urethra or both ureters are involved. Nevertheless, clinically important obstruction to ureters or urethra or both may be associated with normal, supranormal or an intermittent flow of urine. Reference has already been made to the dangers of combined obstruction and infection in the renal tract (Chapter 8, p. 116). Prostatic hypertrophy, pelvic tumours, stones and surgical damage to ureters are the most common causes of postrenal ARF.

Table 16.1 Major causes of acute renal failure

Cause	Examples
Prerenal	
Hypovolaemia	Haemorrhage, severe burns, gastrointestinal losses
Decreased cardiac output	Cardiac failure, cardiac surgery
Septicaemic shock	Gram-negative septicaemia, meningococcal septicaemia
Renal artery occlusion	Cross-clamping during aortic surgery, dissection, renal artery thrombosis
Drugs causing reduction in renal blood flow	See Table 16.3, p. 228
Intrinsic renal	
Vascular	Vasculitides, scleroderma, malignant hypertension, eclampsia, haemolytic uraemic syndrome, thrombotic thrombocytopenia purpura, disseminated intravascular coagulation
Glomerular Tubulointerstitial	Rapidly progressive glomerulonephritis
ATN	
Ischaemia	Prolonged prerenal insults
Toxins	Endogenous: myoglobinuria, haemoglobinuria, Bence-Jones proteinuria
	Exogenous: see Table 16.3, p. 228
Acute interstitial nephritis	Drugs: see Table 16.3, p. 228
	Infections: acute bacterial interstitial nephritis, associated with systemic infection, such as: streptoccoccal, leptospiral, EB virus, *Mycoplasma* pneumonia, *Legionella pneumophilia* pneumonia
Postrenal	
Intratubular crystal formation	Drugs and toxins: see Table 16.3, p. 228
Extrarenal obstruction	Prostatic hypertrophy, pelvic tumours, retroperitoneal fibrosis, stones, papillary necrosis

EB, Epstein–Barr.

Incidence of acute renal failure

The incidence of ARF varies with the clinical setting. Overall, about 50 cases occur annually per million population. Among general medical and surgical patients, the incidence is about 1% of hospital admissions, whilst after major surgery – open heart surgery or major trauma – the incidence rises to 2–5%. In intensive care units, the incidence increases to 15–25%. The spectrum of causes of ARF also varies. After major surgery and in the intensive care unit, ATN due to prerenal and nephrotoxic factors accounts for almost all. In the majority, more than

Table 16.2 Causes of rhabdomyolysis

Trauma	Crush syndrome Extensive burns Extreme exertion Status epilepticus Tetanus
Ischaemia	Aortic aneurysm surgery Leg emboli
Inflammatory	Many infections Polymyositis
Toxic and metabolic	Prolonged coma (especially drug-induced) Carbon monoxide poisoning Severe hypophosphataemia Severe hypokalaemia
Myopathies	Alcoholic Drug-induced (E-aminocaproic acid) Malignant hyperpyrexia Inherited disorders, e.g. carnitine parmityl transferase deficiency

one specific insult can be found. On general wards, the spectrum is more heterogeneous and, although ATN predominates, the aetiology is frequently multifactorial (Fig. 16.1).

Pathogenesis of acute tubular necrosis

The pathogenesis of ATN is complex and not yet fully understood. Oxygen tension in the renal medulla is low, such that this metabolically active site is always relatively anoxic and especially the thick ascending limbs. Thus, when a kidney becomes under-perfused, the medulla suffers disproportionately in comparison with the cortex, and ATN develops in the distal convoluted tubules and the thick ascending limbs of the loops of Henle. Oliguria rapidly develops and GFR falls.

Natural history of acute renal failure

In the majority of patients in whom ARF is due to ATN, the natural history can be described in three phases: the initiating phase, the established (or oliguric) phase and the recovery (or diuretic) phase. In those with primary parenchymal renal disease or obstructive uropathy, the course of the illness is determined by the nature and severity of the underlying process and the effectiveness of treatment.

Initiating phase

In the initiating phase, the kidneys are usually severely under-perfused. Initially, renal autoregulatory mechanisms preserve the GFR and tubular

Table 16.3 Nephrotoxins and acute renal failure

Mechanism	Agents
Diminished renal blood flow	Non-steroidal anti-inflammatory agents Angiotensin-converting enzyme inhibitors Cyclosporin
Direct tubular toxicity (inducing ATN)	Aminoglycoside antibiotics Paracetamol overdose Amphotericin B Polmyxins and colistin Cisplatin Heavy metals Carbon tetrachloride
Acute interstitial nephritis	Non-steroidal anti-inflammatory agents β-Lactam antibiotics Other antibiotics: sulphonamides, rifampicin Diuretics: thiazides, frusemide, ethacrynic acid Miscellaneous: captopril, allopurinol, cimetidine, phenindione, sulphinpyrazone, phenytoin, PAS, carbamazepine, clofibrate, azathioprine, phenylpropanolamine, phenobarbitone
Intratubular crystal deposition	Chemotherapeutic agents (urate) Ethylene glycol (oxalate) Methoxyflurane (oxalate) Sulphonamide (crystals of the drug)
Antianabolic	Tetracyclines
Hypercalcaemia or nephrocalcinosis	Vitamin D intoxication
Unknown mechanisms	Radiographic contrast agents

PAS, Para-aminosalicylic acid.

function. A low volume of concentrated urine is produced. A diuresis may be achieved by rapid restoration of effective circulating volume. If renal ischaemia persists, structural damage to tubular cells occurs and is not immediately reversible by restitution of a normal perfusion pressure. Tubules become incapable of modifying glomerular filtrate. The urine produced resembles an ultrafiltrate of plasma in terms of the concentrations of its constituents. At this stage, ARF (ATN) is said to be established. The length of the initiating phase is variable but is usually less than 24 hours. The borderline between the prerenal, still salvageable, phase and established ATN is often indistinct, and therapeutic efforts may by successful in the ill-defined zone between the two phases.

Phase of established acute tubular necrosis

Many patients with established ATN are oliguric (urine volumes less than 400 ml daily), but non-oliguric ATN is increasingly recognized

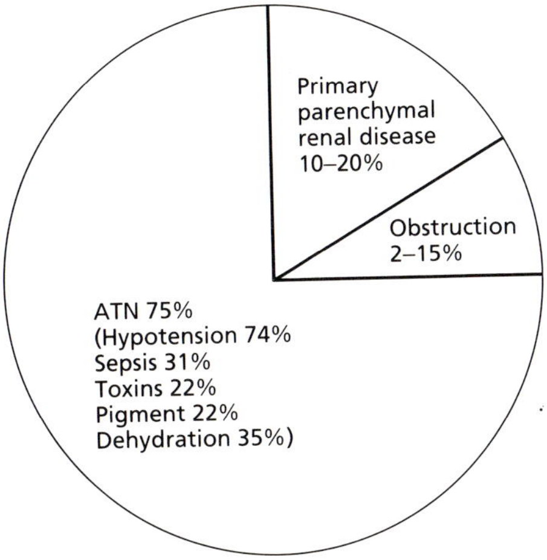

Fig. 16.1 Clinical spectrum of ARF in an adult general medical and surgical population. Factors contributing to development of ATN are shown in parentheses. Note that these figures total >100%, implying that the aetiology of ATN is frequently multifactorial.

and may account for 30–50% of cases. Aetiological factors are similar in both forms of ATN, although nephrotoxins appear to predispose to non-oliguric ATN. Generally, the severity of the precipitating insult and the extent of renal damage is less in non-oliguric ATN, perhaps with up to 10% of nephrons remaining normally functioning, compared with less than 1% in oliguric patients. The duration of established ATN varies from a few days to about 60 days. Persisting or recurrent insults may extend it further. The duration of non-oliguric ATN is usually less than that of the oliguric variety.

Recovery phase

Return of function in oliguric patients is usually heralded by a gradual increase in urine volume. Massive diuresis, once common, is now infrequent because of better fluid balance. Tubular concentrating ability lags behind the recovery of urine volume by a number of days, but is the first sign of improvement in non-oliguric patients. Subsequently, GFR improves over a number of weeks. Follow-up studies years after an episode of ATN indicate that recovery is often incomplete, with persisting minor impairment in GFR and defects of tubular function. Occasionally, and particularly after prolonged episodes of oliguria, GFR may be substantially impaired, due to patchy cortical necrosis.

Diagnosis and management of acute renal failure

The clinical state of patients presenting with ARF ranges from the apparently normal, in whom the condition has been detected biochemically, to the gravely ill, in whom the abnormality is part of a disorder involving the failure of many organs. At diagnosis, the degree of uraemia may be trivial or the patient may be moribund. The crucial first step is a careful clinical assessment, accompanied by preliminary investigations to identify life-threatening conditions requiring emergency action (Fig. 16.2). Only after such conditions have been excluded or treated and the patient's condition rendered safe should other investigations continue.

Shock must be vigorously treated and central venous pressure (CVP) monitoring is essential. Factors precipitating cardiac insufficiency, such as arrythmias, should be corrected urgently. Infections require appropriate intravenous antibiotics and full supportive measures. Drainage of pus is delayed only for resuscitation or dialysis for hyperkalaemia,

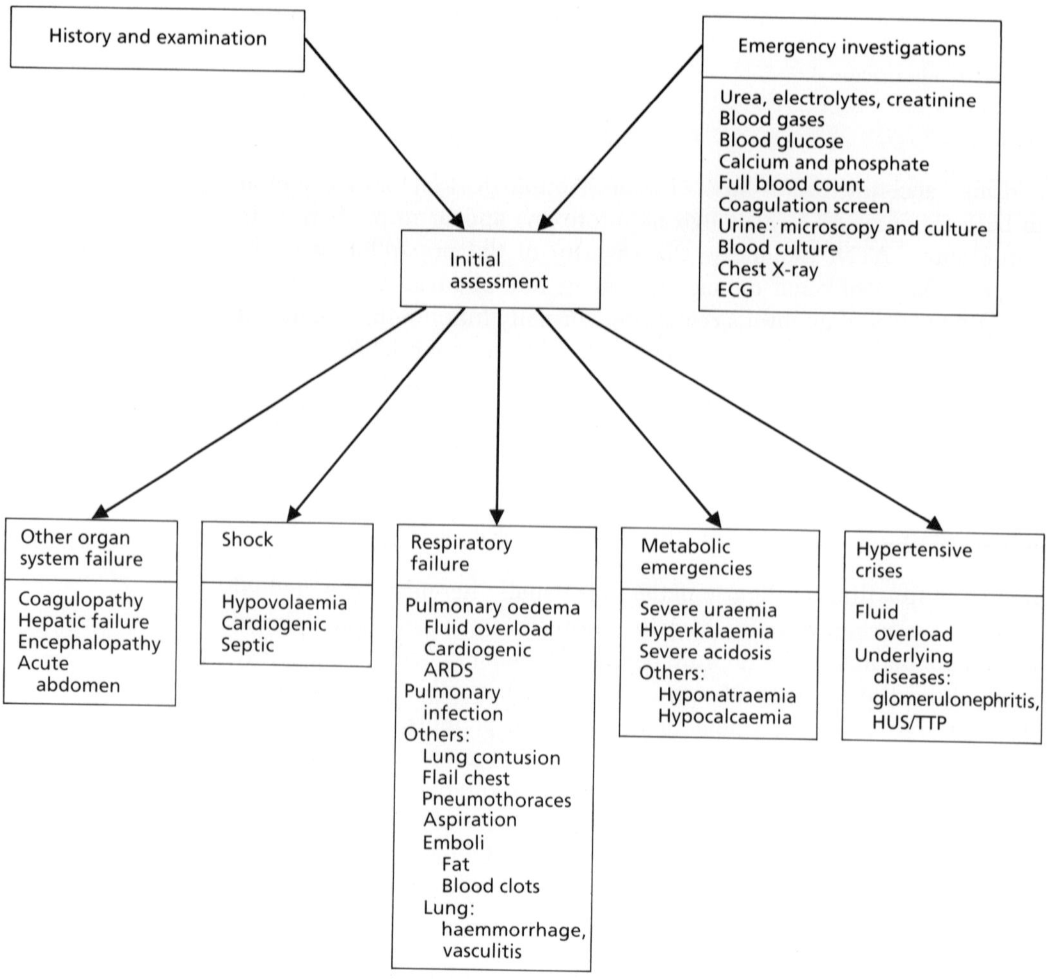

Fig. 16.2 Diagnostic steps, urgent investigations and major complications of acute renal failure. ARDS, Adult respiratory distress syndrome; HUS, haemolytic uraemic syndrome; TTP, thrombotic thrombocytopenic purpura.

uraemia or fluid overload. Other common complications occurring in acutely ill patients with ARF are respiratory failure and coagulopathies. Accelerated-phase hypertension accompanying ARF is usually associated with primary parenchymal renal disease.

Management of acute renal failure, phase I: emergencies

This section will discuss the following steps, all or many of which may need to be instituted in the first hours of active management:

1 Hyperkalaemia.
2 Severe uraemia.
3 Acidosis.
4 Coagulation defects.
5 Respiratory failure.
6 Severe hypertension.

Hyperkalaemia

Hyperkalaemia may cause a cardiac arrest in ventricular fibrillation or asystole and thus requires urgent treatment. A rising plasma potassium concentration produces sequential electrocardiogram (ECG) changes (Table 16.4) but the ECG may not show these features in hyperkalaemia. Two factors are important in assessing plasma potassium concentrations:

1 The current plasma potassium figure.
2 The anticipated rate of rise.

All plasma potassium concentrations above 6 mmol/L need action. In patients who are severely hypercatabolic, in those with extensive rhabdomyolysis, intravascular haemolysis or tumour lysis or in shocked patients with rapidly developing acidosis, lower concentrations should not be set aside because the plasma potassium may rise to a dangerous concentration within hours. Rhabdomyolysis and tumour lysis are particularly dangerous conditions, because the combination of hyperkalaemia and hypocalcaemia is cardiotoxic.

The treatment required depends upon projected risk. In patients with the ECG changes of hyperkalaemia (potassium concentration is usually >7.0 mmol/L), the following measures are suggested:

1 Calcium. Intravenous calcium acts by antagonizing the membrane effects of potassium. It has no effect on plasma potassium concentration. Ten millilitres of 10% calcium gluconate is given over a few minutes. If

Table 16.4 Electrocardiographic changes of hyperkalaemia

Tall peaked T waves
Diminution in amplitude of R wave
Widening of QRS complex
Merging of QRS complex with T wave
Diminution and disappearance of P wave

ECG changes are not reversed, further doses may be necessary. Its protective effect only lasts 30–60 min.

2 Glucose and insulin. Insulin lowers extracellular potassium by increasing cellular uptake of potassium (predominantly into muscle cells). Glucose infusion prevents hypoglycaemia. Fifty millilitres of 50% glucose plus 10 units of soluble insulin are given together as a bolus into a large vein. The doses should by doubled if plasma potassium is >7.0 mol/L. Maximal reduction of the plasma potassium occurs at about 1–2 hours. The electrolyte should be remeasured at this time. Hypoglycaemia is a risk; blood glucose should be monitored hourly. The duration of the hypokalaemic effect is 4–6 hours. If dialysis has not been started by this time, further amounts of glucose and insulin are given, the doses being changed according to the initial response.

3 Sodium bicarbonate. In the presence of acidosis, and providing the patient has no signs of fluid overload or pulmonary oedema, a 50 ml bolus of 8.4% sodium bicarbonate may be given over a 5–10 min period. The potassium-lowering effect is due to intracellular shift of potassium.

4 Definitive measures to remove potassium from the body.

The above treatments are interim measures which only serve to buy time to allow the institution of definitive treatment to remove potassium. In some circumstances, it may be possible to initiate a diuresis by high-dose diuretics. If a urine output of 100–200 ml/hour can be obtained, plasma potassium can usually be controlled with little difficulty. Attempts to provoke diuresis are usually futile in patients with oliguria longer than 24 hours, in whom the respite obtained by interim measures is best used in preparation for dialysis.

In patients with severe hyperkalaemia (>7 mmol/L) without ECG changes, or in patients with lower concentrations in whom it is expected to rise quickly, the above measures may be used, with the exception of intravenous calcium. In more stable patients with lower plasma potassium concentrations, cation-exchange resins are of value. These may also be used as adjuncts in the treatment of severe hyperkalaemia. Resonium A (not used in volume-overloaded patients because the sodium is the exchangeable cation) and Calcium Resonium may be used rectally in doses of 15–30 g up to four times daily. The onset of a hypokalaemic effect is relatively slow (4–6 hours). Oral lactulose or sorbitol to induce diarrhoea may augment gut losses of potassium and increase the effectiveness of oral resins.

Severe uraemia

Patients with ARF may be severely uraemic at presentation, often with hyperkalaemia and acidosis. Urgent dialysis is required. Other complications of severe uraemia, such as disturbances of conscious level, fits, coma and pericardial effusion, are uncommon. When present, they constitute indications for urgent dialysis. In the absence of accompanying features, a precise concentration of blood urea at which dialysis is required is difficult to define, but a blood urea of 40 mmol/L should usually be promptly reduced by dialysis.

Metabolic acidosis

Severe metabolic acidosis affects many organs, particularly the cardiovascular system. It has a negative inotropic effect, blunting responses to inotropic agents, it causes arteriolar dilatation with venoconstriction and it lowers the threshold for ventricular fibrillation.

If arterial pH falls below 7.2 or plasma bicarbonate below 12 mmol/L, intravenous sodium bicarbonate may be given, but fluid overload is a risk. For every 50 mmol of bicarbonate, an equal sodium load occurs. This is equivalent to the expansion of the extracellular fluid volume by about 350 ml per 50 ml of sodium bicarbonate. This treatment is appropriate in patients in whom a diuresis can be obtained, but caution is required in patients with oliguria, even in the absence of signs of fluid overload. The arterial pH should not be restored to normal. A bolus of 50 mmol of sodium bicarbonate should be given over 10–15 min and then artèrial pH and bicarbonate should be remeasured. A further bolus can be given, if necessary, to return the pH to about 7.2, provided that the haemodynamic condition of the patient remains stable. Relatively few patients with ARF and this degree of acidosis are suitable for bicarbonate therapy. Most require urgent dialysis.

Coagulation defects

The major disturbance encountered in ARF is disseminated intravascular coagulation (DIC). When the underlying cause is not readily reversible and the disturbances are severe – elevation of prothrombin time, partial thromboplastin time and thrombin time greater than three times normal with a platelet count $<40 \times 10^9$ per litre, particularly in the presence of bleeding manifestations – supportive therapy with fresh frozen plasma (FFP) and platelet transfusion is indicated. Three units of FFP (a typical dose) constitute a volume of about 1 L. Volume considerations may be unimportant in patients with uncontrollable bleeding but may be crucial in patients with ARF and incipient pulmonary oedema. If such therapy is necessary, a strong argument exists for the institution of early dialysis or haemofiltration to 'make space' for blood products. The role of low-dose heparin infusion in the treatment of DIC is controversial. Its use should be considered in patients in whom a reasonable attempt at supportive therapy has had no effect on laboratory variables.

Patients with ARF may have a bleeding tendency due to acquired platelet dysfunction, as shown by a prolonged bleeding time. Von Willebrand's complex (synthesized by endothelial cells and essential for normal platelet function) may be abnormal in uraemia. Cryoprecipitate and intravenous desmopressin (DDAVP) have both been shown to reduce the abnormal bleeding time in ARF. Uraemic patients with prolonged bleeding times in the absence of other disturbances of coagulation, who have bleeding complications, or who are about to undergo surgery or renal biopsy should receive either cryoprecipitate (10–20 packs) or an infusion of DDAVP (0.3 μg per kg in a 100 ml of normal saline over 30 min).

Respiratory failure

The combination of renal and respiratory failure is increasingly common; up to 40% of patients with postsurgical ARF may also have acute respiratory failure. There are many possible causes (see Fig. 16.2), but it is commonly associated with pulmonary oedema. This may be due to severe fluid overload with normal cardiac function, or lesser degrees of fluid overload in patients with pre-existing cardiorespiratory disease. Profound sepsis produces myocardial depression. Non-cardiogenic pulmonary oedema (adult respiratory distress syndrome (ARDS)) is a common consequence of many of the insults which also produce ARF (Table 16.5).

Management of pulmonary oedema in fluid-overloaded patients with adequate cardiac function and adequate blood-pressure depends on the capacity of injured kidneys to excrete water. If a diuresis of 100–200 ml/hour is not obtained after incremental doses of diuretics – up to 10 mg intravenous bolus of bumetanide or frusemide 500 mg infused over 1–2 hours – dialysis or arteriovenous haemofiltration is required urgently. Diuretics are useless in severely hypotensive patients with pulmonary oedema in whom inotropic support is necessary. It is reasonable to begin with a low dose of dopamine (up to 4 μg/kg/min), which enhances renal blood flow by an action on renal dopamine receptors. Incremental doses of dobutamine (2.5–20 μg/kg/min) may be added. If adequate blood-pressure (90–100 mmHg systolic) is not achieved, higher doses of both inotropes are necessary. Diuretics may be effective once blood-pressure has been restored but, in the absence of a diuresis, dialysis is urgently required.

Table 16.5 Common causes of adult respiratory distress syndrome

Pulmonary
Pneumonia
Aspiration of gastric contents
Lung trauma
Inhaled toxins
Non-pulmonary
Shock of any aetiology
Gram-negative sepsis
Pancreatitis
Fat emboli
Non-thoracic trauma
Disseminated intravascular coagulation
Drugs and toxins – opiates, barbiturates, Paraquat

The major pathophysiological change in ARDS is increased permeability of pulmonary capillaries, which leads to transudation of protein-rich fluid into lung interstitium and alveoli. Differentiation from cardiogenic pulmonary oedema may be difficult and classically depends on the demonstration of a normal pulmonary capillary wedge pressure (PCWP), which reflects a normal left atrial pressure. It should be noted that there is often little correlation between right and left atrial pressures in this condition. Clinical suspicion of ARDS is aroused by the findings of tachypnoea and hypoxia in a recognized clinical setting, especially during resuscitation procedures involving large volume infusions. These clinical features often precede X-ray changes by many hours.

Management of incipient and established ARDS in patients with suspected renal failure depends upon the following:

1 Vigorous measures to control the underlying cause (see Table 16.5).

2 Careful fluid management. Fluid therapy should be guided by measurements of PCWP, although in less than ideal circumstances it may only be possible to monitor right atrial pressure. The objective is to maintain systemic blood-pressure sufficiently to support the perfusion of vital organs, whilst keeping PCWP as low as possible to help resolution of pulmonary oedema. The use of low-dose dopamine, with or without dobutamine, at an early stage may be beneficial. This policy of 'running the patient dry' involves a careful balance between established ARF and worsening ARDS. Both may result, but the outcome may be successful in circumstances in which the underlying disease process can be rapidly controlled. The relative merits of colloid and crystalloid solutions in this condition are still debated. It is common practice to resuscitate initially predominantly with colloid (preferably plasma protein fraction (PPF)). This is especially true in patients in whom the concentration of serum albumin is low. In patients with peripheral oedema, crystalloid solutions should be avoided and the PCWP maintained with PPF.

3 Ensuring adequate oxygenation. Oxygen therapy with a face mask may be sufficient but mechanical ventilation is often required. Positive end-expiratory pressure (PEEP) of 2–10 cm may avoid the need for high concentrations of inspired oxygen. Oxygen toxicity may further aggravate injured alveolar–capillary membrane, although PEEP frequently causes a drop in cardiac output.

4 Steroids. The use of steroids in ARDS is controversial because their efficacy is unproved.

Severe hypertension

The commonest cause of hypertension in ARF is fluid overload, although it may also be caused by the underlying disease process. Severe hypertension (usually diastolic greater than 130 mmHg, with or without retinal changes) in ARF requires urgent treatment. In patients who do not require acute dialysis, therapy should be begun with slow-release nifedipine 10–20 mg two or three times daily. A more potent regimen is minoxidil and 50 mg of atenolol daily. Doses are adjusted to achieve control over a 48-hour period.

Patients with hypertensive encephalopathy, deteriorating vision or microangiopathic haemolytic anaemia require parenteral antihypertensive therapy. Sodium nitroprusside infusion, starting at 0.5 μg/kg/min and increasing by similar increments until control is obtained (maximum dose 8 μg/kg/min), gives good control. Its very short duration of action confers the great advantage that hypotension can be corrected in minutes, by reducing infusion rate. Volume considerations and the possibility of cyanide toxicity prevent prolonged use of high-dose infusions in patients with ARF. An alternative is labetolol (200 mg in 200 ml 5% dextrose), administered at a rate of 2 mg/min until control is achieved. The hypotensive effect lasts 16–18 hours. Diazoxide may be given as intermittent small boluses of 25 mg every 5–15 min. Its duration of action is 3–18 hours. Hydrallazine may be given intramuscularly or intravenously in a dose of 10–20 mg. The hypotensive effect lasts 3–8 hours. Both diazoxide and hydrallazine may produce reflex tachycardia. Whatever agent is chosen, overlapping oral therapy should be started as soon as possible.

Severely hypertensive, fluid-overloaded patients are often resistant to the effect of antihypertensive agents and, if a diuresis cannot be initiated with high-dose diuretics, dialysis is necessary. Prior treatment with antihypertensive drugs with prolonged actions may hinder fluid removal during dialysis. Under these circumstances, nitroprusside infusion has the advantage of rapid reversibility. Ideally, before nitroprusside is infused, the patient should be in an intensive care unit and have his/her blood-pressure measured via an intra-arterial line.

Management of acute renal failure, phase II: investigations

When a patient has presented in a stable condition or after initial emergency management has been undertaken to stabilize the patient's condition, the next phase of management consists of a logical attempt to find the cause of ARF. This is particularly aimed at identifying those patients who require early specific treatment. Four questions need to be answered:

1 Is there a reversible prerenal component?
2 Is there obstruction of the urinary tract?
3 Is there primary parenchymal renal disease?
4 Is there acute-on-chronic renal failure?

The approach is based on a careful history and clinical examination, together with specific investigations.

Is there a reversible prerenal component?

Persistent oliguria despite apparently adequate volume replacement may indicate the presence of established ATN or suggest continuing renal hypoperfusion. Microscopy of urinary sediment and biochemical assessment of urine may clarify matters. Poorly perfused, normally functioning kidneys produce concentrated urine with a low sodium concentration. In established ATN, urine biochemically resembles an ultrafiltrate of plasma and usually contains numerous granular casts and tubular cells. In practice, the two states may merge into each other (Table 16.6). Three points are to be made concerning the use of urinary indices:

1 They can only be applied to the assessment of oliguric patients who have not been treated with diuretics. Figures are uninterpretable:
 (a) in patients with normal urine volumes;
 (b) after diuretic treatment, even if oliguria is persistent.

2 A major reason for their introduction was the identification of patients with occult hypovolaemia. This is now more reliably achieved by measurement of the CVP.

3 The indices may predict the response to diuretic therapy. However, few would withhold careful fluid challenge or a trial of diuretic therapy, whatever the indices suggested.

The clinical value of these indices is limited and they are not often requested.

A practical scheme for the management of patients presenting with oliguric ARF and a potential prerenal component is outlined in Fig. 16.3. It is based on a clinical assessment of the state of hydration, usually supplemented by measurement of CVP. Hypovolaemia requires rapid correction by appropriate fluid administration, with CVP monitoring. This may be sufficient to induce a diuresis which leads to resolution of the renal condition or the emergence of non-oliguric ATN. If the patient remains oliguric, incremental intravenous doses of a

Table 16.6 Discrimination of hypoperfused normally functioning kidneys from established acute tubular necrosis by microscopy of sediment and urine biochemistry

	Hypoperfused normally functioning kidneys	Established ATN
Urinary sediment	Normal	Granular casts ++ Tubular cells ++
Urinary sodium	<20 mmol/L	>40 mmol/L
Fractional excretion of sodium (Fe_{Na^+})	<1	>1
Ratio $\frac{\text{urinary urea}}{\text{plasma urea}}$	>10	<3
Ratio $\frac{\text{urinary osmolality}}{\text{serum osmolality}}$	>1.5	<1.1

$$Fe_{Na^+} = \frac{\text{urinary sodium}}{\text{plasma sodium}} \times \frac{\text{serum creatinine}}{\text{urinary creatinine}} \times 100.$$

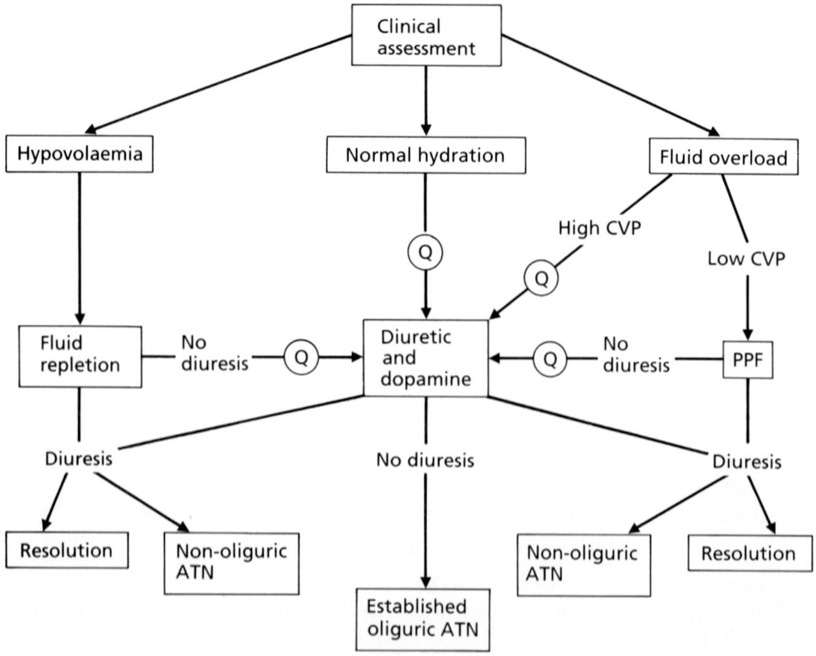

Fig. 16.3 Suggested protocol to detect and treat patients presenting with ARF who have a reversible prerenal component. Q indicates points at which assessment of urinary quality may reasonably be performed. PPF, Plasma protein fraction; CVP, central venous pressure.

loop diuretic or low-dose dopamine infusion, or both, may be tried to initiate a diuresis. The initial dose of diuretic should be low – bumetanide 2 mg or frusemide 80 mg. If this fails, higher doses may be successful – an intravenous bolus of 10 mg of bumetanide or frusemide 500 mg infused over 1–2 hours. Higher doses of frusemide should be infused slowly because rapid administration may result in deafness. Low-dose dopamine (up to 4 μg/kg/min) may also induce a diuresis. The same measures may be used in oliguric patients initially assessed as having a normal state of hydration, in fluid-overloaded patients with an initially elevated CVP and in fluid-overloaded patients with hypovolaemia (usually due to hypoalbuminaemia, caused by prolonged illness, liver disease or nephrotic syndrome) who remain oliguric after volume repletion. A diuresis may commence (more likely in patients with good-quality urine), which indicates resolution of a prerenal failure or the beginning of non-oliguric ATN, which may require additional doses of diuretic. Lack of a diuresis indicates established oliguric ATN and further doses of diuretics are not indicated.

Diuretics and low-dose dopamine infusions may thus prevent some patients with incipient ARF from entering the established phase. In some, renal function may quickly return to normal. Usually, non-oliguric ATN results, which may simplify management by reducing the likelihood of fluid overload and hyperkalaemia. Whether overall mortality is affected is not known.

Is there obstruction of the urinary tract?

The question of obstruction of the urinary tract should be specifically considered in all patients with ARF, irrespective of apparent aetiology. To miss obstruction may be fatal. The following steps are necessary.

Clinical assessment

Prostatic symptoms in males, previous surgery or radiotherapy for pelvic tumours or a history of stone disease suggests possible obstruction. Anuria is very suspicious. An enlarged tense bladder indicates prostatic enlargement, a blocked urethral catheter or urethral stricture. Rectal and vaginal examinations are essential because a pelvic tumour may be found.

Bladder catheterization

Bladder catheterization is important to exclude a distended bladder and confirm oliguria. If obstruction is excluded, the catheter should be removed.

Ultrasound or intravenous urography

All patients with ARF require renal imaging, which should be urgent when there is clinical suspicion of obstruction or no adequate explanation for the ARF. The choice of investigation depends largely on local facilities and expertise. Ultrasound (in combination with a plain abdominal X-ray to detect renal stones) is a safe, reliable, screening method which is sufficient to confirm or exclude a diagnosis of obstruction in most cases. The hallmark of obstruction on ultrasound is dilatation of the pelvicalyceal system (see p. 68). If ultrasound is equivocal or unavailable, high-dose intravenous urography (IVU) is indicated. The disadvantages of this examination have been discussed on p. 71.

The pathognomonic feature of acute obstruction on IVU is a slowly developing, increasingly dense nephrogram, which sometimes requires a 24-hour film to recognize. A 'negative pyelogram' may occur in early films (a rim of opacified renal tissue outlining a distended, non-opacified, collecting system). The collecting system may opacify on late films. If the diagnosis of obstruction remains in doubt, antegrade or retrograde pyelography should be performed.

Relief of obstruction

Once obstruction has been diagnosed, it should be relieved as soon as possible so as to prevent further, possibly irreversible, renal damage.

Bladder outflow obstruction is usually easily relieved by bladder catheterization. Urgent relief of obstruction at a higher level is best performed by the insertion of percutaneous nephrostomy tubes into one or both kidneys, under ultrasound control. Antegrade pyelography may be performed at the same time to delineate the precise site of obstruction, because neither ultrasound nor an IVU can readily demonstrate this. Relief of obstruction may be followed by an intense postobstructive diuresis. Careful fluid and electrolyte management is then essential and intravenous fluids may be required. Once the patient is stable, definitive surgery to deal with the cause of obstruction is planned.

Is there primary parenchymal disease?

The major aim is to detect those conditions that require immediate specific treatment, particularly cases of renal vasculitis, rapidly progressive glomerulonephritis and acute interstitial nephritis. In these conditions, irreversible damage may be caused by delay in diagnosis. All patients with ARF who do not have a clear history of a prerenal or nephrotoxic insult and who have normal-sized, non-obstructed kidneys require a percutaneous renal biopsy. Sometimes a diagnosis of renal vasculitis or rapidly progressive glomerulonephritis is suggested by clinical features, including vasculitic skin lesions, symptoms of multisystem involvement and urinary red cell casts. Patients without such features may have raised titres of antineutrophil cytoplasmic antibodies (ANCAs) or antiglomerular basement membrane (GBM) antibodies (see p. 175). An assay for each should be requested. In drug-induced interstitial nephritis, a history of exposure is sometimes accompanied by features of hypersensitivity, such as fever, rash and joint pains. Nevertheless, clinical features may be subtle or absent and diagnosis is almost always dependent upon biopsy findings.

Renal biopsy is a specialized technique and, if a trained operator and experienced renal histopathologist are not available locally, urgent referral to a specialist centre is essential.

Is there acute-on-chronic renal failure?

Patients presenting with ARF may have underlying chronic renal impairment. This affects subsequent management and prognosis. Evidence of severe underlying chronic renal disease may influence immediate decisions regarding patients who may not be considered as candidates for chronic dialysis because of age or advanced disease of other organs. The presence of underlying chronic renal failure may be obvious from the history or suggested by the presence of complications of chronic renal failure.

The most reliable method of detecting chronic renal impairment is by imaging for renal size, preferably by ultrasound, because in most cases of chronic renal failure the kidneys are small. This subject is dealt with more fully in Chapter 17, p. 257.

Management of acute renal failure, phase III: established acute tubular necrosis

The clinical pictures are very heterogeneous. At one end of the spectrum is the well-nourished, non-oliguric patient with stable cardiorespiratory status in whom the precipitating factors of ATN have been controlled. At the other is the desperately ill, severely wasted, infected, oliguric patient requiring inotropes and mechanical ventilation. Although management is different in these patients, underlying principles are the same:

1 To maintain control of the underlying cause of ARF.

2 To protect the patient from the consequences of renal failure pending the recovery of renal function.

3 To provide adequate nutritional support during this time.

Conservative management

Fluids and electrolytes

Fluid should be restricted to 400 ml daily plus a volume equivalent to the previous day's urine output. This formula accommodates both oliguric and non-oliguric patients. Fluid balance charts are often inaccurate and daily weighing under standard conditions is essential. Even mildly catabolic patients may lose 0.2–0.3 kg body-weight daily. A patient with a steady weight is usually accumulating fluid. In a few patients, regular high-dose oral loop diuretics may allow a more liberal fluid intake. Oliguric patients require dietary restriction of sodium and potassium. A reasonable initial prescription is a diet containing 40 mmol/day of each. Drugs containing sodium or potassium and potassium-conserving diuretics should be avoided. Cation-exchange resins may be useful to help control plasma potassium concentrations if dietary control is inadequate. Non-oliguric patients may require less rigid control of sodium and potassium intake.

Diet

Restriction of dietary protein to control uraemia without recourse to dialysis should only be used in stable, well-nourished patients in whom the duration of ARF is likely to be 6–8 days. Protein restriction of 40 g daily may be prescribed, usually with an energy intake of 2000–3000 kcal daily (8.4–12.6 MJ). Some of this energy may be supplied as polymeric glucose preparations, such as Hycal or Caloreen. Vitamins and mineral supplements are not routinely required. In malnourished patients or those with high catabolic rates, protein restriction is dangerous and ineffective in controlling uraemia. Such patients require dialysis with extra nutrition.

Prevention and treatment of complications

Disturbances of conscious level, pericarditis, hyperkalaemia and acidosis are preventable by adequate control of the uraemic state. Infection is a frequent complication and is the commonest cause of death in patients with ARF. Every effort should be made to avoid infection. Urinary catheterization is not required for monitoring purposes in established ATN. Prolonged catheterization should be performed only if unavoidable. Intravenous cannulae require strict aseptic care if they are necessary at all. Fever requires thorough investigation and any infection needs prompt effective treatment. There is no place for prophylactic antibiotics.

Gastrointestinal haemorrhage is a major complication of ARF, although the incidence has been reduced by dialytic control of uraemia. While there is no firm evidence to suggest a definite benefit, it is reasonable to prescribe a prophylactic H_2 receptor antagonist. If gut bleeding occurs, measures to reverse associated coagulation defects and abnormalities of platelet function should be undertaken (see p. 233).

Anaemia is common and, if severe (less than 10 g/dl), requires a search for causes other than the anaemia of renal failure. Causes include blood loss due to gut haemorrhage or frequent venesections for investigations, haemolysis or folate deficiency. Blood transfusion may be required for an anaemia of less than 8 g/dl. Restoration of haemoglobin to 10 g/dl is sufficient.

Hypocalcaemia is common but rarely severe or symptomatic. Severe hypocalcaemia ($<$ 1.8 mmol/L) occasionally occurs, especially in rhabdomyolysis (due to binding of calcium ions to damaged muscle). Treatment with intravenous calcium gluconate may be required. Treatment with vitamin D analogues or metabolites is very rarely needed. Hyperphosphataemia is invariable and is controlled by dialysis. Hypophosphataemia is an occasional complication of parenteral nutrition.

Drugs in acute renal failure

Potentially nephrotoxic drugs should be avoided where possible in patients with ARF. Renal failure has profound effects on the body's capacity to handle drugs. Apart from major differences in the half-lives and elimination rates of predominantly renally excreted drugs and their metabolites, there are substantial metabolic alterations and changes in receptor sensitivity. These changes and their effects on drug prescribing in renal failure are discussed in Chapter 21, p. 313. Here, it is sufficient to emphasize that doctors inexperienced in drug usage in renal failure should always consult appropriate reference sources before prescribing any drug in ARF. There is a useful section on prescribing in renal impairment in the *British National Formulary*.

Laboratory monitoring

Plasma urea, electrolytes and serum creatinine concentrations should be measured daily and full blood count, serum calcium, phosphate and albumin thrice weekly. Bacteriological surveillance of indwelling catheters and cannulae is performed by daily culture of blood, any other biological fluid and swabs of any potentially infected sites. Other tests are performed as clinically indicated.

Dialysis in acute renal failure

Indications

The major indications for urgent dialysis have been discussed in the section on the management of emergencies in ARF, and are shown in Table 16.7. There is often more than one indication in individual patients.

Patients who are oliguric for more than a few days, even if non-catabolic, will require dialysis to control uraemia and maintain normal fluid, electrolyte and acid–base status. Hypercatabolic patients always require dialysis if oliguric and almost always if non-oliguric. Hypercatabolic ARF is usually secondary to trauma, major surgery, shock, sepsis or rhabdomyolysis. In non-catabolic patients with oliguric ARF, the rate of rise of blood urea is approximately 5 mmol/L per day. In hypercatabolic patients it rises by more than 15 mmol/L per day and may rise by very much more. Hypercatabolism is also associated with rapidly rising potassium concentrations and rapidly developing acidosis (pH <7.2). In these patients it is essential that dialysis is begun early and carried out intensively and daily. All patients with high catabolic rates require parenteral nutrition. 'Space' for this can be made by regular dialysis or continuous arteriovenous haemofiltration. These treatments

Table 16.7 Indications for dialysis in acute renal failure

Urgent dialysis
Severe uraemia (plasma urea >40 mmol/L)
Fluid overload
Hyperkalaemia
Acidosis
Uraemic complications
Impaired conscious level, coma, fits
Pericarditis
Severe hyperuricaemia (especially in tumour lysis syndrome)
Oxalate toxicity (ethylene glycol overdose)
Drug overdose
Routine dialysis, haemofiltration or CAVHD
Prevention of severe uraemia and its complications, when not possible by conservative therapy
Maintenance of normal fluid, electrolyte and acid–base status, when not possible by conservative therapy
'Space-making' for parenteral nutrition, transfusions of blood and blood products
Prophylaxis before surgical procedures

may also be required to allow transfusion of blood, blood products (especially clotting factors) and other infusions.

Available treatments

Peritoneal dialysis is widely available but haemodialysis is usually limited to specialist centres. A third treatment, continuous arteriovenous haemofiltration (CAVH), is now becoming more widely used, especially for the management of ARF in intensive care units.

Peritoneal dialysis

Peritoneal dialysis is a relatively simple technique to begin and to manage: no complex equipment is needed. Many patients with ARF can be managed by this method alone. It may be particularly suitable for patients with cardiovascular instability. Contraindications are mainly relative (Table 16.8) and the technique has been successfully used in patients after recent intra-abdominal surgery. However, if haemodialysis is available, it is better not to embark upon peritoneal dialysis in the presence of the complications listed in Table 16.8

Access to the peritoneal cavity is gained by percutaneous insertion of a semirigid plastic catheter, which remains in place only for the duration of each dialysis. Alternatively, a soft silastic catheter (Tenchkoff) can be inserted surgically. This has a number of advantages. There are decreased risks of perforation of intra-abdominal viscera, fewer difficulties with drainage and no need for repeated semirigid catheter insertion because the catheter remains *in situ* between dialyses.

Bacterial peritonitis is a frequent complication and is often related to poor technique. Leakage of dialysate may occur around the catheter into subcutaneous tissues. Many of the complications of peritoneal dialysis may require transfer to haemodialysis. A detail description of catheter placement and technical aspects of dialysis has been presented by Mion and Beraud (1984).

Table 16.8 Contraindications to peritoneal dialysis

Recent abdominal surgery, especially with drainage tubes *in situ*
Extensive previous abdominal surgery
Ileus
Recent intra-abdominal vascular surgery, especially with vascular prosthesis
Hypercatabolic patients
Severe respiratory disease
Congenital or acquired communication between abdomen and thorax
Cellulitis of abdominal wall
Pregnancy

Continuous arteriovenous haemofiltration

Continuous arteriovenous haemofiltration is rapidly becoming the treatment of choice for ARF in intensive care units. A haemofilter consists of a synthetic membrane of high hydraulic permeability which is capable of producing a high-volume ultrafiltrate of plasma. Up to 24 L of ultrafiltrate may be produced daily. It contains electrolytes and metabolic waste products but no serum protein. Replacement of ultrafiltrate by appropriate volumes of electrolyte solutions allows effective control of the metabolic disturbances in ARF with maintenance of good fluid balance. Parenteral feeding solutions, blood and blood products may be given as part of the replacement regimen.

A schematic representation of the circuit required for CAVH is given in Fig. 16.4. The haemofilter is connected to the circulation, via arterial and venous catheters or an arteriovenous shunt at wrist or ankle. The driving force for filtration is the patient's blood-pressure, plus the negative hydrostatic pressure generated by lowering the drainage bag below the level of the patient. Pump-assisted haemofiltration allows blood to be taken from, and returned to, a central vein. Heparin is infused into the arterial line at a rate of 10 units/kg/hour. Replacement fluid enters the circuit via the venous line. Filtration is adjusted by altering the transmembrane pressure by means of a clamp on the filtrate line. Filtration rates of 10–17 ml/min are required for adequate control of blood urea and creatinine concentrations. The rate of fluid replacement is controlled by the speed of the infusion pump.

Continuous arteriovenous haemofiltration has a number of advantages over other dialysis methods:

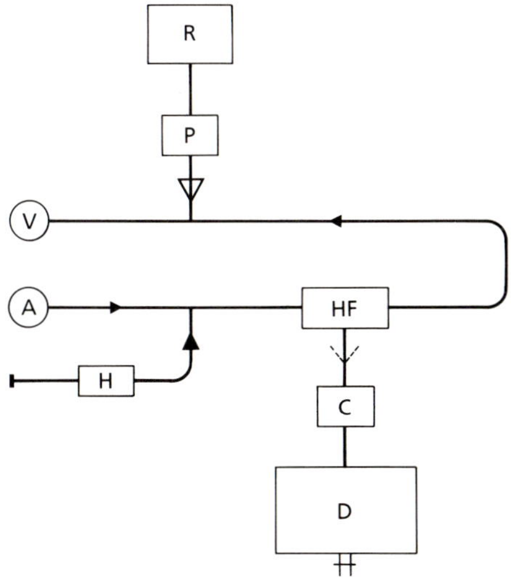

Fig. 16.4 Schematic representation of circuit for continuous arteriovenous haemofiltration. A, Arterial access; V, venous return; HF, haemofilter; C, adjustable clamp; D, drainage bag; R, replacement fluid bag; P, high-volume pump; H, heparin pump.

1 It causes no cardiovascular instability.
2 It can be used in hypotensive patients.
3 No complex equipment is required.
4 Parenteral feeding is easily performed.

The main disadvantages are:
1 The need for continuous heparinization to prevent clotting within the haemofilter.
2 Continuous careful monitoring to avoid potentially fatal imbalances between filtrate output and replacement fluid input.

For details of preparation for and performance of CAVH see Kramer (1985).

A recent modification of this technique – continuous arteriovenous haemodialysis (CAVHD) or venous–venous haemodialysis (VVHD) provides better biochemical control of uraemia than CAVH or VVHD.

Haemodialysis

In spite of the accessibility and convenience of peritoneal dialysis and the increasing use of continuous haemofiltration techniques, a comprehensive service for the management of ARF is based on freely available haemodialysis. It is needed for patients in whom peritoneal dialysis is contraindicated or has failed. Continuous haemofiltration methods are the treatment of choice for ARF in intensive units, but, even so, intermittent haemodialysis may be required for adequate control of uraemia, particularly in hypercatabolic patients. The greatest advantages of haemodialysis are efficiency and wide applicability. The only contraindication is cardiovascular instability. Even in this condition, special techniques such as sequential ultrafiltration and bicarbonate dialysis may allow its use.

Referral for dialysis

Patients with established ARF in hospitals without dialysis facilities often require urgent referral to a specialist centre. Even in non-urgent cases, referral is required soon after diagnosis because there is no sense in observing clinical and biochemical deterioration until dialysis becomes urgent. In centres in which there is expertise in peritoneal dialysis, referral is required for patients in whom the method is contraindicated or has failed.

Experience with continuous haemofiltration is growing and the technique is now routine in intensive care units without haemodialysis facilities. It is important to ensure that the potential benefits of haemodialysis are not neglected; close co-operation with specialist centres is required.

Nutritional support in acute renal failure

The nutritional requirements of patients with ARF vary widely. Some patients may be managed by diet, as described earlier (p. 241). Many have high catabolic rates and require nutritional support by enteral or parenteral routes. The aim of nutritional support in seriously ill patients is to limit tissue breakdown and minimize nitrogen and energy losses during the catabolic phase of injury, by replacement of nitrogen losses and the provision of enough non-protein calories to ensure anabolic utilization. If these aims are approached in patients with ARF, there will be less loss of lean body mass, healing will be promoted and host defence mechanisms will be improved. In addition, the deleterious effects of tissue breakdown on the uraemic state may be reduced. Enteral feeding is usually preferable, provided the patient has a normally functioning gut, but, where enteral feeding is contraindicated or has failed, parenteral feeding is necessary. The techniques of nutritional support in ARF are similar to those employed in other seriously ill patients but there are a number of other important considerations:

1 Whether support is by enteral or parenteral routes, there is a considerable fluid load, which requires frequent dialysis, CAVHD, CAVH or VVHD to accommodate it.

2 Nitrogen requirement is difficult to define. It may be calculated from the following:

$$\begin{aligned}\text{Total nitrogen loss (g/24 hours)} &= \text{urinary nitrogen loss (g/24 hours)}\\ &+ \text{dialysate nitrogen loss (g/dialysis)}\\ &+ \text{change in body urea nitrogen (g/24 hours)}\end{aligned}$$

In oliguric patients in whom the measurement is made between dialyses, the dominant term is the change in body urea nitrogen. This is obtainable from:

$$\text{Rise in blood urea (mmol/L)} \times 0.6\ \text{(kg body-weight)} \times 0.028$$

3 There are increased nitrogen losses in patients on peritoneal dialysis, because serum protein, chiefly albumin, is lost into the dialysate.

4 Potassium and phosphate requirements are difficult to estimate. Blood concentrations of these variables should be measured daily or thrice weekly.

5 There are claims that parenteral nutrition using a mixture of essential amino acids as the nitrogen source (rather than the standard mixture of essential and non-essential) has advantages in patients with acute renal failure, but the evidence for this is inconclusive.

The benefits of nutritional support in ARF may appear obvious but it is difficult to demonstrate even a modest reduction in overall mortality. Nutrition should be considered as an important adjunct to other aspects of management. There may be a small subgroup of patients in whom it may be life-saving.

Management of acute renal failure, phase IV: recovery

In most cases of oliguric ATN, especially if optimal fluid balance has been maintained, the diuretic phase is marked by a gradual increase in urine volume. Fluid restrictions can be gradually relaxed. In a few patients there may be a diuresis of 5 L or more daily. Intravenous fluid replacement may be necessary. Care is required to avoid perpetuating such a diuresis by continuous high-volume infusions beyond the point at which the renal concentrating defects have improved (chasing the diuresis). If this is suspected, urine volumes should be under-replaced for a short period and, if a reduction in urine volume occurs while the patient remains haemodynamically stable, the fluid replacement regimen should be rapidly tailed off.

The onset of a diuresis may precede biochemical improvement by a number of days. Management of fluid and potassium balance may be simplified but dialysis may still be required. Infection is as common in the diuretic phase as earlier. Rebound hypercalcaemia may occur, especially in patients with rhabdomyolysis. It is very rarely severe enough to need specific measures for control.

If the recovery phase is delayed beyond 3–4 weeks, further investigations are required, because the original clinical diagnosis of ATN is then suspect. Plain abdominal X-rays with nephrotomograms of the kidneys may show the diffuse cortical calcification typical of acute cortical necrosis. In this circumstance, a considerable reduction in renal size may have occurred, even over a few weeks. Diethylene triamine pentacetic acid (DTPA) renography is required to confirm renal perfusion, because complete renal infarction may have been missed originally. If the kidneys are normal in size, renal biopsy is indicated to exclude cases of primary renal parenchymal disease, which may have been overlooked and which might respond to specific therapy.

Prognosis in acute renal failure

Mortality from ARF in the years before dialysis approached 90%. After dialysis became available, figures improved to 50–60% but there has been no improvement since, despite technical advances. The probable explanation lies in the dramatic change which has taken place in the type of causes of ARF over this period. Formerly, obstetric complications and septic abortions were common causes of ARF which had a low mortality, but these are now rare. There may also have been a reduction in the number of patients with ARF due to nephrotoxins. The prognosis in such patients with 'uncomplicated' ARF is good. Currently ARF often occurs following major surgical procedures and other medical interventions which were previously technically impossible. In addition, severely ill patients, many of whom formerly died as a result of the original injury or disease, now survive, with modern intensive care, long enough to develop ARF. Such cases of 'complicated' ARF have a very poor prognosis and so overall mortality is unchanged.

The most important factor determining the prognosis of patients with ARF is the severity of the underlying disease process, with particular reference to its effects on other organ systems. Acute renal failure that is uncomplicated by the failure of other organ systems has a good prognosis and a mortality of around 10%. However, when ARF is associated with respiratory failure, circulatory failure, hepatic failure or uncontrolled sepsis, the mortality is high. When there are two or three additional conditions, the mortality approaches 100%. There are obvious, but unresolved, implications regarding patient selection for intensive support. Age by itself is no criterion for selection, having little effect on prognosis.

Prevention of acute renal failure

The high morbidity, mortality and cost of ARF focus attention on attempts at prevention. Because of the diverse and often multifactorial aetiology of ARF, it is not surprising that there is no single effective preventative measure. There are a number of general measures which may reduce the chance of developing ARF:

1 Limiting the use of potential nephrotoxins – avoiding aminoglycoside antibiotics where effective substitutes exist.

2 Maintenance of adequate effective circulating volume before, during and after certain procedures. These include some forms of surgery and nephrotoxic insults – radiographic contrast agents, cisplatin, myoglobin and hyperuricaemia.

3 Ensuring adequate urinary output before, during and after potential renal insults. The induction of a solute diuresis with a loop diuretic may be a useful adjunct to maintaining an adequate urinary volume in the prevention of ARF. A diuresis may be particularly useful in preventing nephrotoxic damage and when used before, during and for 48 hours after surgery for obstructive jaundice. Diuretic-induced hypovolaemia should be carefully guarded against by adequate fluid replacement. The use of low-dose dopamine in these conditions is experimental.

4 To avoid acute urate nephropathy associated with tumour lysis, treatment with allopurinol should be started 3 days before chemotherapy.

5 Alkalinization of urine with intravenous sodium bicarbonate with or without acetazolamide has been advocated, especially in patients at risk of acute urate nephropathy and rhabdomyolysis-associated ARF. However, it is often difficult to achieve and may add little to the measures described above.

There are a large number of agents which may protect renal tubular cells from the effects of ischaemic injury. Calcium channel-blockers may prevent the injurious rise in intracellular calcium levels which follows ischaemic injury and $MgCl_2$-adenosine triphosphate (ATP) may replenish depleted intracellular ATP. Both agents have shown promise in experimental models of ischaemic ARF, but have yet to be shown to be clinically useful.

Summary

A schematic representation of the diagnosis and management of ARF is given in Fig. 16.5.

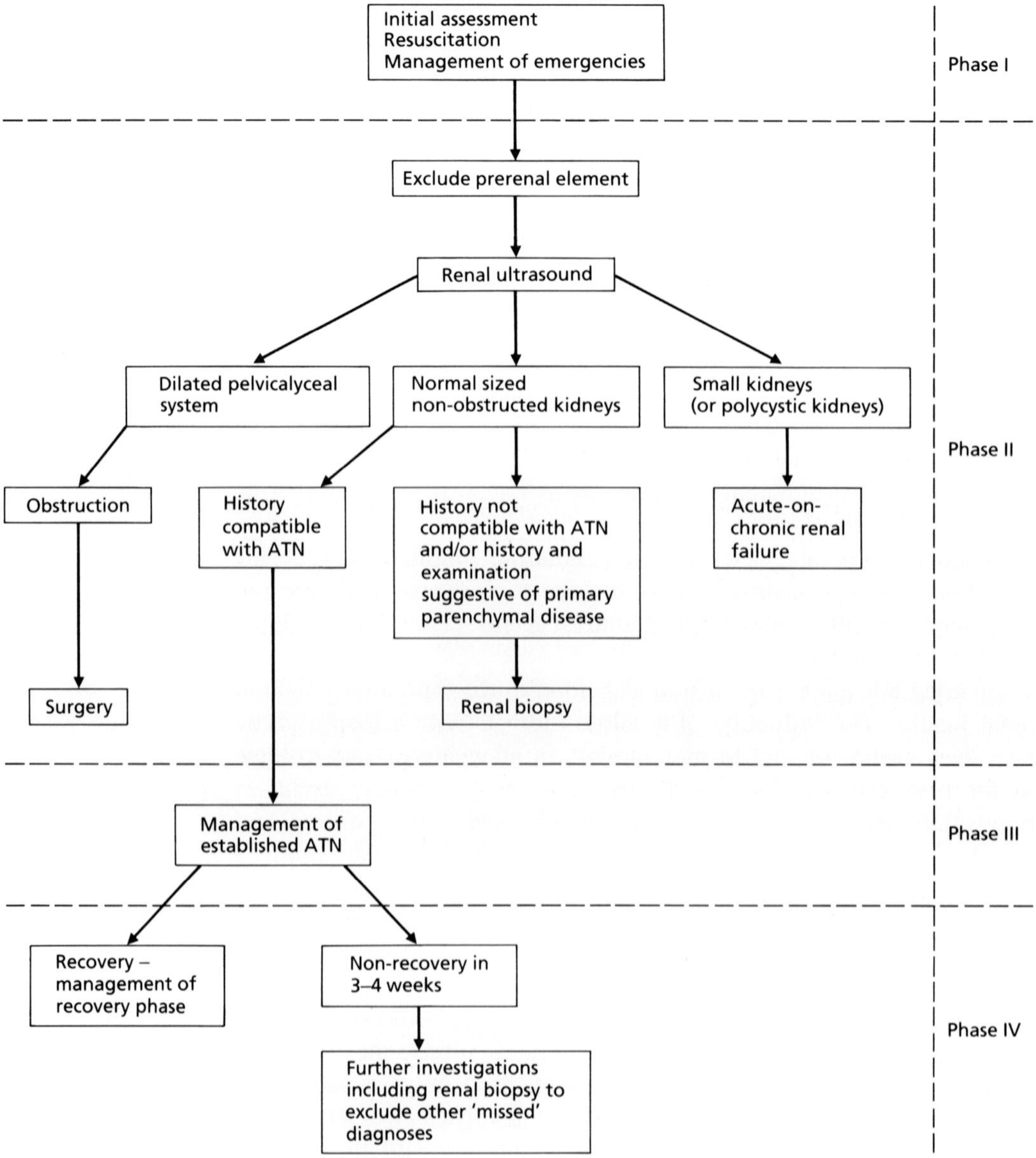

Fig. 16.5 Summary of management of ARF.

Further reading

1 Bone, R.C. (1993) A new treatment for the adult respiratory distress syndrome. *N. Engl. J. Med.* **328**, 431–2.

2 Brenner, B. & Lazarus, M.G. (eds) (1983) *Acute Renal Failure*. Saunders, Philadelphia.

3 Brenner, B. & Stein, J.H. (eds) (1988) *Acute Renal Failure*, 2nd edn. Contemporary Issues in Nephrology 6, Churchill Livingstone, New York, Edinburgh, London and Melbourne.

4 Cameron, J.S. (1986) Acute renal failure – the continuing challenge. *Quart. J. Med.* **228**, 337–43.
5 Chang, R.W.S. (1989) Individual outcome prediction models for intensive care units. *Lancet* **ii**, 143–6.
6 Chew, S.L., Ling, R.L., Daelemans, R. & De Broe, M.E. (1993) Outcome in acute renal failure. *Nephrol. Dial. Transplant.* **8**, 101–7.
7 Gabow, P.A., Kaehny, W.C. & Kelleher, S.P. (1982) The spectrum of rhabdomyolysis. *Medicine* **61**, 141–52.
8 Haag-Weber, M. & Hörl, W.H. (1993) Uraemia and infection: mechanisms of impaired cellular host defence. *Nephron* **63**, 125–37.
9 Henderson, J.A., Beattie, T.J. & Kennedy, A.C. (1980) Dopamine hydrochloride in oliguric states. *Lancet* **ii**, 827–8 .
10 Kramer, P. (1985) *Arteriovenous Haemofiltration: a Kidney Replacement Therapy for the Intensive Care Unit.* Springer-Verlag, Berlin, Heidelberg, New York and Tokyo.
11 Levinsky, N.G. & Barnard, D.B. (1983) Mannitol and loop diuretics in acute renal failure. In Brenner, B.M. & Lazarus, M.G. (eds), *Acute Renal Failure.* Saunders, Philadelphia, pp. 712–22.
12 Lindner, A. (1983) Synergism of dopamine and furosemide in diuretic resistant oliguric acute renal failure. *Nephron* **33**, 121–6.
13 Mion, C.M. & Beraud, J.J. (1984) The treatment of acute renal failure by peritoneal dialysis. In Andreucci, V.E. (ed.), *Acute Renal Failure: Pathophysiology, Prevention and Treatment.* Martinus Nijhoff, Boston, The Hague, Dordrecht and Lancaster, pp. 463–79.
14 Molitoris, B.A. (1991) New insights into the cellular biology of ischaemic acute renal failure. *J. Am. Soc. Nephrol.* **1**, 1263–70.
15 Parsons, V. (1984) The treatment of acute renal failure by haemodialysis. In Andreucci, V.E. (ed.), *Acute Renal Failure: Pathophysiology, Prevention and Treatment.* Martinus Nijhoff, Boston, The Hague, Dordrecht and Lancaster, pp. 447–61.
16 Rainford, D. & Sweny, P. (1990) *Acute Renal Failure.* Farrand Press, London.
17 Routh, G.S., Briggs, J.D., More, J.G. & Ledingham, I.M.A. (1980) Survival from acute renal failure with and without multiple organ dysfunction. *Postgrad. Med. J.* **56**, 244–7.
18 Sachs, S.H. & Ledingham, J.G. (1986) Management of acute renal failure. *Hosp. Update* **12**, 187–204.
19 Silk, D.B.A. (1983) *Nutritional Support in Hospital Practice.* Blackwell Scientific Publications, Oxford, London, Edinburgh, Boston and Melbourne.
20 Smithies, M.N. & Cameron, J.S. (1989) Can we predict outcome in acute renal failure? *Nephron* **51**, 297–300.

Chapter 17
Acute-on-chronic Renal Failure

Ken Farrington

Acute-on-chronic renal failure is defined as an abrupt and potentially reversible deterioration of renal function in a patient with pre-existing renal impairment. It may occur in patients with previously recognized chronic renal insufficiency, in whom it must be differentiated from progression of the disease process originally responsible for the chronic renal failure (CRF). It may also occur in patients in whom chronic renal disease was previously unsuspected, in whom it must be differentiated from acute renal failure (ARF).

Natural history of chronic renal failure

Chronic renal failure occurs as a result of many different disease processes (Chapters 10, 13 and 14; pp. 134, 190 and 198). In some, the underlying disease remains persistently active, such as diabetic nephropathy, while in others renal impairment has occurred as the result of past events that are no longer of consequence – some forms of immune complex glomerulonephritis. Once a critical level of renal functional deterioration has occurred, a gradual loss of remaining function is almost inevitable. The natural history of CRF, almost regardless of cause, is a gradual deterioration towards end-stage renal failure. In a patient with CRF, the rate of progression can often be best appreciated by plotting the reciprocal of serum creatinine against time.

A straight line is obtained (Fig. 17.1), the slope of which reflects the rate of progression. Slopes vary between patients even with the same renal disease, but usually the slope remains fairly constant in a given individual. A sudden increase in slope (Fig. 17.1) reflects an acute deterioration of function: acute-on-chronic renal failure. A search for possible causes is then necessary.

Aetiology of acute-on-chronic renal failure

In CRF the remaining renal function is vulnerable and at risk from relatively innocuous insults. Unlike ARF, where insults are commonly multiple (see Tables 16.1, 16.2 and 16.3, pp. 226, 227 and 228), acute-on-chronic renal failure is more likey to be produced by a single event. Renal function in CRF is also dependent on prostaglandin synthesis,

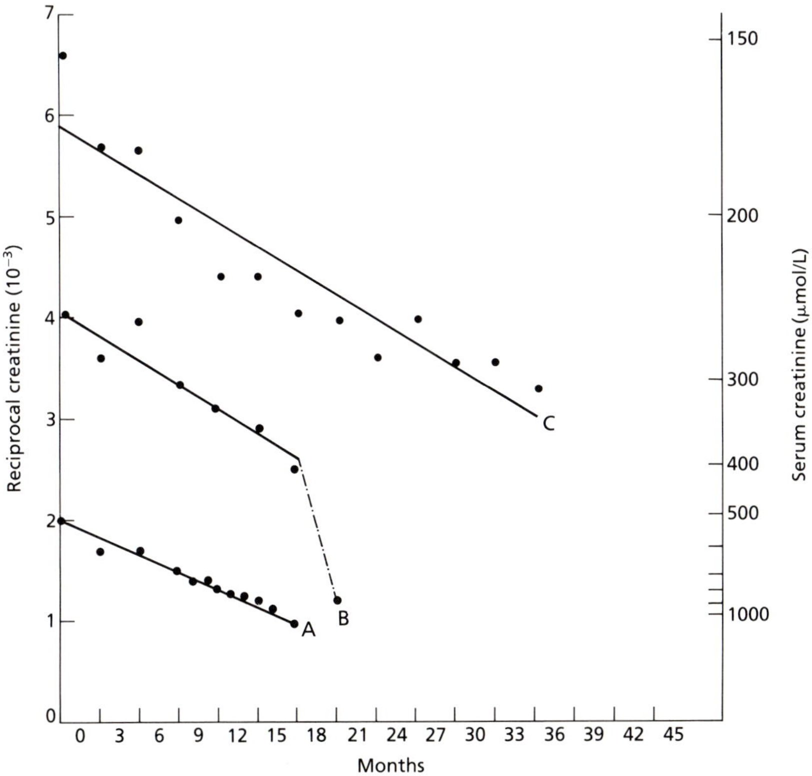

Fig. 17.1 Plots of reciprocal of serum creatinine (left vertical axis) and serum creatinine (right vertical axis) against time. Plot A illustrates the steady decline in renal function in a patient with adult polycystic kidney disease who presented with severe renal impairment (creatinine 500 μmol/L), in whom dialysis was required 17 months later. Plot B shows the initial gradual loss of function in a patient with diabetic nephropathy, culminating in an abrupt deterioration (represented by the sudden change in slope), which was due to a fulminating episode of acute pyelonephritis associated with septicaemia. Plot C shows the slow but inexorable decline in function of a patient with mesangiocapillary glomerulonephritis over a 3-year period.

Table 17.1 Causes of acute-on-chronic renal failure

Renal hypoperfusion	Dehydration Hypotension Gastrointestinal haemorrhage Cardiac failure Inappropriate blood transfusion
Nephrotoxins	Drugs Radiographic contrast materials Hypercalcaemia
Infections	Urinary tract infection Systemic infection
Obstruction	
Complication of underlying renal disease or renal failure	Accelerated hypertension Reactivation or acceleration of underlying disease process Renal vein thrombosis

which explains the potentially serious consequence of prescribing non-steroidal anti-inflammatory drugs (NSAIDs) for patients with renal failure. Major causes of acute-on-chronic renal failure are listed in Table 17.1.

Renal hypoperfusion

Sustained under-perfusion of the kidneys is the main cause. Dehydration may occur as the result of intercurrent illness, especially disturbances of the gastrointestinal tract. Iatrogenic causes are quite common and include over-treatment with diuretics, excessive dehydration prior to an intravenous urogram (IVU) or minor surgical procedure and inappropriate salt restriction in patients with salt-losing states, which comprises 5–10% of patients with CRF. The degree of dehydration required to cause damage is often minor and may be clinically undetectable.

Hypotension may occur as a result of intercurrent illness or due to over-treatment with hypotensive drugs. Hypotension need not be severe or prolonged to produce renal damage in patients with CRF. Gastrointestinal blood loss is not unusual in patients with CRF, because of an increased incidence of peptic ulcers. Substantial blood loss may compromise renal perfusion directly, leading to renal deterioration and an elevated urea:creatinine ratio due to the gut protein load. Cardiac failure may complicate the course of CRF. Hypertension, salt and water overload and anaemia are prominent precipitating factors. Impaired cardiac function compromises renal perfusion and may cause substantial decrements in renal function. Blood transfusion may cause an acute deterioration of renal function. Patients with moderate to severe CRF are usually anaemic. In general, the anaemia is well tolerated. Transfusion is not usually indicated unless the anaemia is severe or symptomatic, and in these circumstances the volume of blood needed is usually modest. Ill-judged transfusions may have serious effects on renal function, probably due to a reduced renal plasma flow as a consequence of too high a haematocrit.

Nephrotoxins

A list of major nephrotoxins is included in Chapter 16, p. 224 (Table 16.3, p. 228). The most common are NSAIDs, ACEIs, aminoglycoside antibiotics and radiographic contrast. Adverse events with these agents are predictable. Difficulties can also be anticipated with less commonly used drugs such as amphotericin B, colistin and cisplatin. Other drugs may cause renal damage, especially those producing acute interstitial nephritis. It is important to emphasize that no list of nephrotoxins is complete and that new nephrotoxic effects of drugs are reported even after well-established use. All drugs taken by a patient with acute-on-chronic renal failure should be regarded critically. Hypercalcaemia is important. Primary or tertiary hyperparathyroidism (the latter arising as a complication of renal failure) and myeloma and other malignancies cause hypercalcaemia, but the commonest cause is iatrogenic and relates to inadequately supervised treatment with vitamin D or synthetic anologues thereof (see p. 206). The toxic effects of hypercalcaemia are magnified by hyperphosphataemia, which frequently coexists in patients with CRF.

Infection

1 Some patients with CRF are particularly susceptible to infection of the renal parenchyma, occurring as a result of ascending infection from the lower urinary tract. Examples include patients with diabetic nephropathy, analgesic nephropathy, polycystic kidney disease and CRF associated with obstruction, renal stone disease or any structural abnormality of the urinary tract associated with poor urinary drainage. Infection may take the form of acute bacterial interstitial nephritis (as in diabetics), acute papillary necrosis (especially in diabetics and those with analgesic nephropathy or obstruction) or intrarenal abscess formation (in polycystic kidneys). Pyonephrosis may complicate obstruction. Any of these infections may be the source of a septicaemia.
2 Systemic infection of any source may be associated with sudden deterioration of function in patients with CRF and is often due to prerenal factors. Occasionally, acute interstitial nephritis may be associated with systemic infection (see Table 16.1, p. 226).

Obstruction

Urinary tract obstruction may complicate CRF and produce a further decrease in renal function. The common causes are:
1 Prostatic hypertrophy.

2 Autonomic neuropathy in diabetics, leading to functional obstruction of the bladder neck.
3 Urethral stricture following instrumentation or catheterization.
4 Renal calculi.
5 Very occasionally, sloughed papillae following acute papillary necrosis.

Other conditions which may abruptly reduce renal function

1 Accelerated (malignant)-phase hypertension may complicate many chronic renal diseases and produced a rapid loss in renal function. Often the lost glomerular filtration rate (GFR) never fully recovers, despite adequate blood-pressure control.
2 Poor control of moderate hypertension increases the rate of nephron loss in CRF and may predispose to the development of the accelerated phase.
3 Some renal diseases are characterized by a relapsing and remitting course, such as lupus nephritis. Other forms of glomerulonephritis may also enter a rapidly progressive or crescentic phase. It is important to differentiate such exacerbations of immunologically mediated disease from other causes of acute-on-chronic renal failure, because specific treatment with immunosuppressive therapy may be indicated. The specific immunological investigations are double-stranded deoxyribonucleic acid binding (dsDNAB) and antineutrophil-cytoplasmic antibody (ANCA) serology (see pp. 51 and 52).

A renal biopsy is necessary in some patients with acute-on-chronic renal failure. The indications include:

(a) Suspected acute interstitial nephritis, polyarteritis nodosa, an exacerbation of lupus nephritis or a disproportionate decline in GFR over time.

(b) All patients with acute-on-chronic renal failure for which there is no obvious explanation, provided that kidneys are not obstructed and not less than 10 cm in bipolar length.

When the creatinine clearance is less than 20 ml/min, it is probable that considerable fibrous replacement of the renal parenchyma has occurred, leading to shrunken kidneys. Renal biopsy is relatively contraindicated and potential benefits for specific therapy in these circumstances are limited. A renal biopsy requires specialized expertise, both for performance and for adequate interpretation; this often necessitates referral to a renal unit (see Chapter 9, p. 125).
4 Renal vein thrombosis is an unusual cause of acute-on-chronic renal failure. It occasionally complicates nephrotic syndrome that is secondary to membranous nephropathy. The diagnosis should be considered if there is a sudden deterioration of function in a patient with this nephritis.

Table 17.2 Investigations of acute-on-chronic renal failure

	Indication
Investigations	
Microscopy of urinary sediment	All patients with acute-on-chronic renal failure
Culture of urine and blood	
Serial plasma urea, electrolytes, serum creatinine, calcium, phosphate and urate	
Urine for Bence-Jones proteinuria and serum immunoglobulins	
Chest X-ray and ECG	
Abdominal X-ray for renal stones or calcification; ultrasound for renal size, position and exclusion of obstruction	
Special investigations	
C-reactive protein, DNA binding, ANCA, complement components	Immunological renal disease such as lupus nephritis and renal vasculitis
Renal biopsy	Patients with acute deterioration of CRF, if obstruction can be excluded
Renal venography	Sudden deterioration of function in patients with membranous nephritis

Diagnosis of acute deterioration of previously diagnosed chronic renal failure

Many of the investigations in acute deterioration of previously diagnosed CRF are straightforward: they are given in Table 17.2. Patients with renal hypoperfusion or accelerated-phase hypertension or those taking drugs with predictable nephrotoxic effects can be diagnosed by history and clinical examination. Nevertheless, a number of the investigations listed in Table 17.2 will be essential in all patients in this category.

Differentiation of acute from acute-on-chronic renal failure

Chronic renal failure usually advances insidiously and symptoms may be absent, minimal or non-specific until late in the disorder. Not uncommonly, the disease only becomes symptomatic after an acute episode has compromised the remaining function (see Case 2, p. 315). These patients present the following ways:

1 As ARF. These are the majority: 20–30% of patients with ARF have underlying chronic renal disease.

2 Quickly developing CRF, as seen in patients with undiagnosed or inadequately treated rapidly progressive glomerulonephritis (see

Chapter 11, p. 170). The distinction between ARF and acute-on-chronic renal failure is an important part of the initial management of patients presenting with ARF (Chapter 16, p. 240) because restitution of function may not occur. Long-term dialysis will then be required. The differentiation is made from a combination of the history, the finding of features specific to CRF and by renal imaging.

The complications of CRF that discriminate most effectively between ARF and acute-on-chronic renal failure are those that take the longest time to develop into easily recognizable conditions.

History of previous renal disease

A history of 'nephritis', oedema or haematuria may be obtained. Enquiry should also be made about episodes of urinary tract infection, particularly during infancy. There may be a history of renal stones. A family history of renal disease suggests polycystic kidney disease, hereditary nephritis or cystinuria. A diabetic, particularly if retinopathy is present, probably has diabetic nephropathy. Patients with rheumatoid arthritis or ankylosing spondylitis may have CRF due to long-term ingestion of NSAIDs. Both the rheumatic conditions predispose to amyloid. Other conditions which may be associated with amyloid have been discussed in Chapter 12, p. 179.

Bone disease

Bone disease is common in CRF. The most prominent features occur in children. They are short and have genu valgus and pseudoclubbing. Bone signs are uncommon when CRF develops in adults. Many patients have radiological features of hyperparathyroidism, osteosclerosis or metastatic calcification. Osteomalacia is uncommon. Radiological signs of bone disease provide firm evidence of underlying chronic renal disease. Hand X-rays are necessary to demonstrate subperiosteal erosions, best seen at the radial aspect of the middle phalanges. Lateral views of the thoracolumbar spine may show osteosclerosis (rugger jersey spine).

A high proportion of patients with CRF have hypocalcaemia, hyperphosphataemia, elevated alkaline phosphatase and raised concentrations of parathyroid hormone. Unfortunately, identical changes are found in ARF.

Skin changes

The dermatological manifestations of CRF are often non-specific. Changes most likely to be helpful in differentiating between ARF and acute-on-chronic renal failure are skin pigmentation and nail changes. Skin pigmentation, thought to be due to deposition of 'urochromes' and melanin, is common in long-standing severe CRF and contrasts with mucosal pallor. The 'half-and-half' nail, which consists of a brown discoloration of the distal portion of the nail (presumably due to melanin deposition), is said to be specific and to occur in 10–30% of patients with severe CRF. Neither skin pigmentation nor the 'half-and-half' nail sign is found in ARF.

Anaemia

Anaemia is an almost invariable accompaniment of severe chronic renal disease – serum creatinine 250 μmol/L or greater or clearance of 20 ml/min or less. Anaemia is also common in ARF and has a variety of causes (see Chapter 16, p. 242). Occasionally, an anaemia of less than 10 g/dl is found in a patient who apparently has ARF. Such an anaemia is suggestive of acute-on-chronic renal failure. Nevertheless, the haemoglobin concentration in these patients has a poor diagnostic value.

Hypertension

A long history of hypertension, a history of hypertensive complications in previous pregnancies or the finding of hypertension, left ventricular hypertrophy or retinopathy suggests possible chronic renal disease. Hypertension or complications thereof provide a poor discriminant between ARF and acute-on-chronic renal failure because of the high prevalence of hypertension within the general population.

Renal imaging

The demonstration, by ultrasound, of small kidneys (bipolar length < 10 cm in adults) is the most reliable indicator of CRF (see Table 6.2, p. 75). Exceptions may include diabetic nephropathy and amyloidosis.

Management of acute-on-chronic renal failure

Management of acute-on-chronic renal failure involves treatment to correct the cause of the deterioration and supportive measures to combat the renal failure. Hypovolaemia and cardiac failure require prompt treatment. Drug therapy should be considered critically, potentially nephrotoxic drugs discontinued and doses of other drugs adjusted proportional to GFR. Infection should be treated aggressively with non-nephrotoxic antibiotics. Bladder outflow obstruction should be urgently relieved by catheterization and upper tract obstruction by percutaneous nephrostomy. In both, definitive surgery can be be planned when renal function has stabilized. Accelerated-phase hypertension requires treatment as discussed in Chapter 16, p. 235. Drug-induced interstitial nephritis usually responds to discontinuation of the offending drug, and steroids are probably beneficial (see p. 172). The management of severe lupus nephritis has been discussed on p. 154 and that of crescentic nephritis on p. 176. These specialized treatments require referral to a renal unit.

Patients with severely compromised renal function (serum creatinine >800 μmol/L) may require supportive treatment to combat the effects of renal failure. In a few patients, decreasing dietary protein to 40 g daily and additional conservative measures (Chapter 16, p. 241) may be helpful, but in others dialysis is required. The indications for dialysis and other measures are broadly similar to those discussed for ARF in Chapter 16, p. 243. In patients with acute-on-chronic renal failure it is difficult or impossible to predict the extent of recovery of function. This is often incomplete and no restitution may ever occur, particularly in patients in whom pre-existing renal function was severely impaired (serum creatinine >500 μmol/L or clearance <10 ml/min). Part of the management of these patients involves early consideration of the prospects of non-recovery of function. Chronic dialysis will be indicated for some. Discussion with a renal physician is necessary. Forearm veins must be preserved because they may be needed for fashioning an arteriovenous fistula.

Prevention of acute-on-chronic renal failure

The renal function of patients with CRF is vulnerable. Relatively trivial events, which would not injure normal kidneys, may cause acute-on-chronic renal failure. Some of the precipitating causes are avoidable.

General

Nephrotoxic drugs should be avoided in CRF patients. Hospital admission and intravenous fluids are necessary in patients with CRF who have vomiting or diarrhoea or both. Care is required to avoid over-treatment with hypotensive drugs, because the required dose may be substantially reduced in the presence of fever or mild dehydration.

Procedures requiring intravenous contrast

Dehydration must be avoided before studies requiring intravenous contrast because the combination of hypovolaemia and X-ray contrast may precipitate acute-on-chronic renal failure. If no oral fluid is permitted before other contrast studies, intravenous fluids are required. Newer non-ionic contrast agents may be less nephrotoxic and therefore preferable in CRF. Induction of a solute diuresis by mannitol or loop diuretic before, during and after the procedure is probably helpful, providing urine volumes are correctly replaced.

Aminoglycoside therapy

Netilicin and tobramycin may be less nephrotoxic than gentamicin. The dose and dosage interval should be adjusted to the degree of renal function and monitored by frequent trough and peak serum concentrations. The duration of therapy should be as short as possible. Dehydration and concurrent administration of other nephrotoxic drugs and frusemide may potentiate aminoglycoside nephrotoxicity. Renal function should be measured regularly during and after treatment. Now that ciprofloxacin and third-generation cephalosporins are available, the indications for aminoglycoside therapy have fortunately diminished.

Surgical procedures

There is no reason to transfuse blood so that the haemoglobin concentration is raised to normal. Dehydration and hypovolaemia must be corrected preoperatively. Intravenous fluids are commenced during the fast before surgery and a diuresis, as described above, is probably protective of renal function.

Methoxyflurane is nephrotoxic and best avoided. Suxamethonium may cause a rise in plasma potassium concentrations and should probably not be used. Plasma potassium should be checked pre- and postoperatively. Adequate hydration should be maintained postoperatively, with daily measurements of serum creatinine, plasma urea and electrolytes.

Some patients with CRF may have an increased sensitivity to opiates; this is important at the postoperative stage.

Summary

Acute-on-chronic renal failure is an abrupt and potentially reversible decline of renal function occurring in patients with pre-existing renal insufficiency, recognized or unrecognized. Common causes include dehydration, hypotension, nephrotoxic drugs, infection and obstruction. In patients with documented CRF, these causes may mimic an exacerbation of the underlying renal disease. Investigations should include renal ultrasound, to exclude obstruction, and renal biopsy, if the cause of the acute deterioration is not clear. The condition may also present as ARF if underlying chronic renal disease was unknown. Here, acute-on-chronic renal failure may be thought of if typical skin pigmentation of CRF or the 'half-and-half' nail sign is present. In most patients the diagnosis is made or confirmed by finding small kidneys at ultrasound examination.

The management of acute-on-chronic renal failure is dominated by the possible requirement for chronic dialysis, because many of these patients do not regain adequate renal function. Even after successful treatment of an episode of acute-on-chronic renal failure, it is unlikely that renal function will return to its previous level.

Further reading

1 Andreucci, V. (1984) Prevention of ischaemic/toxic acute renal failure. In Andreucci, V. (ed.), *Humans in Acute Renal Failure: Pathophysiology, Prevention and Treatment.* Martinus-Nijhoff, Boston, The Hague, Dordrecht and Lancaster, pp. 119–47.
2 Blythe, W.B. (1979) The management of intercurrent medical and surgical problems in the patient with chronic renal failure. In Earley, L.E. & Gottschalk, C.W. (eds), *Strauss and Welt's Diseases of the Kidney.* Little, Brown and Company, Boston, pp. 517–37.

Chapter 18
Pregnancy and Urinary Tract Disease

John Davison

The anatomy and physiology of the kidneys and lower urinary tract change during pregnancy, recognition of which is important for the correct diagnosis and management of renal conditions. In addition, the clinician must be aware of the modern approach to antenatal care, the latest technology for fetal surveillance and the advantages of neonatal intensive care. This chapter will cover renal changes in normal pregnancy, stressing relevance to clinical practice, the problems of chronic renal disease in pregnancy, the effect of pregnancy on remote renal prognosis, and obstetric acute renal failure.

Kidney and urinary tract in normal pregnancy

Anatomical changes

Kidney length increases by about 1 cm, probably the result of increments in interstitial fluid. There is substantial dilatation of the urinary tract, more pronounced on the right than the left at all stages of pregnancy, which is perhaps related to the usual dextrorotation of the uterus. By the third trimester, 97% of women show evidence of stasis or hydronephrosis or both. The changes have important clinical implications:

1 They should not be mistaken for obstructive uropathy.
2 There may be errors in tests based on timed urine collections.
3 Stasis of urine in the ureters may contribute to the tendency for pyelonephritis to develop in pregnant women with covert bacteriuria.
4 Radiological assessment should ideally be delayed until at least 4 months after delivery.

Functional changes

Renal haemodynamics

Effective renal plasma flow and glomerular filtration rate (GFR) increase to about 50–70% above non-pregnant values. These increments occur shortly after conception and are maximal in the second trimester (Fig. 18.1).

Serum creatinine decreases from a non-pregnant value of 73 μmol/L to 65, 51 and 47 μmol/L respectively in successive trimesters. Urea concentrations fall from the non-pregnant figure of 4.3 mmol/L to pregnancy values of 3.5, 3.3 and 3.1 mmol/L, respectively. These precise figures are taken from the classic paper of Kuhlback & Windholm

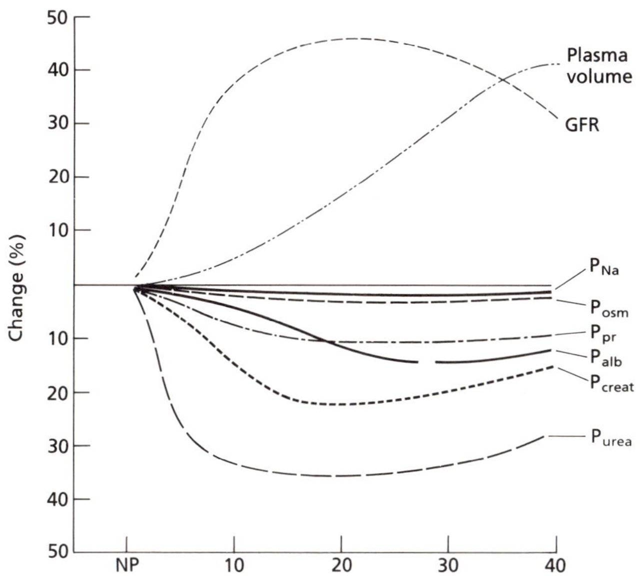

Fig. 18.1 Some of the physiological changes which occur in pregnancy. Variables are expressed as percentage change from normal (non-pregnant; NP) values from early pregnancy to term. P_{Na} = plasma sodium; P_{osm} = serum osmolality; P_{pr}, P_{alb}, P_{creat} = serum, protein, albumin and creatinine respectively; P_{urea} = plasma urea. (From Davison (1983), with permission of author and publisher.)

(1966). Thus values considered normal in non-pregnant women may signify decreased renal function in pregnancy. A serum creatinine of 75 μmol/L or plasma urea of 4.5 mmol/L should alert the clinician further to assess renal function.

Serial assessment of renal function in pregnancy ideally should be based on creatinine clearance rather than on sequential serum concentrations. Formulae have been devised to calculate a value for GFR from a serum creatinine figure but it is illogical to use such calculations in pregnancy where body size or weight does not reflect renal size. Further, these formulae have not been evaluated in pregnancy.

Other renal changes

Normal pregnancy induces relative hypouricaemia but serum concentrations are substantially higher in pregnancies complicated by pre-eclampsia or intrauterine growth retardation. Above a serum concentration of 350 μmol/L there is a considerable perinatal mortality in hypertensive mothers. Serial measurements may be used to monitor progress in pre-eclampsia. Physiological variability is such that some healthy women have high blood concentration without fetal ill-effect. Single random measurements are of no clinical value.

Tubular maximum reabsorption for some sugars, especially glucose, falls. Increased urinary protein excretion may be due to increased glomerular plasma flow. Proteinuria should not be considered abnormal until it exceeds 300 mg in 24 hours. Increasing proteinuria in women with known chronic renal disease does not necessarily imply deterioration.

Volume homoeostasis

Most healthy women gain approximately 12.5 kg during the first pregnancy and 1 kg less during subsequent pregnancies. This increment in weight consists largely of fluid, as total body water increases by 6–8 L, of which 4–7 L are extracellular. There are increases in plasma volume (greatest during the second trimester, when increments approach 50%) and in fluid within fetal and maternal interstitial spaces (greatest in late pregnancy). During most normal pregnancies there is a gradual cumulative retention of about 900 mmol of sodium.

The alterations in maternal intravascular and interstitial spaces produce a 'physiological hypervolaemia'. The meaning of these changes is unknown: women considered 'poor reproducers' have smaller increments in both plasma volume and GFR when compared with those who have delivered normal-sized babies, and often GFR fails to increase in pregnancies of women who subsequently abort.

Blood-pressure in pregnancy

Mean blood-pressure decreases early in pregnancy and, by the second trimester, diastolic pressure is 10 mmHg lower than pre-pregnancy.

The pressure then increases slowly, approaching pre-pregnancy values before delivery. Since cardiac output rises quickly in the first trimester (values are 30–40% greater than pre-pregnancy) and remains relatively constant thereafter, the fall in pressure at this time must be due to a marked decrease in peripheral vascular resistance. The rise of pressure towards non-pregnant levels during the third trimester suggests increasing vasoconstrictor tone. If the clinician is unaware of these changes, diagnostic errors ensue.

Obstetrical implications of renal dysfunction

Conceiving and maintaining pregnancy are related to the degree of functional impairment. Fertility is diminished as renal function falls. When pre-conception serum creatinine and plasma urea exceed 270 μmol/L and 10 mmol/L respectively, normal pregnancy is rare. Successes have been documented in women with moderate to severe disease, including some treated with dialysis.

Ideally, pregnancy is probably best restricted to women whose pre-conception serum creatinine concentration is 200 μmol/L or less and diastolic blood-pressure 90 mmHg or less. Some extend this limit to 250 μmol/L and others believe it should be no higher than 135 μmol/L. Whatever figure is used, one should recognize that degrees of impairment not causing symptoms or disrupting homoeostasis in non-pregnant women may jeopardize pregnancy.

The question has to be asked, 'Is pregnancy advisable?' (Table 18.1). If a woman with chronic renal disease wishes to have a family, the sooner she starts the better because, in some, renal function may continue to decline. Women are not always counselled prior to conception. A

Table 18.1 Pre-pregnancy assessment: is pregnancy advisable?

Type of chronic renal disease (see Table 18.5, p. 273)
General health considerations
Diastolic blood-pressure < 90 mmHg
Renal function
Serum creatinine < 250 μmol/L
Plasma urea < 10 mmol/L
Presence or absence of proteinuria
Review of all drug therapy

Table 18.2 Antenatal assessment: should pregnancy continue?

Type of chronic renal disease (see Table 18.5, p. 273)
General health considerations
Gestational age
Effect of pregnancy on blood-pressure
Effect of pregnancy on renal function
Review of all drug therapy
Past obstetric history

patient with suspected or known renal disease may present as a '*fait accompli*' and then the question has to be asked, 'Should pregnancy continue?' (Table 18.2).

Effects of renal disease on pregnancy versus effects of pregnancy on renal disease

Because of the different obstetrical and remote prognoses in women with different degrees of renal insufficiency, the consequence of pregnancy should be considered by categories of functional renal status prior to conception (Table 18.3).

Normal or mildly impaired creatinine clearance and minimal hypertension

When there is normal or mildly impaired function, there is usually a successful outcome and pregnancy does not adversely affect the course of the disease. This statement has to be tempered somewhat in lupus nephropathy, mesangiocapillary glomerulonephritis and perhaps in IgA/C3 and reflux nephropathies, which appear more sensitive to intercurrent pregnancy.

Most show increments in GFR, but less than those of normal pregnant women. Increased proteinuria is common, occurring in 50% of pregnancies (although rarely in women with chronic pyelonephritis), and it can be of nephrotic range with oedema. When renal failure occurs, it invariably reflects the inexorable course of a particular renal disease.

Moderate renal insufficiency

Prognosis is more guarded when serum creatinine is 125–250 μmol/L. In 50% with initial creatinine concentrations of > 180 μmol/L, further substantial rises occur during pregnancy, and uncontrolled hypertension is an important factor in overall deterioration. In 25%, an accelerated decline in renal function will continue *post partum*.

Severe renal insufficiency

Most women with severe renal insufficiency (serum creatinine > 250 μmol/L) are amenorrhoeic or anovulatory. The likelihood of con-

Table 18.3 Pre-pregnancy categories of renal functional status

Classification	Serum creatinine (μmol/L)
Normal or mildly impaired renal function	⩽125
Moderate renal insufficiency	⩾125
Severe renal insufficiency	⩾250

ception and having a normal pregnancy and delivery is low but not impossible. The risk of severe maternal complications is greater than the probability of a successful obstetric outcome. Ideally, this group of patients should not take additional health risks. The aim should be to preserve renal function or to achieve rehabilitation by dialysis and transplantation. Subsequently pregnancy can be considered.

Pregnancy management

Patients should be seen at 2-week intervals until 32 weeks' gestation, after which assessment should be weekly. Routine serial antenatal observations should be supplemented appropriately (Table 18.4).

Assessment of renal function

If renal function deteriorates, reversible causes should be sought: urinary tract infection, dehydration or electrolyte imbalance; which may be precipitated by diuretic therapy.

Near term, a 15–20% decrease in GFR is acceptable. This decrement hardly affects the concentration of serum creatinine. If there is no reversible cause of a substantial decline, elective delivery is indicated to avoid further deterioration in GFR. When proteinuria persists but blood-pressure is normal and renal function preserved, the pregnancy can be allowed to continue.

Assessment of blood-pressure

Most of the specific risks of hypertension appear to be mediated through superimposed pre-eclampsia. There is controversy about the incidence of pre-eclampsia where there is pre-existing renal disease, largely because a clinical diagnosis cannot be made with certainty because hypertension and proteinuria may be manifestations of the underlying renal disease.

Several special features of hypertension in pregnancy affect decisions on the use of antihypertensive drugs. The hypertension is often short-lived and potentially curable by delivery. The fetus must be considered because it suffers differently from the effects of hypertension and its possible treatment as compared with the mother.

Table 18.4 Supplements to antenatal care in patients with renal disease

Creatinine clearance and protein excretion
Early detection of covert bacteriuria or confirmation of urinary tract infection
Careful blood-pressure monitoring for early detection of hypertension
Early detection of pre-eclampsia
Assessment of fetal size, development and well-being

The level of hypertension to be treated requires a decision that is both physiologically and clinically sensible. While all agree that severe hypertension must be treated, there is a debate as to whether mild to moderate hypertension (here defined as diastolic levels of 90–100 mmHg) requires treatment. A decision to use hypotensive drugs involves knowing the adverse consequences of the level of hypertension under consideration and the potential benefits and adverse effects of treatment.

Drug treatment of raised blood-pressure

Methyldopa remains the safest drug of first choice because of efficacy and the extensive clinical evidence of safety. Beta-blockers have been and are widely used in pregnant women. However, there is good evidence that fetal growth retardation can occur and thus drugs of this group are falling out of fashion. Labetalol has been widely used but because of the β-blocking component its use is declining. It is the drug of first choice in the uncommon hypertensive emergencies requiring parenteral therapy. Possible fetal hazards associated with calcium channel-blocking drugs are unknown. Angiotensin-converting enzyme inhibitors (ACEIs) should not be used.

The aim of treatment is to achieve a diastolic blood-pressure which is never consistently above 90 mmHg.

Mild to moderate hypertension

If hypertension in pregnancy is not severe, or if it has been controlled before pregnancy but drug treatment is required for continued control, the need for further treatment must be decided. Restoring blood-pressure to normal is not sufficient reason for treatment.

Maternal benefits

The risks to the mother of mild or moderate hypertension are unclear. Should a woman be treated with long-term antihypertensive therapy on the same grounds that she would be treated if she were not pregnant? Treatment and potential benefits are long-term considerations and postponing therapy until after pregnancy may be reasonable.

Preventing pre-eclampsia

Patients who develop hypertension in early pregnancy are probably at increased risk of pre-eclampsia. If chronic hypertension has a causal role in the development of pre-eclampsia, treatment of hypertension early in pregnancy might prevent later superimposed pre-eclampsia, as has been claimed. Nevertheless, a critical review of the evidence from controlled trials indicates that, apart from lowering blood-pressure, antihypertensive agents do not affect the development of proteinuria or any of the other features of pre-eclampsia.

Uteroplacental blood flow

The possible effect on the uteroplacental circulation and hence the fetal lifeline are important considerations when deciding whether or not the blood-pressure should be reduced. There are two approaches:

1 If the uterine artery behaves as a rigid conduit (or is maximally dilated), reductions in maternal blood-pressure will concomitantly decrease uteroplacental perfusion. Consequently, large reductions in maternal systemic pressure must be avoided. This is important in relation to the arguments that placental ischaemia is the cause, rather than the consequence, of the hypertension.

2 If uteroplacental blood flow autoregulates rapidly and completely, aggressive lowering of blood-pressure should be the aim. If autoregulation occurs in humans, a critical question is how quickly it occurs, because the fetus may be compromised by trivially brief periods of ischaemia.

Uteroplacental perfusion is normal or even increased with mild to moderate maternal hypertension, only becoming abnormal when severe pre-eclampsia or intrauterine growth retardation or both are present. This endorses the clinical observation that pregnancies complicated by mild to moderate hypertension often exhibit no evidence of fetal compromise.

Fetal benefits

Fetal outcome in later pregnancy is closely linked to the presence of pre-eclampsia. In pregnancies complicated by hypertension without pre-eclampsia, the outcome is no worse than in normal pregnancies. The consensus is that antihypertensive treatment does not produce benefit for fetal outcome. Caution is needed in interpreting results from hypertensive patients who demonstrate improvement over previous pregnancies: superimposed pre-eclampsia with a high incidence of fetal mortality occurs most often in the first pregnancy and a woman is more likely to be compliant if a previous pregnancy was complicated.

Conclusions for mild to moderate hypertension

Antihypertensive drugs can be withheld until diastolic blood-pressure reaches 105 mmHg or more, which takes into account both the mother's safety and the fetal outcome. Non-specific sedation is dangerous and does not control blood-pressure.

Severe hypertension

This section deals with drug treatment when a high pressure climbs further, usually near term or intrapartum. Antihypertensive treatment will only reduce the risk of those complications that are a direct consequence of high pressure. The other complications of severe pre-eclampsia must be specifically managed. The major aim of treating severe hypertension in pregnancy is to prevent acute cerebrovascular injury.

Pressures of 170/110 and 180/120 represent mean arterial pressures of 130 and 140 mmHg respectively, at which vascular decompensation and end-organ damage occur. It is essential to avoid elevations of pressure above these figures, even for short periods. Even when delivery is expedited, a high blood-pressure often does not regress immediately.

A major disadvantage of lowering arterial pressure could be a reduction in perfusion pressure in the systemic vascular beds, especially the uteroplacental circulation. With a careful lowering of pressure by no more than 15%, fetal distress can be avoided. Once control is achieved continuous therapy is more effective and acceptable than repeated injections of depressor drugs. When acute emergencies occur early in the third trimester without marked deterioration in renal function, some attempt might be made to control the hypertension in the short term to enhance subsequent neonatal survival, but other changes of pre-eclampsia may progress. If the pressure becomes uncontrollable, this is an indication to end the pregnancy be elective delivery.

Coagulation abnormalities

During normal pregnancy several clotting factors, including VII, VIII, X and fibrinogen, increase and fibrinolytic activity, as measured by levels of circulating plasminogen, is depressed. This combination of changes suggests a particular susceptibility to the development of intravascular coagulation. There is controversy concerning the incidence and significance of coagulation abnormalities in pre-eclampsia. Some claim that a reduction in platelet count and defects in platelet function are the earliest signs of pre-eclampsia, occurring weeks before clinical signs are evident. Idiopathic thrombocytopenic purpura may be incorrectly diagnosed.

The possibility that coagulation defects and deficient prostaglandin production may be linked has been suggested, since the appropriate balance between vascular prostacyclin (prostaglandin I_2 or PGI_2) and platelet thromboxane synthesis is considered important for normal clotting. It has been suggested that, when the diagnosis of pre-eclampsia is a possibility, an immediate platelet count is necessary to exclude severe thrombocytopenia. There is a subgroup of such patients to which the acronym HELLP (H, haemolysis, EL, elevated liver enzymes, LP, low platelet count) syndrome has been given. Such patients may have extremely high transaminase concentrations ($>$ 1000 IU/L) and platelet counts may decrease rapidly to values $< 40 \times 10^3/mm^3$. This syndrome is a medical emergency and the pregnancy should be terminated rapidly. Fortunately, most patients survive with supporting care, coagulation and liver dysfunction improving a few days after evacuation of the uterus.

Some therapeutic controversies

Role of diuretics

Diuretics do not reduce the incidence of pre-eclampsia or perinatal mortality. Administration of these agents is not without risk: maternal pancreatitis, severe hypokalaemia, neonatal electrolyte imbalance, bleeding diatheses, cardiac arrhythmias and thrombocytopenia can occur. This does not ignore the fact that oedema does occur in pre-eclampsia; it merely emphasizes that, in the mild case, the differentiation between physiological and early pre-eclamptic oedema may not be possible. The only condition where diuretics should be prescribed unhesitatingly is heart failure.

Role of anticoagulant therapy

Anticoagulants in hypertension can be associated with cerebral bleeding and liver haematomata and are too hazardous. A deep venous thrombosis or pulmonary embolus are exceptions.

Role of volume expansion therapy

It has been suggested that the decrease in plasma volume, the occasional low central venous pressure and the vasoconstriction may be due to overcompensation of various pressor systems to the intravascular volume depletion. All are controversial. One view is that decreased intravascular volume is the primary event responsible for the rise in pressure. Another view, that of the traditional hypertension experts, is that decreased volume is secondary to vasoconstriction and treatment with volume expanders is dangerous.

While some of the results of initial studies are impressive, most patients treated had only moderate hypertension. Currently, caution is needed because myocardial performance may be compromised in severe pre-eclampsia and volume expansion, especially with saline, may enhance vascular reactivity. Infusion of crystalloids decreases oncotic pressure, which is already low in most pre-eclamptics and persists *post partum*: pulmonary and cerebral oedema may then develop.

Role of prostaglandin therapy

The incidence of pre-eclampsia is apparently lower in women who take aspirin in pregnancy compared with those who do not. It has been suggested that low-dose aspirin (<100 mg/day), which inhibits the cyclo-oxygenase of thromboxane A_2-generating platelets more effectively than the cyclo-oxygenase of PGI_2-generating endothelial cells, may therefore be beneficial in pre-eclampsia. Aspirin, with or without antithrombotic drugs, has been used successfully from early in pregnancy in women with histories of recurrent fetal loss and hypertension.

Epidural anaesthesia

The use of epidural anaesthesia in the acutely hypertensive patient prior to delivery is controversial. Such patients are vasoconstricted and hypovolaemic. Although autonomic blockade may reverse the hypertension, severe hypotension may ensue because of the hypovolaemia. Avoidance or alleviation of hypotension by intravenous fluid loading may help, but the consequences throughout an already grossly altered cardiovascular system and particularly the perfusion of the uteroplacental circulation are unknown. Epidural anaesthesia provides adequate analgesia without depression of the fetal central nervous system.

Blood transfusion

A pregnant woman with a shrunken intravascular compartment is less tolerant of blood loss than is a normal pregnant woman. Blood replacement needs to be commenced sooner but very carefully, to guard against the dangers of underfilling and overfilling, especially during surgery.

Fetal surveillance and decisions about delivery

Serial assessment of fetal well-being is essential. Antepartum cardiotography and amniotic fluid assessment can be useful. When any complication arises, the correct moment for intervention and route of delivery must be decided with the aim of minimizing the hazards of prematurity and neonatal morbidity and mortality. Most babies weighing >1500 g survive better in a special care nursery than in a hostile intrauterine environment.

Problems with particular renal diseases (Table 18.5)

Chronic and acute glomerulonephritis

It is generally held that renal function only decreases in patients with diffuse glomerulonephritis, in whom hypertension is both more common and severe. Nevertheless, most pregnancies in these women are successful.

Acute glomerulonephritis is a rare complication of pregnancy, but it may be mistaken for pre-eclampsia.

Pyelonephritis (tubulointerstitial nephritis)

As with glomerular disease, outcome in pyelonephritis is most favourable in normotensive women with adequate renal function.

Acute and chronic pyelonephritis have been dealt with in Chapters 7, p. 96, and 8, pp. 108–12. The differential diagnosis includes other

Table 18.5 Pregnancy and specific renal diseases

Renal disease	Effects
Chronic glomerulonephritis	Usually no adverse effect in the absence of hypertension. One view is that glomerulonephritis is adversely affected by the coagulation changes of pregnancy. Urinary tract infections may occur more frequently
Pyelonephritis	Bacteriuria in pregnancy can lead to exacerbation
Polycystic disease	Functional impairment and hypertension usually minimal in childbearing years
Diabetic nephropathy	No adverse effect on the renal lesion, but there is increased frequency of infection, oedema and pre-eclampsia
Systemic lupus erythematosus	Controversial; prognosis most favourable if disease in remission >6 months prior to conception. Steroid dosage should be increased *post partum*
Polyarteritis nodosa	Fetal prognosis is dismal and maternal death often occurs
Scleroderma	If onset during pregnancy, then can be rapid overall deterioration. Reactivation of quiescent scleroderma may occur *post partum*
Permanent urinary diversion	Can be associated with other malformations of the urogenital tract. Urinary tract infection common during pregnancy. Renal function may undergo reversible decrease. No significant obstructive problem but caesarian section often needed for abnormal presentation
After nephrectomy, solitary and pelvic kidneys	Pregnancy is well tolerated. May be associated with other malformations of urogenital tract. Pregnancy dystocia rarely occurs with a pelvic kidney
Urolithiasis	Infections may be more frequent, but ureteral dilatation and stasis do not seem to affect natural history

urinary tract pathology, such as renal calculus or acute hydronephrosis, which may be diagnosed by ultrasound scanning or a limited intravenous urogram. Other causes of fever may be due to pneumonia, viraemia or toxoplasmosis. Causes of acute abdominal pain with fever are most often explained by acute appendicitis, biliary colic, gastroenteritis, necrobiosis of a uterine fibroid or abruption of the placenta. The GFR may be reduced during an acute episode in pregnancy, in contradistinction to the usual lack of change in non-pregnant patients.

Acute pyelonephritis is associated with an increased incidence of premature labour, intrauterine growth retardation and fetal death. It is also a marker for increased risk of sudden infant death of the offspring.

Diabetic nephropathy

Because many patients have been diabetic since childhood, they probably already have subclinical diabetic nephropathy. During pregnancy, these women have an increased incidence of covert bacteriuria (and may be more susceptible to urinary tract infection), peripheral oedema and pre-eclampsia. Most women with diabetic nephropathy demonstrate normal GFR increments and pregnancy does not accelerate renal functional deterioration.

Polycystic renal disease

Polycystic renal disease may remain undetected during pregnancy, but questioning for a family history and the use of ultrasonography can lead to earlier detection. Patients do well when functional impairment is minimal and hypertension is absent, as is often the case in childbearing years. There is an increased incidence of hypertension late in pregnancy, compared with the pregnancies of sisters unaffected by this autosomal dominant disease.

Systemic lupus erythematosus

Systemic lupus erythematosus (SLE) is a relatively common disease in women of childbearing age. Coincidence with pregnancy poses complex clinical problems due to immunological abnormalities, multiple potential organ involvement and the complicated immunology of pregnancy itself. Transient improvement, no change and a tendency to relapse are all recorded. Individual decisions regarding disease activity and the wish to have a baby must be discussed with patient and partner. The majority of pregnancies succeed, especially when the maternal disease is in complete clinical remission for 6 months prior to conception, even if there have been severe structural changes, as shown by renal biopsy. Continued disease activity or increasing renal dysfunction reduces the likelihood of an uncomplicated pregnancy.

Lupus nephritis may sometimes become manifest during pregnancy and, when accompanied by hypertension and renal dysfunction, may be mistaken for pre-eclampsia. Some patients have a tendency to relapse, occasionally severely in the puerperium. It is prudent to prescribe or increase steroids at this time for a few weeks.

Placental transmission of lupus serum factors (perhaps the so-called lupus anticoagulant) occurs. This anticoagulant was first described in patients with SLE but it has since been observed in other conditions and even without any identifiable disorder. Intrauterine death is common in women with lupus anticoagulant, and placentae show extensive thrombotic and arteriosclerotic changes. Because treatment with steroids and aspirin can lead to successful pregnancies, it is important to screen for lupus anticoagulant in all women with SLE in order to identify this particular group and perhaps also in those with a history of recurrent intrauterine death or thrombotic episodes.

An increased incidence of congenital cardiac anomalies occurs in the offspring of women with SLE and other maternal connective-tissue diseases, even when maternal pathology appears quiescent. This association appears to be related to the transplacental passage of a maternal antibody (anti-Ro [SS-A]) and to soluble tissue ribonucleoprotein, which is detectable in almost all cases of isolated congenital complete heart block. Paradoxically, the mother's heart is usually unaffected: the fetal heart may therefore be more vulnerable to antibody-mediated damage than the mature heart.

Polyarteritis nodosa

In contrast to lupus nephritis, the outcome of pregnancy in women with renal polyarteritis nodosa is very poor, largely because of the associated hypertension, which is often of accelerated phase severity. Although a few successful pregnancies have been reported, the fetal prognosis is dismal and there have been many maternal deaths. This is important when discussing a possible pregnancy. Early termination has less maternal risk.

Scleroderma

The combination of pregnancy and scleroderma is unusual because scleroderma occurs most frequently after the fourth decade and younger patients with it tend to be relatively infertile. When it develops in pregnancy, there is a greater tendency for deterioration in maternal renal function. Even after an uneventful and successful pregnancy, postpartum reactivation may occur. Most maternal deaths involve pulmonary complications and infection.

Permanent urinary diversion

Permanent urinary diversion is still used in the management of patients with congenital lower urinary tract defects. Since the introduction of self-catheterization for neurogenic bladders, its use has declined. The most common complication is urinary infection. Premature labour occurs in 20% and the use of prophylactic antibiotics throughout pregnancy may reduce the incidence. Decline in renal function may occur, invariably related to infection or intermittent obstruction or both. With an ileal conduit, elevation and compression by the expanding uterus can cause outflow obstruction and, with a ureterosigmoid anastomosis, ureteral obstruction may occur. Changes usually reverse after delivery.

The mode of delivery is dictated by obstetric factors. Abnormal presentation accounts for a caesarean section rate of 25%, related to minor genital tract abnormalities. Vaginal delivery is safe but, as the continence of a uretherosigmoid anastomosis depends on an intact anal sphincter, this must be protected with a mediolateral episiotomy.

Solitary kidney

Some patients have either a congenital absence of one kidney or unilateral hypoplasia. Most, however, have had a previous nephrectomy because of pyelonephritis, unilateral tuberculosis, congenital abnormalities or a tumour. It is important to know the indication for and the time since the nephrectomy. In patients with infectious or structural renal conditions, pre-pregnancy investigation is needed for detection of persistent infection.

It makes no difference whether the right or left kidney remains as long as it is located in the normal anatomical position. If function is normal and stable, all women with unilateral nephrectomy tolerate pregnancy well, despite the superimposition of GFR increments on already hyperfiltering nephrons (see p. 263). Ectopic kidneys (usually pelvic) are more vulnerable to infection and are associated with decreased fetal salvage, probably because of associated malformations of the urogenital tract. If infection occurs in a solitary kidney during pregnancy and does not quickly respond to antibiotics, then termination may have to be considered for preservation of renal function.

Urolithiasis

The prevalence of urolithiasis in pregnancy is 0.03–0.35%. Renal and uteric calculi are one of the most common causes of non-uterine abdominal pain severe enough to necessitate hospital admission during pregnancy. When there are complications that need surgical intervention, pregnancy should not be a deterrent to intravenous urography. Specific clinical criteria should be met before requesting an IVU, assuming that an ultrasound study has not been diagnostic. They include:

1 microscopic haematuria;
2 recurrent urinary tract infection;
3 sterile urine culture when pyelonephritis is suspected.

The presence of two indicates a diagnosis of calculi in 60% of women and an IVU is advised.

Management should be conservative initially, with adequate hydration, appropriate antibiotic therapy and pain relief with systemic analgesics. The use of continuous segmental (T11–L2) epidural block has been advocated, as in non-pregnant patients with ureteric colic, and this may allow spontaneous passage of a stone or stones. With good pain relief, the patient micturates without difficulty, moves without assistance and is less at risk from thromboembolic complications than if drowsy, nauseated and bedridden with pain.

Nephrotic syndrome

The most common cause of nephrotic syndrome in late pregnancy is pre-eclampsia, which has a worse fetal prognosis than pre-eclampsia with less heavy proteinuria. There are many other causes of nephrotic syndrome (p. 142). Only a minority respond to steroids, emphasizing the importance of a diagnosis before possible steroid therapy.

If renal function is adequate and hypertension is absent, there should be few complications during pregnancy. Several of the physiological changes occurring during pregnancy may aggravate or exacerbate the syndrome. For example, increments in renal haemodynamics as well as increase in renal vein pressure may enhance protein excretion. Serum albumin concentrations usually decrease by 5–10 g/L during normal pregnancy; further decreases in nephrotic patients may enhance the tendency toward fluid retention. Because of decreased intravascular volume, diuretics may compromise uteroplacental perfusion or aggravate the increased tendency to thrombotic episodes.

Counselling patients with chronic renal disease

Patient expectation is higher than ever. Discussion should cover the advisability of pregnancy, the possible complications, the chances of producing a healthy baby and the long-term effects on the woman's kidneys (Table 18.6).

Pregnancy does not adversely affect the natural history of the renal lesion if kidney dysfunction is minimal and hypertension is absent at conception, with the exception of SLE and polyarteritis nodosa. An important factor in remote prognosis is the sclerotic effects that hyperfiltration might already have had in the residual (intact) glomeruli of kidneys of patients with renal insufficiency. Theoretically, further progressive loss of renal function could ensue in pregnancy. Similarly, the superimposition of pregnancy hyperfiltration on the compensatory changes already present in a single kidney could lessen the lifespan of that kidney. The crux of the hypothesis is the implication that increases in glomerular pressure and glomerular plasma flow cause sclerosis within the glomerulus and thus in pregnancy further physiological

Table 18.6 Pregnancy and renal disease: functional status complications and outcome

	Disease severity (see Table 18.3, p. 266)		
Prospects (%)	Mild	Moderate	Severe
Pregnancy complications	22	41	84
Successful obstetric outcome	95 (82)	90 (56)	47 (8)
Long-term sequelae	<5 (8)	25 (77)	53 (92)

These estimates do not include collagen diseases. The figures in parentheses refer to prospects when complications develop before the 28th week of pregnancy.

hyperfiltration augments the damage (see also pp. 199 and 263). More information is needed for women with renal disease.

Acute renal failure specific to pregnancy

This section emphasizes specific conditions in obstetric practice (Table 18.7). Usually, acute renal failure occurs in women with previously healthy kidneys, but it can complicate the course of the disease in patients with pre-existing renal disease. When anuria or oliguria is noted, obstruction to renal outflow must be excluded. It is all too easy unwittingly to damage the urinary tract when performing emergency surgery for obstetric disasters (such as postpartum haemorrhage), which can themselves be causes of acute renal failure.

Acute renal failure in late pregnancy can even be due to obstruction from an enlarging uterus. Practical aspects have been dealt with in detail in Chapter 16, p. 224.

Septic abortion

Liberal abortion laws and antibiotics have led to an apparent disappearance of life-threatening septic abortion. However, the clinician should not be lulled into a false sense of security.

Table 18.7 Acute renal failure in pregnancy

Volume contraction or hypotension	Antepartum haemorrhage due to placenta praevia Postpartum haemorrhage: from uterus or extensive soft tissue trauma Abortion Hyperemesis gravidarum Adrenocortical failure; usually failure to augment steroids to cover delivery in patient on long-term therapy
Volume contraction or hypotension and coagulopathy	Antepartum haemorrhage due to abruptio placentae Pre-eclampsia or eclampsia Amniotic fluid embolism Incompatible blood transfusion Drug reaction(s) Acute fatty liver Haemolytic uraemic syndrome
Volume contraction or hypotension, coagulopathy and infection	Septic abortion Chorioamnionitis Pyelonephritis Puerperal sepsis
Urinary tract obstruction	Damage to ureters: during caesarean section and repair of cervical or vaginal lacerations Pelvic haematoma Broad ligament haematoma

There are many reasons why acute renal failure is associated with septic abortion. Dehydration and hypotension can lead to considerable renal ischaemia. Haemoglobinuria due to haemolysis is often present. Soap and lysol, common abortifacients, have specific nephrotoxic effects. The marked haemolysis caused by bacteria and chemical abortifacients is, however, sufficient to provoke the renal shutdown. Most pregnancy sepsis is due to Gram-negative bacteria; clostridia are responsible for only 0.5% of patients developing shock.

Presentation can be quite dramatic, with an abrupt rise in temperature to 40°C often associated with myalgia, vomiting and diarrhoea, the latter occasionally bloody. Hypotension, tachypnoea and progression to frank shock occur rapidly. The patient is usually jaundiced, with a particular bronze-like colour ascribed to the association of jaundice with cutaneous vasodilatation, cyanosis and pallor. Despite the presence of fever, the extremities are often cold and display purplish areas, which may be precursors of small patches of necrosis on the toes, fingers or nose.

There is laboratory evidence of severe anaemia due to haemolysis, indirect hyperbilirubinaemia, leucocytosis (25 000/mm^3 with marked shift to the left), thrombocytopenia ($<50\,000/mm^3$), disseminated intravascular coagulation and hypocalcaemia, which may provoke tetany. Abdominal X-ray may demonstrate air in the uterus or abdomen, the result of gas-forming organisms, or perforation of the uterus or both. Despite an obvious toxic and septicaemic picture, bacterial identification may be difficult. Matters may be further confused because clostridia are normally present in the female genital tract.

The clinician may be misled by an asymptomatic patient admitted with an incomplete abortion who rapidly develops shock and prostration. Generalized muscular pains, often most intense in the thorax and abdomen may lead to confusion, with an intra-abdominal inflammatory process. This is especially true when a history of provoked abortion is denied or not sought for because heavy vaginal bleeding is often not a prominent feature. Knowledge of recent treatment with antibiotics or other drugs is important if bacterial resistance or suppressed infection is to be diagnosed.

Acute renal failure and pre-eclampsia

Pre-eclampsia is accompanied by a characteristic renal lesion in which the glomeruli enlarge and become ischaemic due to swelling of glomerular endothelial and mesangial cells. Most pre-eclamptic patients have a moderate decrease in GFR. Occasionally acute renal failure develops. Acute tubular necrosis is the most common morphology but acute cortical necrosis may occur. It is possible that acute tubular necrosis is the obligatory outcome of glomerular cell swelling, which can lead to complete obliteration of the capillary lumen.

The patient is vasoconstricted and haemoconcentrated with a reduced intravascular volume. The reduction usually precedes the development of hypertension, and the susceptibility of hypertensive pregnant women to develop prerenal azotaemia when salt-restricted or treated with diuretics is well known. It is therefore possible that these patients (who also have an increased incidence of placental abruption) may be more susceptible than healthy women to the adverse renal effects of antepartum and intrapartum haemorrhage.

Acute renal failure and pyelonephritis

In the absence of complicating features such as obstruction, calculi or papillary necrosis, acute pyelonephritis is an extremely rare cause of acute renal failure in non-pregnant women, but this association appears to be more frequent in pregnant women. It is known that acute pyelonephritis in pregnancy is accompanied by marked reduction in GFR, in contrast to non-pregnant patients. It has been suggested that the vasculature in pregnancy may be more sensitive to the vasoactive effect of bacterial endotoxins.

Acute fatty liver of pregnancy

Acute fatty liver of pregnancy (also called obstetric pseudoacute yellow atrophy) is a rare complication of late pregnancy or the early postpartum period, characterized by jaundice and severe hepatic dysfunction. The renal failure appears to be due to haemodynamic factors, as in the hepatorenal syndrome, but some cases have been associated with DIC.

A typical patient presents with fever, abdominal pain, nausea and vomiting, and then rapidly develops severe jaundice and hepatic encephalopathy. Common misdiagnoses are septicaemia or pre-eclampsia with liver involvement. It has been suggested that acute fatty liver and pre-eclampsia coexist approximately 20% of the time.

Serum transaminases are only minimally increased, if at all, in a patient with marked hyperbilirubinaemia and severe hepatic failure. In contrast to patients with viral hepatitis, serum glutamic oxaloacetic transaminase activity is higher than that of pyruvate transaminase. Alkaline phosphatase and amylase are occasionally raised and hyperammonaemia has been recorded. Serum urate levels may be elevated out of proportion to the degree of renal dysfunction. Hyperuricaemia may precede clinical presentation.

Treatment consists of termination of the pregnancy and supportive therapy for hepatic and renal failure. The efficacy of termination has not been proved. The mortality rate is high, death resulting primarily from hepatic rather than renal failure.

Idiopathic postpartum renal failure

Idiopathic postpartum renal failure (also called postpartum malignant sclerosis, irreversible postpartum renal failure and postpartum haemolytic uraemic syndrome) is rare and usually fatal, characterized by the onset of renal failure in the puerperium. The patient has an uneventful pregnancy and delivery but 3–6 weeks into the puerperium she develops marked azotaemia and severe hypertension, frequently associated with microangiopathic haemolytic anaemia and platelet consumption.

There is uncertainty concerning the management of this condition as many patients succumb despite treatment with dialysis, immunosuppression and heparin, streptokinase, dipyridamole, aspirin or corticosteroids, alone or combined. A supposed lack of prostacyclin (PGI_2), a powerful vasodilator and potent endogenous inhibitor of platelet aggregation, can be counteracted by exchange transfusion or even plasma infusion alone. Prolonged PGI_2 infusions have been tried, with the aim of restoring the deficiency, thus controlling the hypertension and reversing the platelet consumption. It has been argued that DIC is important, with placental thromboplastin being released during labour. Antithrombin III (AT-III) may have a protective effect and can be given as a concentrate to correct the low plasma AT-III concentrations sometimes found at the onset of this syndrome.

Cortical necrosis in pregnancy

Renal cortical necrosis, a pathological entity characterized by necrosis of the cortex with sparing of the medulla, occurs more readily in pregnant than in non-pregnant women. Acute cortical necrosis may develop in patients with DIC and overwhelming septicaemia, but it is more common in the third trimester or the puerperium, when septic complications are less common. Multigravidae over the age of 30 are more likely to develop cortical necrosis, which is particularly associated with placental abruption and, to a lesser extent, unrecognized long-standing intrauterine death and occasionally pre-eclampsia.

While the cortical necrosis may involve the entire cortex, resulting in irreversible renal failure, the 'patchy' variety occurs more often in pregnancy. This is characterized by an initial episode of severe oliguria, which lasts much longer than in uncomplicated cases of acute tubular necrosis. Subsequently, there is a variable return of function and stable period of moderate renal insufficiency. Years later, renal function may gradually decline, leading to end-stage renal failure.

Summary

Changes in plasma and serum variables during normal pregnancy are so marked that non-pregnancy normal ranges cannot be used for obstetric management. Recognition of the changes is essential if kidney conditions in pregnancy are to be diagnosed and managed correctly.

Most women with mild or moderate renal disease tolerate pregnancy well and have a successful obstetric outcome without adverse effect on the natural history of the underlying renal lesion. Crucial determinants are renal function at conception, the presence or absence of hypertension and the type of renal disease. Pregnancy outcome is unpredictable in the presence of focal and segmental glomerular sclerosis, IgA nephritis, mesangiocapillary glomerulonephritis, reflux nephropathy and systemic disorders.

Acute obstetric renal failure occasionally occurs in women with previously healthy kidneys, Pathology peculiar to pregnancy must then be considered.

Further reading

1 Abe, S. (1991) Pregnancy in IgA nephropath. *Kid. Int.* **40**, 1098–1102.
2 Baylis, C. (1987) Glomerular filtration and volume regulation in gravid animal models. *Clin. Obstet. Gynaecol.* **1**, 789–813.
3 Baylis, C. & Rennke, H.G. (1985) Renal hemodynamics and glomerular morphology in repetitively pregnant ageing rats. *Kidney Int.* **28**, 140–5.
4 Brown, M.A. (1990) Urinary tract dilatation in pregnancy. *Am. J. Obstet. Gynecol.* **164**, 641–3.
5 Cietak, K.A. & Newton, J.R. (1985) Serial quantitative maternal nephrosonography in pregnancy. *Br. J. Radiol.* **58**, 405–13.
6 Cox, S.M., Shelburne, P., Mason, R., Guss, S. & Cunningham, F.G. (1991) Mechanisms of hemolysis and anemia associated with acute antepartum pyelonephritis. *Am. J. Obstet. Gynecol.* **164**, 587–90.
7 Cunningham, F.G., Cox, S.M., Harstad, T.W., Mason, R.A. & Pritchard, J.A. (1990) Chronic renal disease and pregnancy outcome. *Am. J. Obstet. Gynecol.* **163**, 453–9.
8 Davison, J.M. (1983) The kidney in pregnancy: a review. *J. Roy. Soc. Med.* **76**, 485–501.
9 Davison, J.M. (1987) Renal transplantation and pregnancy. *Am. J. Kidney Dis.* **9**, 374–80.
10 Davison, J.M. & Dunlop, W. (1984) Renal hemodynamics and tubular function in human pregnancy. *Clin. Obstet. Gynaecol.* **1**, 769–71.
11 Davison, J.M., Dellagrammatikas, H. & Parkin, J.M. (1985) Maternal azathioprine therapy and depressed haemopoiesis in the babies of renal allograft recipients. *Br. J. Obstet. Gynaecol.* **92**, 233–9.
12 Davison, J.M., Katz, A.I. & Lindheimer, M.D. (1985) Pregnancy in women with renal disease and renal transplantation. *Proc. EDTA–ERA* **22**, 439–49.
13 Dekker, G.A. & Sibai, B.M. (1993) Low dose aspirin in prevention of pre-eclampsia and fetal growth retardation: rationale, mechanisms and clinical trials. *Am. J. Obstet. Gynecol.* **168**, 214–17.
14 Editorial (1991) Systemic lupus in pregnancy. *Lancet* **385**, 87–8.
15 Hayslett, J.P. (1982) Effect of pregnancy in patients with SLE. *Am. J. Kidney Dis.* **2**, 223–8.
16 Hayslett, J.P. (1985) Postpartum renal failure. *N. Engl. J. Med.* **312**, 1556–9.
17 Hou, S.H., Grossman, S.D. & Madias, N.E. (1985) Pregnancy in women with renal disease and moderate renal insufficiency. *Am. J. Med.* **78**, 185–94.
18 Imbasciati, E. & Ponticelli, C. (1991) Pregnancy and renal disease: predictor for fetal and maternal outcome. *Am. J. Nephrol.* **11**, 353–62.
19 Jungers, P., Forget, D., Henry-Amar, M., Albouze, G., Fournier, P., Vischer, U., Droz, D., Noel, L.-H. & Grunfeld, J.-P. (1986) Chronic kidney disease and pregnancy. *Adv. Nephrol.* **15**, 103–41.
20 Kincaid-Smith, P., Whitworth, J.A. & Fairley, K.F. (1980) Mesangial IgA nephropathy in pregnancy. *Clin. Exp. Hypertension* **2**, 821–38.
21 Kuhlback, B. & Widholm, O. (1966) Plasma creatinine in normal pregnancy. *Scand. J. Clin. Lab. Invest.* **18**, 654–8.
22 Levey, A.S., Perrone, R.D. & Madias, N.E. (1988) Serum creatinine and renal function. *Ann. Rev. Med.* **39**, 465–9.

23 Lindheimer, M.D. & Davison, J.M. (1987) Renal biopsy during pregnancy. *Br. J. Obstet. Gynaecol.* **94**, 932–6.
24 Lindheimer, M.D. & Katz, A.I. (1991) The kidney in pregnancy. In Brenner, B.M. & Rector, F.C., Jr. (eds), *The Kidney*, 4th edn. W.B. Saunders, Philadelphia, pp. 1762–1837.
25 Lindheimer, M.D. & Katz, A.I. (1985) Hypertension in pregnancy. *N. Engl. J. Med.* **313**, 675–9.
26 Maikranz, P., Coe, F.L., Parks, J.H. & Lindheimer, M.D. (1987) Nephrolithiasis in pregnancy. *Am. J. Kidney Dis.* **9**, 354–8.
27 Meyers, S.J., Lee, R.V. & Munschauer, R.W. (1985) Dilatation and nontraumatic rupture of the urinary tract during pregnancy: a review. *Obstet. Gynaecol.* **66**, 809–15.
28 Mor-Yosef, S., Navot, D., Rabinowitz, R. & Schenker, J.G. (1984) Collagen disease in pregnancy. *Obstet. Gynaecol. Surv.* **39**, 67–83.
29 Naden, R.P. & Redman, C.W.G. (1985) Antihypertensive drugs in pregnancy. *Clin. Perinatol.* **12**, 521–38.
30 Naumann, R.O. & Weinstein, L. (1985) Disseminated intravascular coagulation–the clinician's dilemma. *Obstet. Gynaecol. Surv.* **40**, 487–92.
31 Neilsen, F.R. & Rasmussen, P.E. (1988) Hydronephrosis during pregnancy: four cases of hydronephrosis causing symptoms during pregnancy. *Eur. J. Obstet. Gynaecol. Reprod. Biol.* **69**, 446–50.
32 Patterson, N.S., McKay, E.J., Liggins, G.L. & Lubbe, W.F. (1987) Anticardiolipin antibodies: their presence as a marker for lupus anticoagulant in pregnancy. *N. Engl. J. Med.* **100**, 61–4.
33 Petis, M., Howard, D. & Repke, J. (1991) Frequency of lupus flare in pregnancy. *Arth. Rheum.* **34**, 1538–45.
34 Pertuiset, N., Ganeval, D. & Grunfeld, J.-P. (1984) Acute renal failure in pregnancy: an update. *Semin. Nephrol.* **4**, 232–9.
35 Registration Committee of the European Dialysis and Transplant Association (1980) Successful pregnancies in women treated by dialysis and kidney transplantation. *Br. J. Obstet. Gynaecol.* **87**, 839–45.
36 Reimers, T.J. & Sluss, P.M. (1978) 6-Mercaptopurine treatment of pregnant mice: effects on second and third generations. *Science* **201**, 65–7.
37 Sturgis, S.N., Lindheimer, M.D. & Davison, J.M. (1992) Treatment of hypertension during pregnancy: drugs to be avoided and drugs to be used. In Andreucci, V.E. & Fine, L.G. (eds), *International Year Book of Nephrology*. Springer-Verlag, Heidelberg, pp. 163–96.
38 Taylor, P.V., Taylor, K.F., Norman, A., Griffiths, J. & Scott, J.S. (1988) Prevalence of maternal Ro (SS-A) and La (SS-B) autoantibodies in relationship to congenital heart block. *Br. J. Rheumatol.* **27**, 128–32.
39 Thacker, S.B. & Berkelman, R.L. (1985) Assessing the diagnostic accuracy and efficacy of selected antepartum surveillance techniques. *Obstet. Gynaecol. Surv.* **41**, 121–41.
40 Wallenburg, H.C.S., Dekker, G.A., Makovitz, J.W. & Rotmans, P. (1986) Low-dose aspirin prevents pregnancy-induced hypertension and pre-eclampsia in angiotensin-sensitive primigravidae. *Lancet* **i**, 1–3.

Chapter 19
Renal Stones

G. Alan Rose

Urinary stones have been found in Egyptian mummies and were well known to Hippocrates, receiving special mention in the oath that bears his name. In general, two main types of stone are recognized:

1 Bladder stones in children.

2 Upper urinary tract stones in adults.

The former are common in many developing countries. They are usually composed of a mixture of calcium oxalate and ammonium urate. Several factors contribute to their production:

1 A low-phosphate diet leads to acid urine with high ammonia content, conditions which favour precipitation of ammonium urate.

2 High intake of vegetables rich in oxalate causes hyperoxaluria and precipitation of calcium oxalate.

3 Recurrent acute enteritis causes chronic dehydration and low urinary volumes.

These stones gradually disappear as economic development advances. They disappeared from East Anglia, where they had been rife, at about the turn of the present century and have recently been diminishing in Sicily. In the undeveloped countries bladder stones in children are diagnosed much more frequently in poor villages than in more affluent towns.

In developed countries, while bladder stones in children diminished, upper urinary tract stones of adults have steadily increased in frequency and the prevalence is apparently still increasing. Over 5% of the population of West Germany, Sweden and the USA have or have had urinary stones. Because the incidence increases with age and stones are more common in males, a remarkably high proportion of elderly men will be found to have this condition. The more affluent sections of the community are especially affected, but the reason for this is still not clear.

Medical investigation of urinary stones

History

The history should reveal not only the number of stone episodes and whether the condition is unilateral or bilateral but also possible clues to the cause of stone formation. The following should therefore be included:

1 *Family history*. Some causes of stone formation, such as cystinuria, primary hyperoxaluria and uric acid stones, are familial or inherited.

2 *Dietary history*. This is especially important in the case of calcium oxalate stones. One should ask about intake of:

(a) Calcium-rich foods – milk, cheese, yoghurt and milk puddings. Calcium-rich medicaments such as calcium-aspirin or certain antacids.

(b) Oxalate-rich foods – rhubarb, spinach, beetroot, strawberries, nuts, chocolate, celery, tea and instant coffee.

(c) Ascorbate-rich foods – fruit juices and vitamin C tablets.

Note that it is the diet during the period that stones were being formed that is important. Frequently patients have modified their diet by the time the dietary history is taken.

3 *Drinking history*. Does the patient drink water with meals and at other times during the day or does he/she dislike water-drinking?

4 *Occupational history*. Has the patient's past or present occupation resulted in chronic dehydration? This might be because of exposure to heat or the difficulty of micturition, as in the case of a man who spent all his working day high up on a crane.

5 *Social history*. Certain sports such as sailing, skiing and jogging result in chronic dehydration. If the patient indulges in these, does he/she take active steps to avoid dehydration?

6 *Travel history*. Long-distance air travel is dehydrating because of the low humidity of the pressurized air. Arrival unacclimatized in a hot climate can lead to remarkably high loss of water in sweat. Hence the frequency of travel as well as the destination is important.

Thus one should aim at obtaining a complete picture of the patient's way of life and time spent so doing may be very rewarding.

Physical examination

There are few physical findings but certain signs may be helpful when seeking a cause for urolithiasis:

1 Asymmetry. Hemihypertrophy of the body is seen in about 30% of cases of medullary sponge kidney (MSK). Compare sizes of both arms and legs. In the case of the arms, one must know which is dominant.

2 Corneal calcification. This may be seen in long-standing hypercalcaemia. It can be seen readily with an auroscope, using the detached eyepiece as a magnifying glass.
3 Features of Cushing's syndrome, which can cause osteoporosis and hypercalciuria.
4 Hyperthyroidism.
5 Paget's disease of the bone, which can present with stones due to hypercalciuria.
6 Stigmata of old rickets (bow-legs, Harrison's sulcus), which might indicate renal tubular acidosis.

Laboratory investigations

Certain biochemical investigations are mandatory in all cases of urolithiasis unless the cause is already known.

Stone analysis

It is essential that the chemical nature of the stones is established by experienced laboratory staff. If not, cystinurics and uric acid stone-formers may be wrongly treated for calcium stone disease for years. Analysis should be by quantitative methods as the qualitative methods may give misleading results. Any district general hospital laboratory should be able to analyse stones quantitatively by wet chemistry, although most do not do so. Sophisticated methods are not essential but can be used if the equipment is available:
1 Thermogravimetric analysis.
2 Infra-red spectroscopy.
3 X-ray diffraction.

Twenty-four-hour urine

Twenty-four-hour urine is best collected as an out-patient while normal occupation and diet are pursued. It is best to ask the patient to bring with him/her the collection at his/her first appointment before he/she has been questioned about diet and water-drinking. Eating and drinking habits may be very different when working from when not working at the weekend. It is probably best to have the collection mid-week during a working-day, but it may be useful to have another collection over a weekend when not working. A collection made during a hospital admission may be highly misleading and should not be relied upon. The urine should be analysed for creatinine (as a guide to completeness of the save), calcium, oxalate, urate, sodium, citrate and magnesium. Of these, oxalate may well be the most important, but unfortunately it cannot be measured reliably in most laboratories at present. However, the position is changing and laboratory staff should be encouraged to try to make this measurement. If the urine becomes alkaline or even neutral during the collection period, any ascorbate present will spontaneously convert to oxalate. It is therefore best to collect into a bottle which contains 100 ml of 1 M HCl. This in turn causes other difficulties:

1 Uric acid may precipitate. If it is important to have reliable figures for urinary urate, either the sample should be thoroughly mixed in the laboratory and an aliquot for uric acid assay rendered alkaline, or a separate 24-hour save should be made with thymol substituted for acid. The latter is better because precipitated uric acid may stick to the walls of the container and be difficult to redissolve.

2 Urine pH of acidified urine has no physiological meaning. Because citrate excretion rises with urine pH, the value of the urinary citrate measurement is considerably reduced by not having the corresponding pH. Citrate is therefore measured on a random urine sample (see below).

In interpreting the urinary calcium measurement it is important:

1 To know the normal range in the locality in which one is working.

2 To realize that the upper limit of normal is not sharply defined in adult males. A small proportion of apparently healthy males have remarkably high urinary calcium values. It is still not clear if these are individuals who will make stones later. The following working rule is suggested. In a calcium stone-former the 24-hour urinary calcium should be below 9.0 mmol/24 hours in adult males or 7.5 mmol/24 hours in adult females.

Blood studies

A single sample of blood can be used for the following determinations:

1 Calcium, total proteins, albumin, sodium, potassium, bicarbonate, chloride, creatinine, alkaline phosphatase, urate and magnesium.

2 Sedimentation rate.

3 Serum immunoglobulins and light chains if there is any possibility of myeloma.

The serum calcium result should be corrected for protein abnormalities, using a formula based either upon total protein or upon albumin. It must be realized that these can only be approximate corrections and no one formula will always give the best results because all serum proteins bind calcium to some extent. The following may be used:

1 When serum proteins as a whole are altered due to constriction of the arm at venepuncture, allow 0.19 mmol of calcium for every 10 g/L of total proteins.

2 When albumin is low due to steatorrhoea or nephrotic syndrome, allow 0.25 mmol/L of calcium for every 10 g/L of albumin.

Random sample of urine

A random sample of urine is readily obtained in the out-patient department or an early morning sample may be collected in hospital. It is convenient and useful for the following:

1 *pH.* Uric acid stone-formers often have highly acidic urine and if the pH is below 5 the probability that a stone-former has uric acid lithiasis is high. A pH above 7.5 is strongly suggestive of urea-splitting bacterial infection as the cause. The urine pH is also helpful in interpreting the citrate result.

2 *Citrate:creatinine ratio.* In normal men the ratio is 0.08–0.5 and in women it is 0.15–0.7. The ratio is strikingly low – below 0.05 – in type I renal tubular acidosis (RTA) and is a useful way to recognize this condition. However, it must be remembered that the concentration of urinary citrate is low in renal failure and in steatorrhoea, so that one should exclude these conditions before concluding that RTA is present.

3 *Cystine screen test.* The cyanide/nitroprusside test is very easily performed on a random sample of urine and will identify or exclude cystinuria.

4 *Osmolality.* This is the most reliable measure of concentration of urine. It can be quite revealing. When performed on an out-patient random sample, it may expose inadequate water intake in a patient who says he drinks a lot of water. If osmolality cannot be measured, creatinine concentration is almost as good.

Imaging techniques

A KUB (kidneys, ureters and bladder) film is necessary for investigation of urolithiasis. The stones may be:

1 Clearly denser than nearby bones, indicating calcium oxalate/phosphate composition.

2 Radiolucent and not seen on the KUB, indicating uric acid, ammonium urate, xanthine, dihydroxyadenine or small cystine stones.

3 Visible on the KUB but not as dense as expected for calcium oxalate stones. These may be larger cystine stones or infection stones made of calcium phosphate/magnesium ammonium phosphate (MAP), or the very rare silica stones. Cystine stones are usually homogeneous in appearance whereas infection stones are usually striated with varying density in different layers.

The distribution of stones may be of interest. Clusters of small stones distributed through both kidneys suggests a metabolic cause:

1 Primary hyperparathyroidism (HPT).

2 Hyperoxaluria.

3 Renal tubular acidosis.

4 MSK.

Hemihypertrophy of the body may show up on the KUB film, suggesting MSK. An intravenous urogram (IVU) is necessary to reveal radiolucent stones and to confirm the diagnosis of MSK. The IVU will give an approximate idea of the degree of function in the kidneys and whether there is obstruction to urine flow from or one or more renal calyces, which might be a reason for urgent surgical or lithotriptic intervention. Renal stones are not well demonstrated by ultrasound; hence the need for an IVU in this context.

Special investigations

Urinary crystal studies

A random sample of urine is passed directly into a Dewar flask and examined as soon as possible. The same sample may be used for the 'random sample of urine', as above. Crystals may be examined on the intact urine by Coulter-counter, or examined in the deposit after centrifugation of a standard volume (25 ml). The crystals in the deposits may be demonstrated by suspending in a small standard volume and microscopy with a 37°C stage and measured by redissolving in acid and assaying the phosphate and oxalate. If the urine is dilute and there are no crystals, it can be quickly concentrated on a rotary evaporator *in vacuo* to standard osmolality (1250 mmol/L) and re-examined for crystals.

Urine acidification test

If urine pH is repeatedly at or above neutral, there may be a suspicion of RTA. To confirm or exclude this diagnosis an ammonium chloride load (0.1 g/kg body-weight) is given orally. This may induce nausea or vomiting and should therefore be given in gelatine capsules. If enteric-coated tablets are used, they should be well scored before use. The normal response is a fall in urinary pH to 5.3 or less within 4 hours.

Serum parathyroid hormone assay

The serum parathyroid hormone (PTH) assay is useful in the differential diagnosis of hypercalcaemia because assays for the intact PTH molecule are now available. The assay is expensive but has a high sensitivity and specificity.

Although most malignant hypercalcaemias are accompanied by low concentrations of serum PTH, occasional tumours do secrete this hormone. Furthermore, since primary HPT is now a rather common condition, it can occur in combination with tumour. Hence, there is still considerable scope for clinical skills in identifying these patients.

Parathyroid tumour localization

Because finding a parathyroid tumour may be difficult it would be useful if the position of the adenoma could be identified preoperatively. A number of techniques for doing so have been tried and found wanting; they work for large tumours, which are usually easy to find at operation, but fail to find the small ones which prove surgically difficult. The most useful procedure is probably catheterization of the neck veins, with measurement of PTH in blood from various sites. This is an invasive technique and subject to some risk and it is expensive because it requires a large number of PTH assays. It should be reserved for use after a first neck exploration has failed and before a second operation.

Chronic dehydration stone disease

It is often forgotten in the search for a metabolic cause of stone formation that low urinary volume is the most important risk factor and that chronic low urine volume is a common cause. About 16% of stone-of formers referred to my stone clinic prove to have no metabolic abnormality, but have a history of chronic dehydration due either to living in a hot climate or to working in a locally hot environment. It is important to recognize this group of patients because the treatment is so simple: water-drinking. It has been shown by prospective trial in Israel that immigrants to desert areas have higher urinary flow rates and make fewer stones if previously taught the importance of water-drinking.

Water-drinking as basic therapy for all urinary stone-formers

It is essential to advise all stone-formers to drink sufficient water to raise urinary volume to 3 L/24 hours (per 70 kg man) and for the flow to be distributed equally through each 3-hour period. If this were achieved, further stone formation would be most unlikely, but unfortunately it may fail, for a number of reasons:

1 The treatment is so simple and cheap that the patient does not believe it can be effective.
2 Daytime drinking is prevented by the patient's occupation.
3 Night-time micturition and drinking may be unacceptable.
4 Diurnal rhythm may prevent night-time excretion of a water load.
5 Hard water may be thought of as unacceptable because of its calcium content. This is incorrect. It is easily shown that, at least in a temperate climate where sweat losses are small, hard water is better than no water.

Patients require repeated reminders and encouragement to drink water until the habit is firmly established. They should bring a 24-hour urine collection at each hospital visit and the doctor should measure and discuss the volume with them.

In the specific conditions described below, it should be taken for granted that high water intake is invariably recommended.

Calcium oxalate/phosphate stones

The large increase in upper urinary tract stones in the developed countries in the last 90 years is due to calcium oxalate/phosphate stones. Calcium oxalate may be virtually the sole mineral or it may be associated with up to about 50% of calcium phosphate (apatite, brushite or octocalcium phosphate). Sometimes these stones form on Randall's plaques of calcium phosphate, even though the rest of the stone may be calcium oxalate. There is general agreement that urinary phosphate is normal in this type of stone disease. Urinary calcium may be raised, but there is little agreement on the magnitude and frequency of the rise. Some well-established centres find hypercalciuria frequently and other equally well-known centres find it rarely. Referral patterns of patients may vary from clinic to clinic. In recent years many groups have been recognizing hyperoxaluria as a characteristic of this stone type, probably as a result of improved methods for oxalate assay.

The following causes of calcium oxalate/phosphate stones will be considered:

1 Idiopathic hypercalciuria.
2 MSK.
3 Primary HPT.
4 RTA.

Idiopathic hypercalciuria

In the idiopathic hypercalciuria type of stone formation, there is no metabolic abnormality other than raised urinary calcium and perhaps low serum phosphate due to low Tm_{PO_4} (maximum tubular reabsorption of phosphate) in proximal renal tubules. This condition occurs predominantly in males. These patients do not develop bone rarefaction, are therefore in calcium balance and must be over-absorbers of dietary calcium. Some have attempted to divide the primary lesion into:

1 Over-absorption of dietary calcium.
2 Renal leak of calcium.

However, such attempts are probably misconceived and in any case do not help in choice of treatment. All respond well to thiazide diuretics with a fall in urinary calcium without any long-term large change in calcium balance.

Idiopathic hypercalciuria is accompanied by over-absorption of dietary oxalate and mild hyperoxaluria due to reduced faecal calcium. The hyperoxaluria is probably much more important than the hypercalciuria as a cause of stone formation. It is necessary to restrict oxalate intake as well as calcium. Reduction in dietary calcium alone will lead to hyperoxaluria and oxalate stone formation. The following dietary advice is therefore given:

1 Stop all cheese, milk, milky drinks, yoghurt, custard and milk puddings.
2 Milk allowed in tea and coffee from a daily allowance of 6–7 cups per day.
3 Stop all rhubarb, spinach, beetroot, strawberries, nuts, chocolate and celery.
4 Stop calcium-rich medicaments such as fizzy tablets or antacids

containing chalk or aluminium hydroxide. Milk of magnesia is allowed.

If urinary calcium remains too high, then thiazide diuretics may be added. Bendrofluazide is recommended, 2.5 mg/day for 4 days and thereafter 5 mg/day. However, caution is required if there is a family history of diabetes mellitus or gout and, in all patients, plasma concentrations of glucose, urate and potassium should be measured regularly. Other treatments have been used. Milk of magnesia in the highest dose tolerated without causing loose stools is probably helpful; the same applies to neutral phosphate. The latter involves a considerable load of sodium and potassium, which may be unacceptable with renal damage or hypertension or both.

Medullary sponge kidney

Medullary sponge kidney is a sporadic congenital condition with multiple cystic dilatations of the collecting tubules of the kidneys. It affects about 10% of stone-formers, males and females equally. Usually both kidneys are involved but sometimes only one or even one segment of one kidney may be affected. Urine stagnates in the cysts, leading to

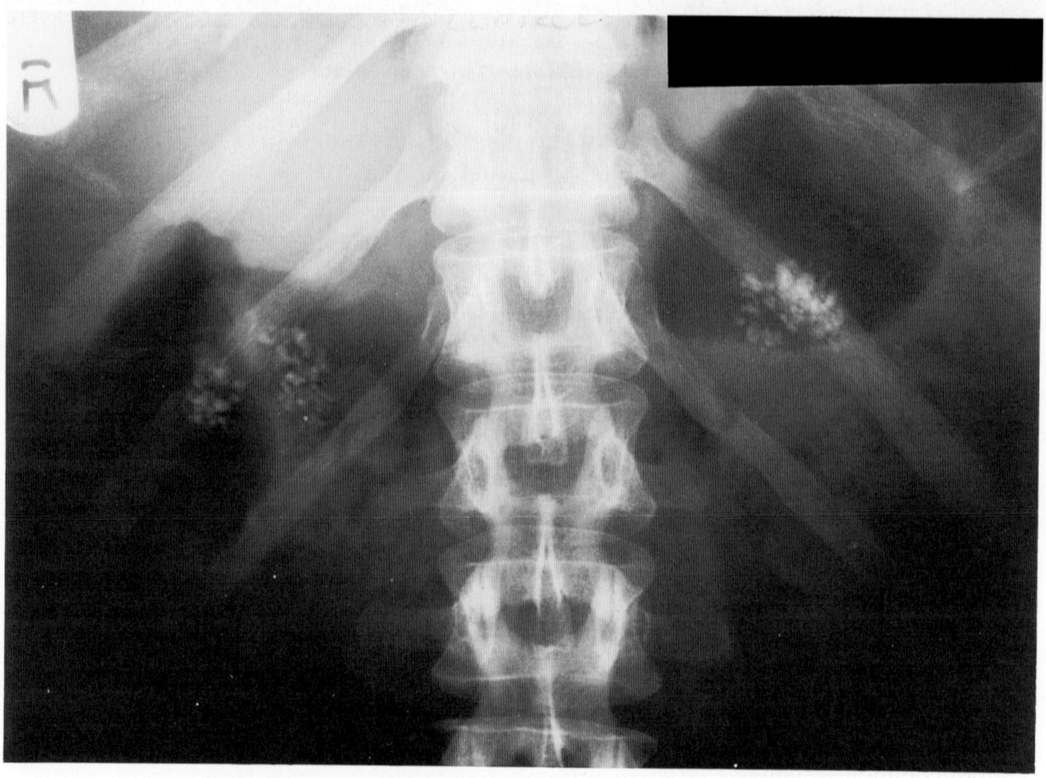

Fig. 19.1 Plain X-ray film from a man with medullary sponge kidney affecting upper segments of both kidneys. The distribution of opacities suggests the diagnosis but does not prove it.

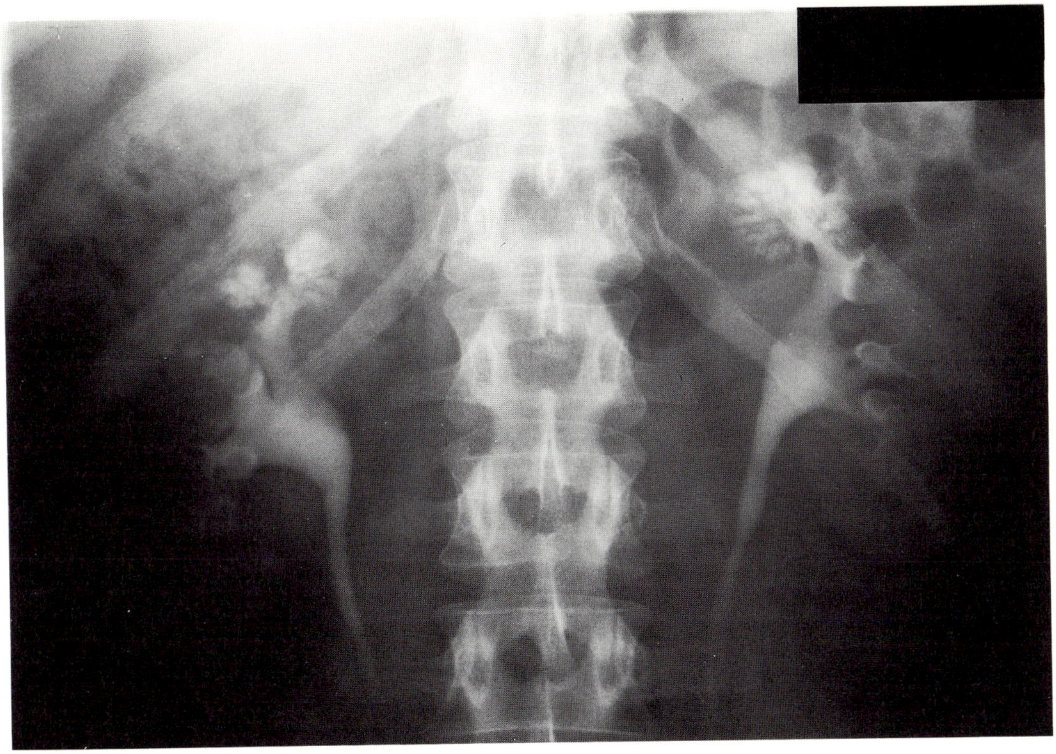

Fig. 19.2 An IVU from the same man as in Fig. 19.1. First, there are more cysts than there are opacities in Fig. 19.1. Secondly, the relationship of the cysts to the calyces is clearly seen. Thirdly, only the upper segments of the kidneys are affected in this particular case.

infection (mainly in females) or multiple stones related to the calyces, or both. Diagnosis may be suspected on a KUB film but can only be confirmed by demonstrating the cystic dilatations on an IVU film (Figs 19.1 and 19.2). Rather curiously, about 40% of cases also have hypercalciuria. It is important in this condition to reduce urinary calcium and oxalate as much as possible, using both diet and thiazides (see above). The condition does not usually lead to renal failure but can cause severe recurrent stone formation, with pain and suffering.

Primary hyperparathyroidism

Primary HPT is not uncommon and is often asymptomatic. It accounts for 5–10% of all stone-formers in many developed countries. It is a disease of 'bones, stones and abdominal groans', the latter being due not only to renal colic but also to acute pancreatitis and peptic ulcer. It is more common in females. The diagnosis depends upon the findings from laboratory and X-ray investigations:

1 Raised serum calcium.

2 Low serum phosphate.

3 Raised serum alkaline phosphatase.
4 Osteitis fibrosis cystica.

Bone disease is not usually present in patients with stones and thus numbers 3 and 4 are not seen. Serum phosphate is not invariably low, even where glomerular function is normal, and may be low in idiopathic hypercalcuria, with which it is most likely to be confused. Other measurements of renal tubular handling of phosphate are no more helpful. The most useful guide is the serum calcium concentration. It is not possible to make the diagnosis of HPT without finding an elevated serum calcium (after correction for serum proteins if necessary). A possible exception is when corrected serum calcium is repeatedly at the upper limit of normal. Measurement of plasma ionized calcium is difficult and rarely more helpful than a well-measured corrected total serum calcium. Measurement of serum PTH may be helpful when taken in conjunction with serum calcium. If PTH is low and the calcium concentration high, HPT can be excluded and the cause of the hypercalciuria will be malignancy, vitamin D overdose or sarcoid. Malignant tumours do occasionally secrete PTH. Hyperparathyroidism usually has a long clinical course while malignant hypercalciuria has a rather short course.

Treatment for HPT which is causing recurrent urinary stones is by surgical removal of the over-active parathyroid(s). Usually this is a single adenoma, but occasionally there is more than one adenoma or hyperplasia of all four glands. In the latter case the surgeon has a dilemma. Removal of all four leaves the patient dependent upon vitamin D therapy for life, while leaving 100 mg of one parathyroid behind will probably lead to recurrence of HPT. Reimplanting 100 mg in the arm muscles is currently under evaluation. If the surgeon fails to find an adenoma, localization studies are then required, as described on p. 289.

Renal tubular acidosis

Renal tubular acidosis is an uncommon condition in which there is inability or reduced ability of the renal tubules to generate acid urine in response to acidaemia. There are two main subtypes:

1 Distal tubular reduced ability to sustain a pH gradient between urine and epithelial cells. This is the more common of the subtypes. It is usually inherited but can be acquired. Even when challenged with an ammonium chloride load, urinary pH cannot fall below 5.3. Patients may present with sodium or potassium depletion, osteomalacia or nephrocalcinosis and urinary stones. The latter are probably largely due to low urinary citrate, which is a hallmark of this condition. Treatment is with a mixture of sodium bicarbonate 1 g tds and potassium citrate 1 g tds. Occasionally the stone formation is exacerbated by this treatment.

2 Proximal tubular bicarbonate leak. Bicarbonate which leaks from the proximal renal tubules swamps the acidification mechanism in the distal tubules. As plasma bicarbonate falls, the load presented to the distal tubules also falls and response to the ammonium chloride can then be a normal fall in urinary pH. Urinary citrate is normal in this condition and nephrocalcinosis and stone formation do not occur. This subtype is not inherited but is due to substances which damage the proximal tubules, including PTH. Large doses of alkali are needed to raise the plasma bicarbonate concentration to normal but fortunately it is not usually necessary or even desirable to attempt such vigorous treatment.

Infection stones

When the urine is infected with urea-splitting organisms, the urine pH rises into the alkaline range with high ammonia content. Under these conditions, mixed calcium phosphate and MAP stones form. These are porous and bacteria can survive inside the pores, making it very difficult to eradicate the infection as long as the stones are present. The standard treatment is first to give a course of antibiotics and then to remove the stones by lithotripsy while continuing antibiotics for a further 10 days. In theory the infection should be eradicated but unfortunately the relapse rate is rather high. The infecting bacteria are usually easy to identify as *Streptococcus faecalis*, *Proteus* or *Escherichia coli*, but occasionally the organism may be difficult to grow without special culture medium and prove to be *Ureaplasma urealyticum*. This should be suspected when stones rich in MAP are accompanied by alkaline urine and pyuria but the urine is 'sterile' on routine culture.

When inadequately treated, infection stones may grow into stag-horn calculi of great size, leading to obstruction of calyces and pyonephrosis.

Uric acid stones

Only 2% of urinary stones from the indigenous population of the UK are of uric acid. The figure is higher in France, about 25% in Germany, 50% in Israel and some 75% in Leningrad. In Japan, the figure is again 2%. There are two main causes of uric acid stones:

1 *Excess uric acid production*:
   (a) Metabolic errors.
   (b) Some myeloid tumours.
2 *Low urinary pH*:
   (a) Reduced ability to secrete ammonia.
   (b) Chronic diarrhoea.

Most cases are due to low urinary pH, which should be measured as soon as uric acid lithiasis is suspected. Gout is often linked with uric acid stone formation, which leads to measurement of serum uric acid. The link is due to reduced production of ammonia from glutamate in certain cases of gout and hence again to low urinary pH.

Sodium biurate is much more soluble than uric acid. Hence uric acid stones are readily prevented and often dissolved by raising urinary pH. As in RTA, sodium bicarbonate with potassium citrate is given in a dose sufficient to raise urinary pH to 6.5. If the value rises beyond this point, calcium phosphate may coprecipitate on to uric acid surfaces and render medical stone dissolution impossible. The dose of the alkalis may be 3–6 g/day but should be slowly increased, checking urinary pH at each stage.

If alkalis are contraindicated (renal failure, fluid retention, hypertension), allopurinol may be very helpful, but if the condition is due to low urinary pH this does not treat the underlying abnormality.

Cystinuria

Cystinuria is an inborn error of metabolism in which there is a transport defect for four amino acids: cystine and the basic amino acids lysine, arginine and ornithine. Each has two NH_2 groups separated in space by about the same distance, and it is thought that a single transport system therefore operates for each compound. All four amino acids appear in the urine but the condition would be harmless were it not for the limited solubility of cystine. Urine can hold 2.1 mmol (500 mg) cystine per litre and since the usual output is about 6 mmol (1.5 g) per day, 3 L of urine per day should be sufficient to prevent stone formation. When patients fail to drink sufficient water, other remedies are available:

1 *Alkalis.* Sufficient sodium bicarbonate to raise the urinary pH to 7, but no higher, increases the solubility of cystine. However, the therapeutic pH range is rather narrow. Too low a value may be ineffective and too high a value may cause calcium phosphate to precipitate on the existing cystine surfaces. Consequently, this treatment is not much used. Recently, a weak correlation has been shown between urinary sodium and cystine. Perhaps alkali treatment should now be abandoned.

2 *Penicillamine.* This is dimethylcysteine, an analogue of cysteine. Penicillamine-cysteine disulphide appears in the urine in place of cystine and fortunately the former has a higher solubility. The D-isomer is used. It can lead occasionally to nausea, anorexia, fever, rash, thrombocytopenia, neutropenia, proteinuria, nephrotic syndrome and haematuria. It is best to begin with a small dose of 200 mg three times a day, increasing to a maximum of 3 g daily in divided doses. It may be useful to give a single dose or an increased dose at times of high risk, as when recumbent overnight. Other similar compounds have been tried, the best known of which is Triopronine (α-mercaptopropionylglycine, or 'Thiola'), but these have little or no advantage over D-penicillamine.

3 *Ascorbic acid.* It has recently been claimed, but not yet independently confirmed, that 5 g/day of vitamin C reduces urinary cystine to normal.

4 *Low salt diet.* It has been shown recently that there is a correlation between urinary cystine and sodium. Thus, in difficult cases, it may be of value to restrict dietary sodium.

If treatment is pursued vigorously, it is possible to dissolve cystine stones.

Hyperoxaluria

Primary hyperoxaluria is a rare disease, more common in males than females and transmitted by two autosomal recessive genes. In the usual type, there is excessive production and urinary excretion of glycollic and oxalic acids. Calcium oxalate stone formation often starts in the early years of life. Progressive renal damage causes azotaemia with rising plasma oxalate and oxalosis with further renal damage. In about half of the cases, pyridoxine (up to 800 mg/day per 70 kg body-weight) results in a fall in urinary oxalate and glycollate. The other patients benefit from a low-oxalate diet with high water intake and either milk of magnesia or neutral phosphate.

All patients with primary hyperoxaluria develop terminal renal failure. Unfortunately, in such patients a renal graft will fail due to oxalate stone formation and recurrent graft obstruction, oxalosis and infection. The definitive treatment of primary hyperoxaluria is a liver transplant; the healthy liver corrects the excessive oxalate biosynthesis. There are reports of a few patients who have received both liver and kidney transplants and are faring well.

Hyperoxaluria may also be due to steatorrhoea or over-indulgence in oxalate-rich foods (see p. 310). Both of these conditions are treated with low-oxalate diets.

Summary

Low urinary volume is the most important risk factor for stone formation. Chronic dehydration due to hot environment, either from occupation or climate, causes an appreciable proportion of stones. High water intake with production of 3 L/day of urine will usually prevent stones and should be advised for all patients.

While bladder stones in children have virtually disappeared in the developed countries, upper urinary tract stones in adults have become very common. These usually consist of calcium oxalate/phosphate. Many patients (mainly men) have over-absorption of dietary calcium, with hypercalciuria, but the resultant mild hyperoxaluria is probably more important in stone formation. Low-calcium diet treatment should always be accompanied by low-oxalate diet. Other causes of calcium-rich stones are primary HPT (mainly in women), MSK and RTA. The diagnosis of primary HPT is mainly biochemical and that of MSK radiological.

The problem of infective stones due to urea-splitting bacteria is still not completely solved, but the principle of treatment is antibiotics, lithotripsy and surgery to clear the urinary tract completely of stones.

Uric acid stones are not common in the UK but more common in Central Europe and the Middle East. They are usually due to low pH urine and are treated by alkalis.

Cystinuria is treated with high fluid intake, supplemented, if and when necessary, with penicillamine or perhaps ascorbic acid.

Further reading

1 Chisholm, G.D. & Fair, W.R. (1990) Urolithiasis. In Chisholm, G.D. & Fair, W.R. (eds), *Scientific Foundations of Urology*, 3rd edn. Heinemann Medical Books, Oxford, pp. 170–223.
2 Coe, F.L., Parks, J.H. & Asplin, J.R. (1992) The pathogenesis and treatment of kidney stones. *N. Engl. J. Med.* **327**, 1141–52.
3 Embon, O.M., Rose, G.A. & Rosenbaum, T. (1990) Chronic dehydration stone disease. *Br. J. Urol.* **66**, 357–62.
4 Lemann, J. (1993) Composition of the diet and calcium kidney stones. *N. Engl. J. Med.* **328**, 880–2.
5 Rose, G.A. (1982) *Urinary Stones: Clinical and Laboratory Aspects.* MTP Press, Lancaster.
6 Rous, S.N. (1987) *Stone Disease: Diagnosis and Management.* Grune & Stratton, Orlando.
7 Vahlenseick, W., Gasser, G., Hesse, A. & Schoeneich, G. (eds) (1990) *Proceedings of 1st European Symposium on Urolithiasis, Bonn,* 1989. Excerpta Medica, Amsterdam.
8 Van Reen, R. (1977) *Idiopathic Urinary Bladder Stone Disease.* Fogarty International Centre Proceedings, no. 37. Department of Health, Education and Welfare, Washington.
9 Walker, V.R., Sutton, R.A.C., Cameron, E.C.B., Pak, C.Y.C. & Robertson, W.G. (eds) (1989) *Urolithiasis.* Plenum, New York.
10 Wickham, J.E.A. & Buck, A.C. (eds) (1990) *Renal Tract Stone Disease: Metabolic Basis and Clinical Practice.* Churchill Livingstone, Edinburgh.

Chapter 20
Dietary Treatment in Renal Disease

Malcolm E. Phillips

Diet and nutrition are subjects which increasingly preoccupy the public as well as doctors. Much current interest is placed on the use of various dietary programmes, the aim of which is to prevent disease. There are a substantial number of diseases which may be wholly or partly caused by eating habits and the list is extended year by year. It is not surprising, therefore, that more attention is now being given to the role of diet in the treatment of renal disease. The topic is not new for renal physicians, who have used therapeutic diets for more than a century, but there has been a reawakening of research and clinical activity in this field.

This chapter will deal with those renal diseases in which dietary management is most commonly used. Much of the discussion will be about patients with renal failure, irrespective of the causes. The use of low-protein diets in patients with chronic renal failure not on dialysis is well established. Recently, the emphasis of such treatment has changed from that of a purely symptomatic role to a therapeutic one. There is evidence that the progression of renal disease in some patients may be slowed or halted by using low-protein diets. The potential to delay the time at which dialysis is required, whilst maintaining the patient in good health, is advantageous.

The use of diets for renal patients is not esoteric – general physicians may well wish to manage chronic renal failure for a period of time until dialysis is required, and will also treat patients with nephrotic syndrome or with renal stones. The relevance of dietary treatment in these conditions will be discussed. Most of the dietary measures which may be employed are within the scope of a good general dietitian.

Chronic renal failure

Protein

Reduction in dietary protein intake has been used to improve the wide variety of symptoms of patients with end-stage renal disease. As symptomatic treatment, this approach is successful. A wide variety of diets have been formulated – some practical, some almost intolerable. When the alternative to diet was, or is, death, this symptomatic approach is acceptable, even if the result is protein depletion, muscle-wasting and drastic weight loss. The availability of dialysis has necessitated that low-protein diets used prior to commencing dialysis must meet two requirements: control of uraemic symptoms and maintenance of protein balance.

Protein intake to meet these requirements will vary from patient to patient. In a stable patient, a protein intake of 0.4–0.5 g/kg body-weight/day is the conventionally accepted formula. The diet should contain protein of high biological value and must be adequate in respect of energy (35–55 kcal/kg body-weight/day), vitamins and minerals.

Extensions of the principle of low-protein diet therapy have been made by the use of essential amino acids and keto-acid analogues of essential amino acids. The use of diets with a nitrogen content that is mainly or partially derived from these substances may be more effective in reducing nitrogen retention in comparison with a low-protein diet. The patient may feel better and his/her nutritional status be maintained. These diets may be unpalatable, relatively expensive and require more dietary surveillance. Such regimens are probably only appropriate in the hands of specialists with access to an experienced renal dietitian.

For many years, the view of clinicians using the diets discussed above was that, whilst symptoms were controlled, the diet did nothing directly to affect renal function. From both animal and human studies there is now increasing evidence that a reduction in dietary protein intake may prolong useful renal function in conditions where renal failure has occurred experimentally or pathologically.

Patients who have lost more than 50% of their glomerular filtration rate (GFR) usually continue to lose the remainder at varying rates. Sometimes primary renal conditions, such as polycystic renal disease or active glomerulonephritis, are naturally progressive and are responsible for this deterioration. Nevertheless, in other patients, even when the primary disease process has been halted, the same progression of renal failure is seen. A typical example is reflux nephropathy. Despite correction or disappearance of reflux and control of infection and hypertension, progressive loss of renal function may occur. This is usually characterized by the presence of substantial proteinuria – in a disease not noted as a cause of proteinuria. Glomerular sclerosis is found, superimposed on any histological changes attributable to the primary disease. The glomerular lesion may also be found in the contralateral kidney not affected by reflux. A similar pattern of events has been described in unilateral renal agenesis, following bilateral renal cortical necrosis and after postinfectious glomerulonephritis.

A number of explanations of these observations have been proposed. Because high protein intake seems to have an adverse effect on renal function in the presence of reduced nephron mass, a protein-derived nephrotoxin may exist. A reduced protein intake would lower the amount and therefore the effect of this substance. It is unknown whether an actual nephrotoxin exists but it is clear that a physiological mechanism occurs, perhaps triggered by a 'toxin', which leads to an increase in GFR and hypertrophy of remaining nephrons.

This adaptive response, as studied in the rat, consists of changes in glomerular arteriolar pressure, increased glomerular plasma flow and increased GFR. Such changes are directly proportional to the reduction in renal mass when surgically induced. While the increase in GFR may be considered beneficial, the subsequent development of sclerosis of remaining glomeruli is believed to be a consequence of hyperfiltration. Reduction of protein intake results in a reversal of histological changes and improvement in the glomerular damage. These findings, accompanied by persuasive observations in human renal disease, have stimulated investigations in man into the therapeutic rather than the symptomatic effects of low-protein diets. Measurement of renal plasma flow and GFR in relation to protein intake shows that high protein intake leads to hyperfiltration. There is increasing evidence, from some prospective controlled studies, to show that a reduced protein diet can halt or slow progression of renal disease in patients with chronic renal failure.

Case 1 (Fig. 20.1)

A 41-year-old Caucasian was found at life insurance examination to be hypertensive and to have proteinuria. There was no significant past or family history. Examination revealed a blood-pressure of 169/105 mmHg and no other physical signs.

Investigations showed the following: midstream urine (MSU) no cells, sterile; 24-hour urine protein excretion 1.2 g; serum creatinine 210 μmol/L; ^{51}Cr-EDTA (ethylenediamine tetra-acetic acid) clearance 41 ml/min. An intravenous urogram (IVU) showed a left kidney 5 cm in length with changes suggestive of reflux nephropathy; the right kidney was normal and 11 cm long. Renal biopsy was not attempted. The patient was started on antihypertensive drugs. During subsequent years, his blood-pressure remained well controlled and drug compliance appeared to be excellent. Initially, his renal function remained stable, but then started to decline. After approximately 3 years, the following results were obtained: serum creatinine 430 μmol/L; 24-hour urine protein excretion 3.6 g; EDTA clearance 19 ml/min; IVU was unchanged. A low-protein diet (0.5 g/kg) was instituted. After a further 3 years, urine

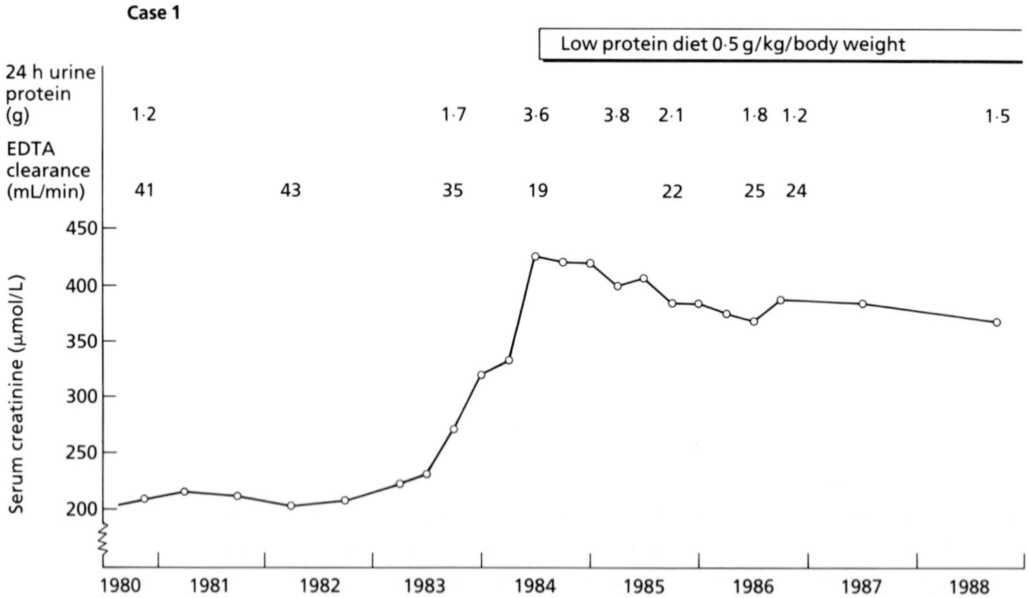

Fig. 20.1 Improvement in GFR (EDTA clearance) and serum creatinine in a patient with chronic renal failure, during treatment with a low-protein diet. In 1988 he was lost to follow-up and no further data are available.

protein excretion was 1.2 g/24 hours and the EDTA clearance 24 ml/min.

No obvious reason was found for the deterioration in renal function in 1983–4. Subsequent stabilization appeared to be associated with reduced protein intake and less proteinuria.

A number of practical considerations arise when considering the introduction of a low-protein diet to prolong renal function:

1 In which patients is it suitable?
2 When should the diet be started?
3 How much protein restriction is necessary?

These questions are not yet fully answered. A wide variety of renal diseases causing renal failure have been reported to respond beneficially to a low-protein diet, whether used relatively early (serum creatinine <300 µmol/L) or late (serum creatinine >500 µmol/L) in the course of the disease. Because the process of hyperfiltration and progressive glomerular sclerosis starts soon after the initial renal injury, it appears logical that, when serum creatinine has reached 200 µmol/L, indicating a loss of more than 50% of renal function, protein intake should be reduced.

Diets used have involved protein restriction of varying degrees alone, or protein and phosphate restriction, or protein restriction plus supplements of essential amino acids or keto acids. Practicality is essential. A diet must be palatable or patient compliance will be poor; complicated diets require close medical and dietary supervision. The well-tried formula of approximately 0.5 g protein/kg body-weight/day will provide protein and phosphate restriction, is palatable and adequately nutritious and will not require extra dietetic monitoring.

Lipids

Lipid abnormalities are common in patients with renal disease. Renal failure *per se* and nephrotic syndrome are frequently associated with different types of hyperlipoproteinaemia. Because some primary lipid diseases are associated with renal failure, it has been suggested that the lipid abnormalities seen in primary renal diseases may further directly impair GFR. Some lipoproteins can bind glycosaminoglycans, which are major constituents of the glomerular basement membrane. This process may alter membrane permeability and allow lipoproteins to enter the mesangial region of the glomerulus and produce cell proliferation and ultimately sclerosis. In experimental animal studies, high-cholesterol diets may lead to glomerular damage and diets low in certain essential fatty acids may protect against glomerular damage. Lipid-lowering drugs have also been shown to ameliorate glomerular damage in experimentally induced nephrotic syndrome in rats. Supplementation of the diet with other fatty acids may also protect against glomerular damage. In particular, the fatty acids linoleic and eicosapentanoic acid seem to protect against immunological glomerular damage and glomerular sclerosis after subtotal nephrectomy. Diabetic retinopathy in the human may also be retarded by the use of linoleic acid. Whether these effects are mediated through metabolic pathways, such as prostaglandin synthesis, or by an effect of fatty acids on platelet function and coagulation is not yet clear. Nevertheless, the possible role of lipids in progressive renal damage should be borne in mind, and may direct future dietary management.

There has been much controversy over the incidence of vascular disease in renal patients. The bulk of evidence supports the view that patients with renal failure, especially those on dialysis and renal transplant and nephrotic patients, all have a higher than average incidence of serious vascular disease. These complications may be contributed to in varying degrees by the lipid disorders found in many of the patients.

Calcium, phosphate and vitamin D

Disturbances in calcium and phosphate metabolism may cause both progression of renal failure and skeletal and vascular complications. It is usual for patients with renal disease to develop phosphate retention when the GFR falls below 50%. This may be one of the mechanisms leading to the well-recognized changes in calcium, vitamin D and parathyroid hormone (PTH) in such patients. Phosphate retention leads to reduced renal synthesis of 1,25-dihydroxy-vitamin D_3, which causes hypocalcaemia by impairing gut absorption: secondary hyperparathyroidism results. Various dietary measures may be taken to interrupt or slow this progression of events. Phosphate intake (particularly dairy products) may be reduced and phosphate absorption from the gut reduced by using phosphate-binders. Calcium supplements, of which calcium carbonate is the cheapest and most effective, may also be used to increase serum calcium concentrations and suppress PTH.

There is no place for cholecalciferol or ergocalciferol in the treatment of hypocalcaemia in chronic renal failure unless the serum concentration of 25-hydroxy-vitamin D is low. The use of these parent compounds may lead to hypercalcaemia, which can be prolonged and result in further loss of GFR. There is more reason to use calcitriol (1,25-dihydroxy-vitamin D_3) since this metabolite of vitamin D is diminished or absent in patients with seriously impaired renal function. Hypercalcaemia occurs if this drug is used incautiously (see p. 206).

Apart from controlling hyperparathyroidism, mention has already been made of the possibility that control of phosphate intake may slow progression of renal failure. In animal studies and probably in humans, it is thought that renal impairment leads to phosphate retention and subsequent deposition of calcium and phosphate in the kidney. This produces interstitial nephritis, fibrosis and nephrocalcinosis. Some early animal studies in which phosphate depletion was used to protect against progressive experimental renal failure did not distinguish the effects of protein depletion from those of phosphate depletion. This was because the anorexic effects of phosphate deficiency caused a reduction in total food intake. Subsequent work suggested that phosphate restriction achieved without producing anorexia and protein depletion did not have this beneficial effect on renal function. Recently, further studies have been reported in animals with renal failure, produced by five-sixths nephrectomy, in whom phosphate depletion was produced solely by the use of phosphate-binders. Nutrition in the phosphate-depleted group of animals was otherwise the same as the control group. Renal failure was progressive in the latter animals and was associated with glomerular sclerosis, interstitial nephritis, fibrosis and tubular damage. These animals were also found to have higher calcium content in the heart, aorta and kidney. In the phosphate-depleted group, renal function was maintained, renal histopathological changes were less severe and tissue calcium content was lower.

As well as reducing calcium-phosphate deposition in tissues, phosphate depletion may have other effects which may help preserve renal function. These include amelioration of hypertension, alteration of lipids and, by reducing cellular energy production, reduction of the hypertrophy and hyperfiltration that is seen following nephron loss.

While aspects of dietary management and the slowing of the progression of renal impairment remain controversial, there is a broad consensus, which includes:

1 Palatability and practicality of a diet are essential.

2 Protein reduction to 0.5 g protein/kg body-weight/day provides protein and phosphate restriction. This amount of protein restriction reduces phosphate intake to about 550 mg daily.

3 An adequate calorie intake is essential to prevent muscle protein from being mobilized for gluconeogenesis. An inadequate evergy intake in uraemic patients causes calorie malnutrition and a negative nitrogen balance.

4 Calcium carbonate is the gut phosphate-binder of first choice: a number of palatable preparations are available. The correct dose is that which maintains a normal serum phosphate concentration. It is logical to commence calcium carbonate when serum phosphate is persistently above 1.8 mmol/L.

5 The diet is begun when serum creatinine reaches 200–250 μmol/L, at which stage the serum phosphate concentration also tends to become abnormal.

6 When the diet is started, the patient will have no symptoms, so a full explanation by physician and dietitian as to why the diet is necessary is essential.

7 The diet is maintained until dialysis is commenced.

Acute renal failure

Acute kidney failure usually occurs as a result of a serious disease or injury. Most patients are extremely ill and oliguric and some are hypercatabolic. They frequently have multisystem failure and their renal and nutritiitional management is complex. Occasionally, a patient will present in a less parlous state and management is more straightforward.

A simple and useful method of assessment of severity can be made from the rate of rise of plasma urea. Where the increase in blood urea is 4–8 mmol/L/day, conservative management may be possible. Hypercatabolism is characterized by a much greater urea production, causing rises in excess of 16 mmol/L/day. Patients in this category require continuous arteriovenous haemofiltration, with or without dialysis, or perhaps haemodialysis.

Moderate acute renal failure

Patients with a purely renal cause for acute renal failure, such as acute interstitial nephritis or acute obstruction, may not require dialysis. Similarly, patients with known pre-existing renal failure may lose renal function more rapidly from dehydration or the injudicious use of nephrotoxic drugs and may also be managed without dialysis.

Corrective measures including rehydration, relief of obstruction and withdrawal of nephrotoxins. In the absence of an immediate improvement of renal function, conservative dietary management can be used, along with measures to control electrolyte and fluid balance. Restriction of protein intake to 0.5 g/kg body-weight/day should be made. Lower protein intakes than this may also be used to reduce the concentrations of urea and other nitrogenous compounds, as a short period of protein depletion is acceptable.

Patients must also receive at least 40 kcal/kg body-weight/day to reduce endogenous protein breakdown for gluconeogenesis. If this cannot be achieved, dialysis may be necessary.

Potassium is a major electrolyte, to be controlled by a dietary intake of 30–50 mmol/day and by the use of ion-exchange resins, such as calcium or sodium polystyrene sulphonate. After correction of dehydration, fluid intake should not exceed 500 ml plus the volume of the previous day's urine output.

If the patient cannot eat the prescribed diet and if gut function is normal, enteral feeding by means of a nasogastric tube may be used. A number of proprietary preparations are available from which the physician may choose one that combines the correct protein and energy supply according to body-weight and assessed needs, with fluid allowance. These feeds contain vitamins and minerals.

This conservative approach can be used while the patient remains well and can tolerate a diet and if biochemical and fluid balance is satisfactory. Careful daily monitoring is necessary. Dialysis should be introduced when uraemia, hyperkalaemia or fluid overload occurs. This topic is discussed fully in Chapter 16, p. 224.

Severe acute renal failure

The majority of patients with acute renal failure are usually too ill to be managed with oral feeding. They may remain in renal failure, dependent on dialysis, for long periods. Maintenance of nutrition is essential.

Hypercatabolism arises as a result of the primary 'injury' to the patient – sepsis, trauma or burns – and also as a result of secondary hormonal changes. There may be elevated concentrations of glucocorticoids, glucagon, catecholamines, growth hormone and antidiuretic hormone, which are all catabolic and cause a high rate of urea production. Energy and protein requirements are high. There is a danger that nutritional and fluid requirements will be underestimated if losses due to nasogastric suction, diarrhoea, fistulae and sweat are not taken into account.

Nitrogen and energy requirements must be promptly supplied if rapid body-wasting is to be avoided. Artificial enteral therapy may be possible but parenteral nutrition is often necessary. Either regimen may involve large volumes of fluid which, in the presence of oliguria, must be dealt with by regular dialysis, daily if necessary, or by continuous haemofiltration. These procedures introduce their own effects on nutrition, such as loss of amino acids in dialysate, requiring adjustment of supply. In practice, total parenteral nutrition (TPN) becomes the only adequate method of dealing with the severely ill patient with acute renal failure.

Many TPN regimens have been described. Some include only essential amino acids, while others have individual amino acid contents varying from patient to patient. These regimens are unnecessarily complicated.

It has been demonstrated that careful management of the patient with regular dialysis, using an uncomplicated intravenous regimen and insulin, can lead to a significant reduction in mortality in acute renal failure associated with trauma. Energy requirements should be met, using 50% glucose ± 10% or 20% emulsified fat. Nitrogen supply is best given as a mixture of essential and non-essential amino acids. A wide range of products exist providing between approximately 5 and 25 g of nitrogen per litre, with variable caloric and mineral content. Such amino acid solutions should not be given while the patient is on dialysis since the amino acids are easily dialysable and thus wasted. The electrolyte content must be taken into account to prevent excess administration of potassium, phosphate or magnesium. Details of the range and constituents of products used for TPN are excellently set out in the *British National Formulary*. A wider discussion of TPN can be found in Dickerson and Lee (1978).

Nephrotic syndrome

Two of the main features of nephrotic syndrome are salt and water retention and protein depletion. Accordingly, it would seem logical to restrict salt and to increase protein intake. However, it is unrealistic to expect patients to eat a high-protein diet with no salt. Secondly, even with massive oral protein intake, hypoproteinaemia and oedema always persist until the disease is no longer active or renal failure ensues.

Case 2 (Fig. 20.2)

A 51-year-old woman developed massive oedema and proteinuria. Investigations showed the following: serum albumin 27 g/L; 24-hour urine protein 9.4 g; serum creatinine 97 μmol/L. A renal biopsy showed minimal-change glomerulonephritis. The patient declined steroid therapy. Treatment was started, using a 120 g protein, no added salt diet with diuretics. After 6 months, albumin was 25 g/L, 24-hour urine protein 11.4 g and serum creatinine 108 μmol/L. The patient's weight had fallen but she was still oedematous, despite quite large doses of diuretics. At this point, she agreed to a course of steroid therapy (prednisolone 60 mg/day, reducing slowly over 4 months). After 3 weeks of steroids, urine protein had fallen to 4.7 g/24 hours and serum albumin was 31 g/L. After 3 further weeks of treatment, there was only a trace of protein in the urine and serum albumin was 42 g/L.

The bulk of evidence indicates that, in patients with nephrotic syndrome, negative nitrogen and protein balance is due to protein and amino acid losses in the urine and to protein catabolism predominantly in the proximal renal tubule, or a combination of both.

To replenish protein stores and serum albumin concentration, a nephrotic patient would have to make up the deficit of protein which had occurred since the onset of his illness, and to compensate for the

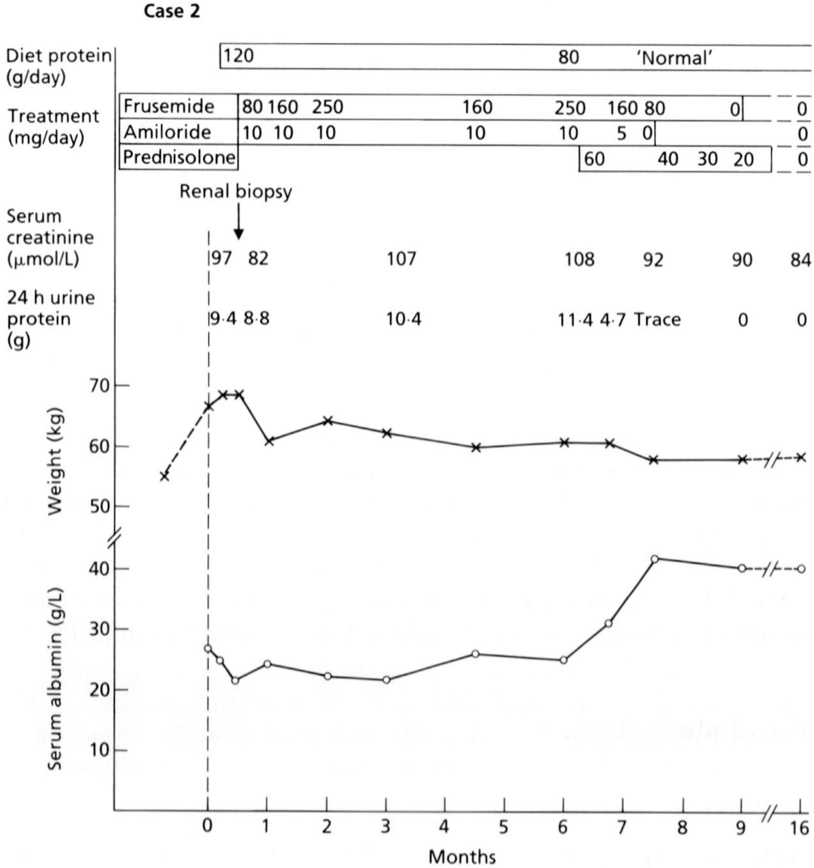

Fig. 20.2 Nephrotic syndrome – failure of high-protein diet to correct serum albumin. Response of serum albumin and proteinuria to prednisolone treatment.

continuing urinary nitrogen losses. It has been calculated that restoration of albumin stores in a patient with a serum albumin of 15 g/L would require the consumption of 2.7 kg protein.

The uphill struggle to replenish protein stores is limited by the capacity of the liver to synthesize albumin, the maximum rate being 25–30 g/day in a 70 kg man. Nephrotic patients have a normal or slightly enhanced albumin synthesis rate, provided they are otherwise well. The presence of infection, renal failure or systemic disease – especially with liver involvement (systemic lupus erythematosus (SLE) or amyloid) – will impair albumin synthesis and increase protein breakdown.

It is fruitless to press patients to eat large amounts of protein – up to 200 g/day have been suggested. A diet containing 1.2–1.5 g/kg bodyweight is reasonble. A recent study has shown that a higher protein intake (1.6 g/kg) whilst stimulating albumin synthesis was associated with greater albuminuria and a lower serum albumin and albumin mass. Conversely, a reduced protein intake (0.8 g/kg) was associated with lower albumin synthesis but less albuminuria, a higher serum albumin and maintenance of albumin mass. This short-term study seriously questions the value of high-protein diets and tends to support reduction in protein intake. Nevertheless, patients with long-standing nephrotic syndrome are often severely wasted and protein repletion is important whilst attempting to suppress glomerular protein loss. Currently, a diet containing a protein intake of 1.2–1.5 g/kg bodyweight is appropriate; this should help in the repletion of total body protein.

If a nephrotic develops chronic renal failure, protein intake must be reduced to prevent uraemic symptoms and hyperfiltration. As glomeruli sclerose and become obsolescent, urine protein excretion falls and the concentration of serum albumin rises. Body protein stores return to normal but at the cost of chronic renal failure.

In some patients hypovolaemic acute renal failure may occur, whilst the tissues remain waterlogged. In this state diuretics alone are often ineffective and intravenous salt-poor albumin may also be required. This combination therapy may achieve a diuresis (see also pp. 131–41).

Lipid disorders occurring in nephrotic syndrome have already been discussed in the section dealing with chronic renal failure (p. 303).

Renal stone disease

Cystinuria

Dietary attempts have been made to lower urinary cystine excretion, thus reducing the likelihood of stone formation. Methionine is the most important precursor of cystine: both low-methionine and low-protein diets have been used. Results have been variable and there are misgivings about the use of protein restriction in children. A fluid intake of 3–4 L, evenly distributed throughout a 24-hour period, is the main treatment. If a patient cannot tolerate habitual nocturia, he/she will reduce the fluid intake at night. Sodium bicarbonate, 5–10 g at least, may also be taken at bedtime. D-Penicillamine is used if stones recur (see also p. 296).

Uric acid stones

A small number of patients who have uric acid stones associated with hyperuricosuria may respond to dietary management. These include grossly obese subjects and those who eat foods containing large amounts of purines. Weight-reducing diets or low-protein and low-purine diets may then be used without need for drug therapy. Allopurinol with a high fluid intake is the treatment of choice to lower uric acid excretion and prevent stone formation.

Foods with a high purine content include all forms of offal, meat broths, sardines, most shellfish and wholemeal bread.

Oxalate calculi

Oxalate stone formation can arise from three sources:
1 Inborn errors of metabolism of oxalate.
2 Excess intake or absorption of oxalate.
3 Excess intake or accumulation of oxalate precursors.

Untreated primary oxalasis will cause early recurrent stone formation with renal failure. Dietary oxalate must be reduced. Pyridoxine treatment may help by converting the oxalate precursor glyoxalate to glycine. Magnesium supplements, to produce soluble magnesium oxalate in the urine, should be tried (see also p. 297).

Excess gastrointestinal absorption of oxalate leading to renal stones is seen in a variety of diseases, including Crohn's disease, blind-loop syndrome, chronic pancreatitis, small bowel bypass resections and biliary disease. These patients should all be treated with a high fluid intake and a low-oxalate diet. Foods with a high oxalate content include: rhubarb, beet, green beans, carrots, celery, parsley, spinach, various fruits, nuts and chocolate products. Very rarely, ingestion of excess oxalate-containing food – usually rhubarb – causes hyperoxaluria.

Ascorbic acid is one of the main precursors of endogenous oxalate. Very large doses of ascorbic acid can produce hyperoxaluria. In addition, pyridoxine deficiency leads to accumulation of glyoxalate and hyperoxalauria, though rarely to stone formation. Correction of vitamin excess or deficiency is the appropriate treatment.

Role of a dietitian

Few, if any, doctors have the knowledge, interest or skill to advise patients adequately regarding diet. Diets are essential to perhaps more than 60% of patients with renal disease, so the renal dietitian is an essential member of the renal unit staff. Her/his duties include:
1 In- and out-patient consultation and advice regarding modification of food and fluid intake.
2 Providing additional menus to help with dietary compliance.
3 Attending renal unit meetings where biochemical figures are reviewed.
4 Having her/his own clinics for follow-up, preferably in parallel with renal out-patients. In this way, the patient receives the benefit of two complementary opinions at one hospital visit.

In the out-patient setting, it is essential that the dietitian has access to blood results. This may be via the departmental computer or she/he should be provided with copies of laboratory reports. She/he can thus assess how well patients are adhering to reduced protein diets and avoidance of excess animal fats.

Involvement of the dietitian in direct clinical events is most important for good clinical practice.

Summary

Many patients with renal disease require dietary supervision, particularly those with renal failure, whether or not on dialysis. Prior to dialysis, a reduced protein intake, 0.4–0.5 g/kg body-weight/day, improves uraemic symptoms and is now used as a therapeutic manoeuvre to prolong renal function in a wide variety of renal disorders. This role for dietary therapy is supported in both human and animal studies, and is thought to relate to a reduction in glomerular capillary damage due to hyperfiltration occurring in residual nephrons. It is probably correct to start this treatment when creatinine clearance falls to 50 ml/min.

In nephrotic patients, protein depletion should be avoided but there is little evidence of a beneficial effect of high-protein diets on the nephrotic process. There is recent evidence that some aspects of the protein status of nephrotic patients are improved by a protein intake of 0.8 g/kg body-weight/day.

Lipid abnormalities are common in renal failure, nephrotic, dialysis and transplant patients. These abnormalities may accelerate vascular disease and contribute to progressive nephron loss. Control of obesity and of fat intake and adjustment of saturated to polyunsaturated fat in the diet are the main therapeutic procedures.

Changes in calcium, phosphate and vitamin D metabolism in renal failure lead to bone disease and, prior to dialysis, may cause interstitial fibrosis and nephrocalcinosis, which accelerate the loss of glomerular function. Serum concentrations of calcium, phosphate and metabolites of vitamin D should be controlled by diet, dietary supplements and phosphate-binders.

A major advance in the management of acute renal failure in recent years has been the use of intensive nutrition, usually parenteral, supported by as much dialysis as required to accommodate the fluid volume of the diet. Dietetic and clinical assessment is required daily.

Further reading

1 Anderson, S., Meyer, T.W. & Brenner, B.M. (1985) The role of haemodynamic factors in the initiation and progression of renal disease. *J. Urol.* **133**, 363–8.

2 Dickerson, J.W.T. & Lee, H.A. (1978) *Nutrition in the Clinical Management of Disease.* Edward Arnold, London.

3 El Nahas, A.M. (1986) Management of progressive renal failure: the role of dietary manipulation. *Postgrad. Med. J.* **63**, 611–15.

4 Kaysen, G.A., Gambertoglio, J., Jimenez, I., Jones, H. & Hutchison, F.N. (1986) Effect of dietary protein intake on albumin homeostasis in nephrotic patients. *Kidney Int.* **29**, 572–7.

5 Klahr, S., Buerkert, J. & Purkerson, M.L. (1983) Role of dietary factors in the progession of chronic renal disease. *Kidney Int.* **24**, 579–87.

6 Lee, H.A. (1980) What are the nutritional problems in renal failure? *Acta Chirurgica Scand. Suppl.* **507**, 318–26.

7 Lumlertgul, D., Burke, T.J., Gillum, D.M., Alfrey, A.C., Harris, D.C., Hammond, W.S. & Schrier, R.W. (1986) Phosphate depletion arrests progression of chronic renal failure independent of protein intake. *Kidney Int.* **29**, 658–66.

8 Maschio, G., Oldrizzi, L., Tessitore, N., D'Angelo, A., Valvo, E., Lupo, A., Loschiavo, C., Fabris, A., Gammaro, L., Rugiu, C. & Panzetta, G. (1982) Effects of dietary protein and phosphorus restriction on the progression of early renal failure. *Kidney Int.* **22**, 371–6.
9 Mitch, W.E. (1984) The influence of the diet on the progression of renal insufficiency. *Ann. Rev. Med.* **35**, 249–64.
10 Moorhead, J.F., Chan, M.K., El Nahas, A.M. & Varghese, Z. (1982) Lipid nephrotoxicity in chronic progressive glomerular and tubulo-interstitial disease. *Lancet* **ii**, 1309–11.
11 Rainford, D.J. (1980) Nutritional management of acute renal failure. *Acta Chirurgica Scand. Suppl.* **507**, 327–30.
12 Rosman, J.B., Ter-Wee, P.M., Meijer, S., Piers-Becht, T.P.M., Sluiter, W.J. & Donker, A.J.M. (1984) Prospective randomised trial of early dietary protein restriction in chronic renal failure. *Lancet* **ii**, 1291–6.
13 Walser, M. (1983) Nutrition in renal failure. *Ann. Rev. Nutr.* **3**, 125–54.

Chapter 21
Drug Treatment of Patients with Renal Disease

Roger Gabriel

Patients with renal diseases have a higher than average chance of an adverse drug reaction. These are usually of the type A variety: those which can be predicted from the pharmacological properties of the drug. Generally, an adverse reaction is more likely to occur with increasing degrees of renal impairment. Thus, in all patients, increasing uraemia leads to greater complexities when prescribing and a reduced chance of therapeutic efficacy.

Accelerated-phase hypertension and hypoalbuminaemia may present difficulties when prescribing. Severe or accelerated-phase hypertension may be treated badly, either with failure adequately to control the pressure (see p. 219) or by over-treatment in the early hours after diagnosis, such that under-perfusion of brain, retinae, heart or kidneys occurs, with possible irreparable ischaemic damage. Hypoalbuminaemia is a risk factor because some drugs are transported, in plasma, bound to serum albumin. Many of the drugs listed in Table 21.1 are commonly prescribed. Hypoalbuminaemia is not uncommon in patients with renal disease: the principal examples are nephrotics, patients with septicaemias and those receiving chronic peritoneal dialysis. In acute use, warfarin, salicylates and other non-steroidal anti-inflammatory drugs (NSAIDs) are the most dangerous.

Drug treatment

Most general medical patients receive several drugs. The individuals at greatest risk of receiving an inappropriate drug or dose thereof are

Table 21.1 Commonly prescribed drugs in which the binding is decreased in both hypoalbuminaemia and chronic renal failure

Benzodiazepines	Penicillins
Bumetanide	Phenytoin
Clofibrate	Propranolol
Diazoxide	Salicylates
Disopyramide	Sulphonamides
Frusemide	Tricyclic antidepressants
NSAIDs	Warfarin

those with unrecognized renal impairment or hypoalbuminaemia in general medical or surgical wards. Dialysis patients and transplant recipients are least likely to incur drug-related injury because their degree of renal function is known and they receive prescriptions from practitioners of renal medicine. Nevertheless, accidents occur, as the following case history shows.

Case 1

A woman aged 53 years was satisfactorily established on continuous ambulatory peritoneal dialysis (CAPD) in mid-1985; her renal failure was due to mesangiocapillary glomerulonephritis, diagnosed 15 years previously. Six months later, she underwent five separate coronary artery bypass grafts (CABG). From theatre, she went to an ITU where all patients after CABG surgery are given intramuscular digoxin 0.25 mg twice daily for 1 day and then 0.25 mg daily. The renal unit medical staff were not aware of this policy. The patient's renal failure, whilst in ITU, was managed by continuous-cycle peritoneal dialysis, which has a urea clearance of about 10 ml/min – proportional to advanced CRF. Digoxin is eliminated primarily (>90%) by the kidney.

This patient received 8 days of digoxin treatment; the error in prescribing was discovered when she developed ECG signs of digoxin toxicity. Blood sampled 18 hours after the last dose of digoxin contained digoxin at a concentration >8 nmol/L (therapeutic range 0.6–2.5 nmol/L).

The patient was transferred to a coronary care unit where, without any specific treatment, the 48-hour trough concentration of digoxin was 2.7 nmol/L: the patient recovered from a potentially fatal digitalis poisoning.

This case history illustrates two points:

1 It is difficult to communicate adequately between two groups of doctors prescribing for the same patient.

2 It is probably wise never to prescribe any 'routine' drug for a patient with renal failure, except by doctors trained in renal medicine.

Pharmacokinetics in renal failure

The principles of prescribing for renal patients are elementary and depend primarily on four points:

1 The renal excretion of the drug and its metabolites.
2 Is the main route of excretion via the bile?
3 Albumin-binding of the drug (Table 21.1).
4 Nephrotoxicity of the drug.

These points appear straightforward but renal unit staff often have to work extra hours attempting to rescue patients who have been damaged iatrogenically by incautious or incorrect prescribing. The following case history chronicles a typical example.

Case 2

A man of 66 years was nephrotic, due to idiopathic membranous glomerulonephritis, with a creatinine clearance of 20 ml/min. He had been treated with clofibrate in an effort to control hyperlipidaemia. A deep venous thrombosis developed in his left calf. He was admitted to his local hospital, where the diagnosis was verified by venography and he received 5 days of intravenous heparin. Clofibrate was continued. Twenty-four hours before ending heparin, 15 mg of warfarin was given, followed by 5 mg after the infusion line was taken down. The following day, he passed melaena with fresh blood, before experiencing a series of major haematemeses. The prothrombin time was greater than 120 sec. Control of bleeding was only achieved by a partial gastrectomy. Before and during surgery, there were prolonged periods of hypotension and not surprisingly the patient became oliguric, with acute-on-chronic renal failure – from which he did not recover. He began chronic haemodialysis, perhaps 4 or 5 years prematurely. His mismanagement was probably actionable in law.

The use of two drugs, both of which are protein-bound, in a hypoalbuminaemic patient requires thought and skill.

To the four principles of prescribing mentioned above, the following pharmacokinetic observations should be added for completeness.

Absorption

As renal failure advances, it is probable that all drugs are less rapidly absorbed and the therapeutic response is either delayed or less than expected, or both. This decrease in bioavailability is due to the following reasons:

1 Anorexia or nausea.
2 Delayed gastric emptying.
3 Oedema of the mucosa of stomach and gut wall secondary to:
  (a) hypoalbuminaemia;
  (b) fluid overload;

(c) congestive cardiac failure.

In emergencies, if absorption appears to affect therapy adversely, the drug is administered parenterally, with appropriate dose modification.

First-pass effect

Drugs which are absorbed from the gut first pass through the liver, where metabolism of the drug may occur. This extraction of the drug before it reaches the systemic circulation is called the first-pass effect.

It is probable that the first-pass effect is impaired in uraemia, particularly for propranolol and propoxyphene. Thus the first dose should be lower but the dosage interval unchanged.

Protein-binding

Many drugs are transported in the circulation, some bound to plasma protein, especially albumin, and some as unbound drug. The unbound, or free, percentage of a drug is available to receptors to produce pharmacological effects and is available to liver and kidney for metabolism or secretion, or both. Reference to the clinical importance of these events has been made on p. 313 and drugs competing for binding are mentioned in Case 2.

Renal clearance

Drugs enter the ultrafiltrate dependent upon:

1 The molecular size.

2 The percentage unbound which is available for excretion.

3 Plasma concentration.

4 The electrical charge.

Proximal tubular cells transport organic acids or bases from peritubular capillaries into tubular lumens by active mechanisms. Examples are listed in Table 21.2.

Tubular secretion is especially important for the renal elimination of drugs that are highly protein-bound and of negatively charged compounds. The rate at which secretion occurs depends on:

1 Renal blood flow.

Table 21.2 Examples of acidic and basic drugs secreted by active mechanisms across proximal tubular cells into tubular lumens

Acidic	Basic
Acetazolamide	Codeine
Bumetanide	Dopamine
Frusemide	Morphine
Hydrochlorthiazide	Procaine
Penicillins	Quinine
Probenicid	
Salicylates	

2 Saturability of the transport system.
3 The presence of other drugs competing for the same transport mechanism.

The clinical importance of the above observations is that renal elimination can be:
1 Increased by promoting a diuresis.
2 Modified by altering urine pH. Alkalinization of urine enhances excretion of weak acids and acidification enhances the loss of weak bases (see Table 21.2).

Renal failure decreases the elimination of drugs by the reduction in glomerular filtration rate (GFR) and loss of tubules for secretion. The clinical importance of reduced renal function for the pharmacokinetics of a given drug depends, to a major extent, on the route by which the drug and its active metabolites are removed, either by renal or extrarenal mechanisms. Those drugs cleared by the liver are given in normal dose and dosage intervals. Conversely, those drugs which are excreted by the kidney must be given in smaller doses or with longer dose intervals, or both. Prescribing in renal failure is thus similar to prescribing for elderly patients, in whom GFR is naturally reduced with increasing age. Table 21.3 lists some important drugs which should not be prescribed if serum creatinine is greater than 250 μmol/L unless the practitioner has experience in this area. The list is not comprehensive; a good résumé can be found in the *British National Formulary*.

Table 21.3 A short list of drugs for which the prescriber requires experience before prescribing for a patient with renal impairment. The exclusion of a drug from this list does not necessarily imply that it may be used safely in patients with chronic renal failure

Analgesics	*Gastrointestinal*
Aspirin	Magnesium carbonate
NSAIDs	Magnesium trisilicate
Narcotics	Sodium bicarbonate
	Carbenoxolone
Antibiotics	
Aminoglycosides	*Diuretics*
Nitrofurantoin	Amiloride
Tetracyclines	Chlorthalidone
	Triamterene
Antituberculous drugs	Thiazides
Cycloserine	
Pyrazinamide	*Hypoglycaemics*
Streptomycin	Chlorpropamide
	Metformin
Cardiovascular drugs	
Digoxin	
Procainamide	
Chemotherapy	
Cisplatin	
Methotrexate	

Drug effect

Matters are made more complicated because renal failure may enhance the pharmacological effect of certain drugs. This appears to be particularly true for hypotensive, sedative, hypnotic and narcotic drugs.

Prescribing in renal failure

A section on prescribing in renal failure cannot be comprehensive: only selected areas will be discussed. No drug should be prescribed for any patient if the degree of renal impairment is not known. Serum creatinine alone will suffice but an estimated clearance (see p. 42) is also helpful. The concentration of plasma urea is not an adequate measure of GFR: this assay need not be requested in this context.

Infections

Surprisingly, there are only three antibiotics which may be used without dose reduction in renal failure: erythromycin, sodium fusidate and rifampicin. They are predominantly excreted via the liver. The dose of all other antibiotics must be reduced proportional to the creatinine clearance (Table 21.4). Peak and trough serum concentrations should be measured whenever possible and repeatedly.

The principles of treating systemic infection in the presence of renal failure are no different from those in treating infected patients with normal renal function. Nevertheless, sepsis is substantially more difficult to eradicate in the presence of CRF. In particular, renal function frequently declines in the presence of sepsis; the patient requires precise management (see Chapter 16, p. 224).

Urinary tract infection

Treatment of urinary tract infection, which is common, is covered in Chapter 7, p. 90, and Chapter 8, p. 108.

Table 21.4 Necessary modification of dose of common antibiotics in patients with persistently impaired renal function. See also Table 8.3, p. 111

Normal dose	Slight modification of dose	Major modification of dose	Avoid
Erythromycin	Aztreonam	Aminoglycosides	Nitrofurantoin
Rifampicin	Cephalosporins		Sulphadiazine
Sodium fusidate	Co-trimoxazole		Tetracyclines
	Metronidazole		
	Penicillins		
	Semisynthetic penicillins		

Tuberculosis

General principles with tuberculosis are no different from conventional therapy. However, ethambutol, isoniazid and pyrazinamide must be given with particular care because they are all eliminated by the kidney. It is very desirable that serum concentrations of these antibiotics be measured to ensure appropriate doses and dose intervals. Rifampicin is given in standard doses, preferably before breakfast.

The correct duration of therapy is probably 9–12 months, as in other patients without CRF.

Cardiovascular disease

Diseases of the heart and the arterial vascular tree and hypertension are very common in patients with renal insufficiency. Generally, as creatinine clearance falls, the arterial pressure rises.

Angina

Nitrates or dinitrates, administered sublingually, by inhalation, transdermally or intravenously, are used without dose modification. Nitroglycerine is metabolized in the liver and excreted in bile. Isosorbide dinitrate is usually excreted in urine as isosorbide glucuronide but in CRF is probably eliminated in bile.

Atenolol and sotalol are amongst the most water-soluble of the β-blockers. They are therefore less likely to enter the brain and lead to depression, sleep disturbance or nightmares. Both are given as single daily doses and are best started as a nocturnal dose. The maximum dose of atenolol is 50 mg daily and that for sotalol 80 mg.

Arrhythmias

Procainamide is frequently used to control ventricular arrhythmias. This drug and a pharmacologically active metabolite are both excreted in the urine. The half-life of the metabolite is substantially increased in CRF. It follows, therefore, that the dose of procainamide should be reduced and the dose interval increased in the presence of renal impairment. The same caveats apply to disopyramide, flecainide and tocainide.

If possible, digoxin is never used in renal failure.

Hypertension

Hypertension has been covered in Chapter 15, p. 214. It should be emphasized that the initial dose of any hypotensive should be small and, if there is a substantial degree of CRF, individual doses ideally should be prescribed for the first 48–72 hours.

Analgesics

Pethidine (meperidine) is metabolized to norpethidine (normeperidine), which accumulates in renal failure and may precipitate fits. Repeated doses of pethidine or infusions thereof are better avoided. Uraemic patients are more sensitive to opiates than people with normal renal function. Metabolites of morphia are retained in CRF and such patients are more likely to be unduly drowsy or suffer respiratory depression following repeated doses or infusions. Codeine is metabolized to morphia and may be used at all levels of renal function. Nevertheless, when creatinine clearance is less than 10 ml/min, the dose interval should be increased and preferably a different compound should be chosen.

Aspirin is partially excreted into urine, especially so when a dose is greater than 500 mg. In advanced renal failure (creatinine clearance <10 ml/min), regular doses of aspirin enhance uraemic platelet dysfunction, may cause gastric bleeding and cause extra fluid retention. A single daily dose of 300 mg of aspirin may be acceptable but repeated doses are potentially dangerous.

Paracetamol (acetaminophen) is the analgesic of choice for mild to moderate pain in patients with varying degrees of CRF. Metabolites of paracetamol do accumulate in the presence of CRF but appear to be non-toxic. Not infrequently, patients request prescriptions for the compound analgesic (Co-proxamol; Distalgesic) which contains 325 mg paracetamol and 32.5 mg dextropropoxyphene per tablet. Dextropropoxyphene is retained as clearance falls below 10 ml/min and leads to drowsiness and respiratory centre depression. Thus, while this compound analgesic is welcome to many patients, it must be used with care in advanced renal failure and should be avoided by those who do not regularly prescribe for patients with CRF.

Non-steroidal anti-inflammatory agents are best avoided for two reasons:

1 When creatinine clearance is below 50 ml/min, fluid retention may occur.

2 Many of the NSAIDs have been documented in inducing an acute renal failure (ARF), some with an associated nephrotic state, both of which are reversible upon withdrawing the NSAID.

Nevertheless, many patients depend upon NSAIDs to control chronic pain, and drugs in this group will remain widely prescribed because their benefits outweigh their disadvantages. However, if possible, they should be avoided when creatinine clearance is 20 ml/min or below because at this stage NSAIDs may accelerate loss of GFR.

Psychotherapeutic treatments

Patients with advancing renal failure may have major anxieties and fears, which often express themselves as depression, difficulty in reaching decisions and insomnia. Matters may worsen when dialysis is perceived as a chronic therapy.

Benzodiazepines are safe for mild to moderate symptoms, but treatment should be begun with a small dose and the patient warned regarding excessive sedation. Temazepam is probably the best drug for insomnia; the advantages over nitrazepam include less morning sedation and much less propensity to accumulation. Diazepam is widely used to treat daytime anxieties, but abuse is a risk.

Benzodiazepines have variable degrees of binding to serum albumin, which is relevant to nephrotic and subnourished patients (Table 21.1, p. 314). All benzodiazepines are excreted via the liver; the dose in renal failure is unchanged. Probably not more than 1 week's treatment should be prescribed because of the dangers of habituation, dependence and addiction.

Tricyclic antidepressants are the main drugs used in renal failure for depression. They are prescribed at standard dose because these drugs, after hepatic oxidization, are excreted in bile conjugated with glucuronic acid. Amitriptyline is useful in patients who are both depressed and insomniac because it is a moderately potent sedative, best taken shortly before retiring.

Lithium salts can be used in CRF if essential, but very regular checking of serum lithium concentrations, together with measurement of early morning urine (EMU) osmolality at monthly intervals, is essential. It is probably easier to judge the correct dose of lithium in a dialysis patient than in advanced renal failure. There is a nephropathy specific to lithium.

Hypoglycaemic agents

Diabetic nephropathy (p. 190) is the second commonest cause of CRF in Western Europe. The majority of those who develop nephropathy are insulin-dependent. Insulin requirements tend to decrease as CRF advances; this is judged from plasma glucose concentrations.

Glibenclamide, gliquidone, tolbutamide and tolazamide are safe to use in uraemia. Other sulphonylureas should not be prescribed. Metformin is contraindicated because it may precipatate lactic acidosis.

Diuretic therapy

There are three main indications for diuretics in renal medicine:

1 Partial control of peripheral oedema, secondary to salt and water retention, which is very common in CRF.

2 Management of nephrotic oedema. This has been discussed in detail in Chapter 10, p. 134.

3 As an agent in hypertension either alone or combined with a hypotensive drug. This indication is now becoming limited as long-term elevation of serum lipid concentrations occurs.

Thiazides

Thiazides become ineffective when creatinine clearance falls below 25 ml/min. Potassium-sparing combinations of thiazide with amiloride, spironolactone or triamterine should be avoided in renal failure because they are ineffective and may cause fatal hyperkalaemia. Other aspects of thiazide therapy are discussed on p. 219.

Metolazone

Metolazone is a thiazide-related drug which may be used at all levels of renal function. Alone it is barely effective but when prescribed with a loop diuretic it often induces a useful diuresis previously not induced by an equivalent dose of bumetanide or frusemide (see pp. 137 and 139).

Loop diuretics

A surprising and as yet inadequately explained phenomenon is the need to increase the dose of bumetanide or frusemide substantially to induce a diuresis in CRF. Both drugs function as sodium reabsorption inhibitors in the thick ascending limb of the nephron (Table 21.5). There is a reduced number of nephrons in CRF of all causes. It is therefore surprising that, in the presence of many fever binding sites for bumetanide or frusemide, the dose of these drugs must be increased by a factor of 10–12. This is so even in hypoalbuminaemia (Table 21.1, p. 314).

Care must be taken in using high doses of loop diuretics when clearance is less than 20 ml/min because of the following possibilities:

1 Extracellular volume contraction may occur in the presence of peripheral oedema. The diuretic then becomes ineffective and fluid accumulates.

2 Volume contraction is frequently associated with increased metabolic

Table 21.5 Sites of action of different diuretics upon the nephron

Proximal tubule
Acetazolamide
Thick ascending limb
Bumetanide
Frusemide
Cortical diluting segments
Metolazone
Thiazides
Collecting ducts
Amiloride
Spironolactone
Triamterine

acidosis and hyperkalaemia. In this circumstance the diuretic is withheld and the patient treated as in the following case history.

Case 3

A man of 27 years was admitted for control of worsening peripheral oedema. He had a mesangiocapillary glomerulonephritis with a clearance of 19 ml/min and urine protein excretion 2–4 g/day. He had been taking 500 mg of frusemide daily at breakfast. On admission (day 1; Table 21.6), he was fluid-restricted to 1000 ml fluid daily and ate a diet containing 100 mmol sodium daily. On the ninth day of admission, the dose of frusemide was doubled to 1 g daily.

This extra and too great a dose had a rapid and deleterious effect on all seven parameters, as shown in Table 21.6 days 10 and 11, with oliguria, fall in clearance, hyponatraemia, hyperkalaemia and worsening acidosis. The patient became hypotensive, confused and incoherent. Because drinking had become difficult, normal sodium chloride was infused at varying rates to ensure adequate hydration but avoiding fluid or salt overload. This was continued over days 12 and 13, when no diuretic was given. On the morning of day 14, the drip was taken down and a modest dose of frusemide with 5 mg of metolazone was prescribed. By the evening of the 14th day, it was clear that a diuresis had been re-established. Without change in fluid allowance or diuretics, the patient continued to make good progress, as shown by the data of days 20 and 25 (Table 21.6).

This case history illustrates four points:

1 In the presence of severely reduced clearance and peripheral oedema, an increase in the dose of a loop diuretic does not necessarily lead to an enhanced diuresis.

Table 21.6 Weight, urine volume, biochemical variables and doses of diuretics in a man of 27 years with chronic renal failure. For details see text (Case 3)

Day	Weight (kg)	Urine volume (ml/day)	Serum creatinine (μmol/L)	Creatinine clearance (ml/min)	Sodium	Plasma potassium (mmol/L)	Bicarbonate	Frusemide (mg/day)	Metolazone (mg/day)
1	72	1200	520	19	139	5.0	17	500	0
7	76	1000	536	17	137	5.2	17	500	0
8	77	1100	529	18	138	5.0	16	500	0
9	79	950	545	17	140	4.9	18	1000	0
10	82	670	756	13	133	5.8	14	1000	0
11	83	710	768	9	129	6.3	11	1000	0
12	84	635	794	8	127	6.4	9	0	0
13	83	980	740	9	132	6.1	12	0	0
14	82	1150	680	11	134	5.8	14	250	5
15	81	1480	596	11	135	5.9	13	250	5
20	69	1250	481	18	139	4.8	18	250	5
25	64	1080	478	19	136	4.5	17	250	5

2 When this error is recognized, elementary principles of management must be instituted:

(a) Withdraw all diuretics.
(b) Maintain fluid input.
(c) Keep accurate fluid balance.
(d) Make regular biochemical observations.

3 If this man had continued to receive inappropriate high-dose frusemide, he would:

(a) either have died of hyperkalaemia and acidosis, or
(b) have required urgent referral for dialysis.

4 Metolazone, presumably by functioning at a different site on the nephron from loop diuretics (Table 21.5, p. 322), is able to enhance a loop diuretic-driven diuresis.

Acetazolamide

Acetazolamide, a carbonic anhydrase inhibitor, is a weak diuretic which works on proximal tubules (Table 21.5, p. 322) and the trabecular meshwork by the peripheral iris. Within the eye, acetazolamide, given by mouth, will rapidly lower intraocular tension in patients with acute closed-angle glaucoma. Glaucoma is a disease of the elderly and CRF is not uncommon in this age-group. Sometimes they occur together. In CRF, acetazolamide induces a metabolic acidosis, which leads to decompensated CRF. The carbonic anhydrase inhibitor should be avoided when serum creatinine is greater than 400 μmol/L. In these circumstances, glaucoma is treated with topical carbachol, pilocarpine or timolol maleate and perhaps iridectomy.

Treatment of epilepsy

While there is no direct relationship between a propensity to epilepsy and a likelihood of developing CRF, fits are not uncommon in renal patients. They occur in ARF in association with fluid and salt overload, many develop if a patient is dialysed too acutely, are a central feature of hypertensive encephalopathy and occur in acutely deteriorating CRF.

Intravenous diazepam is the drug of first choice for any of the above emergencies and is used without modification of dose. Intravenous phenytoin sodium is also a suitable drug to control a fit or status epilepticus. Phenytoin has three additional advantages:

1 An oral form is available.
2 Dose modification for renal impairment is not needed.
3 Most clinicians are able to have plasma phenytoin concentrations measured. This ensures that the correct dose is prescribed.

The main antiepileptic which should be avoided in renal failure is phenobarbitone, as shown in the following case history.

Case 4

A man of 48 years became very hypotensive when his inferior vena cava was torn during removal of a kidney thought to contain a clear cell carcinoma. Twelve hours after surgery he was oliguric, hyperkalaemic (plasma potassium 7.2 mmol/L) and acidotic (arterial pH 7.1; 80 nmol $[H_a^+]$/L). During an emergency, overnight dialysis, he suffered several fits, probably as a result of over-aggressive haemodialysis. The fits were suppressed by intravenous paraldehyde, and prophylactic phenobarbitone 30 mg tds was begun. Three weeks later, the patient had reached the diuretic stage of ARF but was persistently drowsy.

After a few days, it was appreciated that up to 25% of phenobarbitone is eliminated by pH-dependent renal excretion and the remainder is inactivated by hepatic microsomal enzymes. Phenobarbitone was withdrawn and the patient made an unremarkable recovery.

Drugs for the gastrointestinal system

Gastric symptoms are not uncommon in CRF: there is an increased incidence of peptic ulcer. When creatinine clearance is less than 20 ml/min, an additional sodium load cannot easily be eliminated. Thus sodium bicarbonate and Gaviscon should be avoided, otherwise peripheral oedema will increase. Similarly, ingesting magnesium carbonate or trisilicate leads to additional sodium and the possibility of magnesium toxicity.

Carbenoxolone enhances fluid retention if prescribed in the presence of advanced CRF.

Cimetidine appears to cause a reversible confusional state if used in renal failure. Ranitidine is less likely to cause this effect but a dose reduction is advised. The proton pump inhibitor, omeprazole, may be used without modification of dose. The proprietary compound Fybogel has a high sodium content and is best avoided. Lactulose is probably the laxative of first choice in CRF.

Drugs to control nausea

Nausea is one of the most unpleasant symptoms of advanced CRF. The best treatment is to perform a series of dialyses, which almost invariably control nausea. Some compounds are of some benefit. If used in CRF, the side-effects must be known and single doses given. Ideally, the drug is given before nausea occurs – such as 1 hour before a meal (p. 34). It is futile to prescribe an oral antiemetic for a nauseated patient: usually the tablet is recovered from the vomitus.

Three main drugs are available, but there is substantial need for more effective antiemetics to be developed.

Prochlorperazine is available in different prescriptions to be taken by mouth, by intramuscular injection or as suppositories but has only moderate antiemetic properties.

Metoclopramide hydrochloride is widely used in renal units. The dose is 10 mg by mouth or by intramuscular or slow intravenous injection. Unfortunately, metoclopramide is retained in renal failure and causes reversible extrapyramidal signs, especially in young women. These neurological features are not noted after a single dose, only following chronic treatment in advanced CRF.

Domperidone is probably the most potent antiemetic available. It has advantages over metoclopramide and prochlorperazine in that it is less likely to cause sedation and dystonic movements, because very little crosses the blood–brain barrier. Nevertheless, it is retained in CRF, such that if prescribed regularly the dose must be reduced by up to 50%.

Ondansteron was released in 1990 for the prophylaxis of cisplatin-induced nausea and vomiting. It is very effective in other regimens also. Ondansteron is a highly selective 5-hydroxytryptamine$_3$ (5-HT$_3$) receptor antagonist. It has no dopamine antagonist activity and consequently produces no extrapyramidal signs. Mental performance is not affected. In renal impairment, retention of metabolites occurs, the clinical consequences of which remain to be defined.

Contraception

As renal failure advances, there is a decline in fertility in women. Further, if a woman with CRF conceives, she is very likely to miscarry. Contraception may be discussed under four headings:

1 *Vasectomy or tubal ligation.* For the husband and wife who have completed their family, one of these procedures is the measure of first choice.

2 *Barrier methods.* This involves the use of condoms and diaphragms, preferably used in conjunction with a spermicide introduced into the vagina before copulation or with a condom coated on its outer surface with a spermicidal agent. Used intelligently, barrier methods are very effective but are beyond the scope of some couples.

3 *Intrauterine devices.* These are not a first choice in the woman with CRF because of the risks of heavy or prolonged periods, worsening the pre-existing anaemia of CRF, and because of pelvic sepsis, which might be difficult to eradicate.

4 *Combined oral contraceptives.* Oral contraceptives containing an oestrogen and a progesterone are very effective but not without some risks in CRF, including the following:

(a) Vomiting is not uncommon as renal function declines; thus tablets may be lost in vomitus.

(b) Antibiotics are used quite frequently in CRF: ampicillin may reduced absorption of a contraceptive within the small bowel, or ampicillin-induced diarrhoea may increase gut transit time and thus further reduce absorption.

(c) In any woman, oral contraceptives carry a minor risk of thrombo-embolic and myocardial complications. These events are increased in the presence of hypertension, diabetes and cigarette-smoking. Hypertension is almost invariable as renal function declines, diabetes is the second most common cause of CRF in Western Europe and many dialysis patients are heavy smokers.

Despite the above, oral contraceptives are widely used in women with advancing renal failure. Any increase in hypertension requires an increase in hypotensive medication. It is prudent to discuss these matters with individual patients.

If possible and ethical, sterilization is best; barrier methods are the contraception of second choice.

Anticoagulants

Heparin infusions are used in full therapeutic doses. The same is true for epoprostenol. Likewise, warfarin and other coumarins are given in standard loading and maintenance doses according to the international normalized ratio. It must be remembered that warfarin is one of the most likely drugs (p. 313) to produce an adverse event when used incautiously. In plasma, warfarin is carried 99% bound to serum albumin. There is a risk of displacement from albumin by other compounds which are also protein-bound (see Case 2, p. 315). The principal drugs which may be prescribed or taken inadvertently are as follows:

1 Oral contraceptives and primidone, which diminish anticoagulation.
2 Alcohol, cimetidine, many antibiotics and thyroxin, which potentiate warfarin.
3 Allopurinol, some NSAIDs, paracetamol and cholestyramine may potentiate warfarin.
4 Phenytoin may either potentiate or inhibit anticoagulation.
5 Aspirin and dipyridamole increase the risk of bleeding due to their anti-platelet effects.

This is a complex area and accidents may easily occur.

Renal osteodystrophy

Many patients require treatment for secondary hyperparathyroidism when their creatinine clearance is about 20–10 ml/min, especially if their CRF is protracted over years. This has been discussed on pp. 206 and 304. The only point that needs emphasis is the probability of hypercalcaemia when 1-α-hydroxycholecalciferol (1-α-HCC) and calcium carbonate are prescribed and taken together. Patients with renal osteodystrophy are in negative calcium balance; they therefore require calcium supplementation. Calcium absorption is impaired in CRF; hence the need for 1-α-HCC to enhance absorption. Patients should be seen initially at weekly intervals and serum calcium assayed on each occasion, and they should be asked to telephone if nausea or vomiting occurs.

In renal medicine, there is now no place for either cholecalciferol (vitamin D) or dihydrotachysterol, because hypercalcaemia induced by either may last for weeks and perhaps only be controlled by many hours of haemodialysis.

Hyperuricaemia

All patients with CRF have raised concentrations of serum urate. Only a small minority – perhaps 5% – have symptoms of gout. These individuals are presumably those who have a gouty diathesis and probably some others have an enhanced hyperuricaemia due to a thiazide preparation and very occasionally pyrazinamide. There are four preparations available:

1 *Allopurinol.* This is the drug of first choice for long-term prophylaxis. Nevertheless, when the creatinine clearance falls to 20 ml/min, the dose should be reduced to 200 mg daily. When the clearance halves, the dose is halved to 100 mg daily. If dose reductions are not observed, side-effects, which include fever, rashes and gastrointestinal disorders, may occur. Allopurinol should not be prescribed during an acute attack of gout because it may itself precipitate acute gout. Allopurinol may potentiate warfarin and does potentiate azathioprine, leading to enhanced marrow suppression.

2 *Colchicine.* This is indicated for relief of acute gout and for short-term prophylaxis during initial therapy with allopurinol or a uricosuric drug. If creatinine clearance is 10 ml/min or less, colchicine is best avoided, because the toxic effects on the gut become very prominent.

3 *Probenicid.* This uricosuric drug is used in the prophylaxis of gout by enhancing urate clearance by blocking reabsorption in nephron segments antegrade to the distal convoluted tubule, increasing the fractional excretion of urate and reducing the concentration of serum uric acid. Like allopurinol and for the same reason, probenicid should not be prescribed during an acute attack of gout.

Because probenicid functions at nephron level, its effectiveness is diminished when clearance falls below 20 ml/min, and toxic events, mainly gastrointestinal, occur.

The principal drug interactions of probenicid are:

(a) an increase in bioavailability of ketoprofen and naproxen;
(b) an interaction with acyclovir, leading to diminished urinary excretion and hence raised plasma concentrations of acyclovir;
(c) a similar delay in the excretion of methotrexate;
(d) increased plasma concentrations of indomethacin.

4 *Sulphinpyrazone.* This uricosuric agent is perhaps less frequently used than probenicid but, like probenicid, may be used with allopurinol in refractory cases. It shares the contraindications of probenicid, which include concurrent salicylate therapy and a tendency to marrow suppression, and it should not be used during an acute attack of gout.

Sulphinpyrazone potentially has a number of drug interactions, which include:

(a) potentiation of the anticoagulant effects of warfarin;
(b) potentiation of sodium phenytoin;

Table 21.7 The main immunoregulatory drugs used in renal medicine

Alkylating agents
Cyclophosphamide*
Chlorambucil*
Cytotoxic immunosuppressants
Azathioprine*
Other immunosuppressants
Cyclosporin*
Corticosteroids
Prednisolone
Methylprednisolone

* The dose of those bearing an asterisk has to be adjusted according to creatinine clearance.

(c) enhanced hypoglycaemia if administered with any sulphonyluria;
(d) it is antagonized if prescribed with pyrazinamide.

The efficacy of sulphinpyrazone declines with increasing degrees of CRF, such that when the clearance is 20 ml/min no uricosuric activity remains and it should be discontinued.

In all patients with hyperuricaemia who require treatment, aspirin should not be used, partly because of its toxicity in CRF (p. 320) and also because it antagonizes the uricosuric drugs discussed above. Likewise, NSAIDs should not be used to treat a gouty arthropathy in a patient with CRF.

Immunoregulatory drugs

The main agents used in renal medicine are listed in Table 21.7.

Cyclophosphamide

Cyclophosphamide is quite widely used in renal medicine, the initial doses often being given intravenously. The main indications are:

1 *Severe proliferative lupus nephritis* (pp. 154 and 176). There is good evidence that 500 mg doses of intravenous cyclophosphamide, in conjunction with other immunosuppressive drugs, substantially improve the prognosis.

2 *Microscopic polyarteritis and Wegener's granulomatosis.* Control of acute manifestations of these two conditions can be achieved as described in number 1 above.

The haemorrhagic cystitis which may complicate the use of cyclophosphamide can be avoided by inducing and maintaining a diuresis (> 10 ml/min) whilst the drug is infused. After control of the acute features of immune inflammation mentioned above, cyclophosphamide is then continued in tablet form. The toxicity of this alkylating agent is increased in the presence of renal failure. If the clearance is less than

20 ml/min, the oral dose must be reduced by at least 50% and later dose changes made in the light of white blood cell and platelet counts.

The decision to prescribe cyclophosphamide is serious in patients who may later wish to reproduce, because of potential impaired fertility of parent and offspring. In long-term use, cyclophosphamide is mutogenic.

Chlorambucil

Alternated with methylprednisolone, chlorambucil is used to control idiopathic membranous glomerulonephritis (p. 146). The same attention to dose and renal function must be paid as for cyclophosphamide.

Azathioprine

Outside transplant medicine, the main use of azathioprine, a cytotoxic immunosuppressant, is in combination with prednisolone in many of the nephritides of systemic lupus (p. 153). In addition to anti-inflammatory effects, azathioprine acts as a corticosteroid-sparing agent.

Generally, azathioprine is straightforward to use but the dose must be adjusted to renal clearance. When creatinine clearance is below 20 ml/min, the dose should not exceed 1 mg/kg body-weight because of the distinct risk of marrow suppression. Leucopenia and thrombocytopenia may last for more than 10 days: fatalities have been recorded.

In the absence of renal failure, the daily dose of azathioprine is about 2 mg/kg body-weight, given in divided doses. White cell and platelet counts must be performed regularly during the first months of therapy in order to reduce the dose if necessary. Host defence is impaired by azathioprine. Other than enhancing marrow toxicity if given with an alkylating agent, the only interaction of importance is that allopurinol potentiates the marrow toxicity of azathioprine.

Cyclosporin

The use of cyclosporin in transplant medicine is well defined and its position in the glomerulonephritides is under evaluation. Cyclosporin should only be prescribed by those experienced in its use and with access to an assay for dose monitoring. It may be used either as a primary therapy in glomerulonephritis or to permit a reduction in steroid dose. Cyclosporin-dependent nephritis is a recognized event, the term being equivalent to steroid dependence.

It has been shown to be of benefit in two nephritides which also respond to corticosteroids – minimal-change and lupus nephritis. It is of considerable benefit in 20–30% of patients with focal and segmental glomerulosclerosis and is being evaluated in selected patients with other nephritides.

Cyclosporin is usually taken twice daily. The dose is about 3–5 mg/kg body-weight but is adjusted so that the 12-hour trough concentration

Table 21.8 A brief list of drugs which affect plasma concentrations of cyclosporin

Increase	Decrease
Erythromycin	Carbamazepine
Ketoconazole	Phenobarbitone
Metoclopramide	Phenytoin
Methytestosterone	Rifampicin
Nicardipine	
Norethisterone	
Verapamil	

is within a therapeutic range of about 100–150 ng/L. The drug is presented in 100 mg and 25 mg capsules. There are a number of interactions:

1 With angiotensin-converting enzyme (ACE) inhibitors, potassium supplements and potassium-sparing diuretics, there is an increased risk of hyperkalaemia.

2 There is an added risk of cyclosporin-induced nephrotoxicity when used with aminoglycosides or amphotericin.

3 The plasma concentration of cyclosporin may be substantially altered by other drug interactions, as shown in Table 21.8.

Cyclosporin is both nephrotoxic and hepatotoxic.

Corticosteroids

Drugs of the corticosteroid group are the most powerful anti-inflammatory agents available but they have many dose-dependent, unpleasant side-effects, which include adrenocorticoid, glutocorticoid and gastric effects and suppression of signs of sepsis or tuberculosis. For these reasons, the dose must be kept as low as possible and the length of therapy as short as feasible.

Prednisolone is the most widely used corticosteroid. Those taking the drug should carry a steroid treatment card. Unfortunately, there is an enteric-coated preparation of prednisolone available. This should be avoided for the following reasons:

1 There is a wide range in amount per tablet that is absorbed, which may be as great as 50%.

2 If a patient has been prescribed, say, 20 mg of enteric-coated prednisolone, one should assume that effectively 10 mg is being absorbed.

3 There is a danger, if a patient obtains prednisolone from two or more sources, that inadvertent alteration of dose may occur because of the enteric-coated preparation.

4 Evidence is not available that enteric-coated prednisolone is less likely to produce gastric bleeding than non-enteric-coated.

Methylprednisolone is a very potent parenteral corticosteroid. Within general nephrology, it is perhaps most frequently used in treatment of acute phases of rapidly progressive renal failure (p. 176).

Summary

The principles of drug treatment in patients with different degrees of renal failure are straightforward. The basic information required is the route of elimination – renal or other routes. If renal elimination is the case for a specific drug and its metabolites, the following steps are essential:

1 In most cases the loading dose is unchanged.
2 Subsequent doses are either reduced, or
3 are given with an increased dose interval.

It is usually necessary to have some measure of renal function. Generally, the dose is related to clearance. If possible, peak and trough plasma concentrations are measured to adjust subsequent doses.

In renal impairment, there are often altered pharmacokinetic variables, including volume of distribution, protein-binding and drug interactions. It is quite easy to give too large a dose; under-dosing occurs in some patients. Perhaps diminished protein-binding is the single variable which, if forgotten, may lead to severe difficulties.

The *British National Formulary* has a valuable section on prescribing for patients who have renal failure; it should be consulted regularly.

Further reading

1 Bennett, W.M. & De Broe, M. (1989) Analgesic nephropathy – a preventable disease. *N. Engl. J. Med.* **320**, 1269–71.
2 Bennett, W.M., Hosenpud, J., Pantley, G., Starr, A. & Norman, D.J. (1990) *Drug Prescribing in Renal Failure: Dosing Guidelines for Adults*, 2nd edn. BMA Publications, London.
3 Calhoun, D.A. & Oparil, S. (1990) Treatment of hypertensive crises. *N. Engl. J. Med.* **323**, 1177–83.
4 Cupps, T.R. (1990) Cyclophosphamide: to pulse or not to pulse. *Am. J. Med.* **89**, 399–402.
5 Davis, K.B.K. *et al.* (1993) Prescribing in renal impairment. In *British National Formulary*, p. 515.
6 Maderazo, E.G., Sun, H. & Jay, G.T. (1992) Simplification of antibiotic dose adjustments in renal insufficiency: the DREM system. *Lancet* **340**, 767–70.
7 Oparil, S. (1993) Antihypertensive therapy – efficacy and quality of life. *N. Engl. J. Med.* **328**, 959–61.
8 Parker, S.E. & Davey, P.G. (1993) Once-daily aminoglycoside dosing. *Lancet* **341**, 346–7.
9 Puschett, J.B., Greenburgh, A., Holley, J. & McCauley, J. (1990) The spectrum of cyclosporin nephrotoxicity. *Am. J. Nephrol.* **10**, 296–309.
10 Reynolds, D.J.M. & Aronson, J.K. (1993) Making the most of plasma drug measurements. *Br. Med. J.* **306**, 48–51.
11 Shetty, H.G.M., Fennerty, A.G. & Routledge, P.A. (1989) Adverse effects of anticoagulants. *Adverse Drug React. Bull.* **137**, 512–15.

Chapter 22
Renal Disease: a Tropical Perspective

Margaret Z. Borok

In any country the pattern of disease will be determined by the interplay of genetic, geographical and environmental factors with socio-economic influences and cultural practices. All this will normally be within the grasp of a practitioner in his own country. Now that international travel has become commonplace, it has also become necessary for a familiarity with the patterns of disease in other countries to be part of a practitioner's skills.

This chapter will deal with diseases likely to be imported from the tropics, with particular reference to Africa. Standard clinical principles of diagnosis and management apply both to residents of the tropics and to travellers returning from these regions. Differences in the approach to these patients and to their management will be emphasized.

A separate section is devoted to the discussion of typhoid, malaria and schistosomiasis. The last two are parasitic diseases of global importance and all of them have a propensity for causing renal damage.

Acute renal failure

The broad categories of prerenal, renal (intrinsic) and postrenal (obstructive) causes of acute renal failure (ARF) have been defined in Chapter 16, p. 224. Tables 22.1, 22.2 and 22.3 are not exhaustive and should be used in conjunction with the standard list of causes of ARF. The clinical picture will depend on the underlying cause of the ARF. Principles of management do not differ from standard practice.

In the tropics a combination of infection and haemolysis is frequently associated with ARF. *Salmonella typhi* infection is very common in this context. Glucose-6-phosphate dehydrogenase (G-6-PD) deficiency

Table 22.1 Prerenal renal failure (renal hypoperfusion)

Causes	Comments
1 Loss of circulating volume	Diarrhoeal illnesses are common in tropics
2 Fall in blood-pressure	Marked fluid loss can occur in:
Combination of factors usually exists	gastroenteritis (often of undiagnosed aetiology)
Uncorrected, prerenal failure progresses to renal (intrinsic) failure	acute dysenteric illness (shigellosis, amoebiasis)
	salmonellosis
	cholera
	Dehydration is exacerbated by:
	fever
	high ambient temperature
	Stool microscopy and culture are essential
	Apart from rehydration, specific therapy may be indicated

is not invariable in these patients, despite the haemolytic episodes (see Table 22.2).

Septic abortion may be the commonest cause of ARF in some parts of Africa. The precise mechanisms are obscured by the fact that many patients will have taken potentially nephrotoxic traditional remedies.

Chronic renal failure

Accurate records are not available from most tropical countries but chronic renal disease is estimated to be much more common than in Europe and North America. The incidence of new cases of terminal renal failure is unknown but is probably as high as 200 or more new patients per million of population per annum.

The list of causes of chronic renal failure (CRF) in a patient indigenous to a tropical area is similar to that pertaining to Western Europe but the incidence of the various causes is different. For example:

1 The high incidence of nephritis which progresses to CRF. In Nigeria and Uganda, this is linked to the prevalence of chronic *Plasmodium malariae* infection. Other infections, including schistosomiasis and hepatitis B virus (HBV), also contribute.

2 *Schistosoma haematobium* is widespread in many African countries. This trematode has a predilection to infect the bladder wall and ureters. Chronic infection leads to distortion of ureteric orifices and to ureteric strictures. Reflux of infected urine is common and renal failure develops. *Schistosoma haematobium* infection is the third most common cause of CRF in Zimbabwe.

3 Malignant-phase hypertension is common, is often detected late and is either the first or second commonest cause of CRF in Zimbabwe and many other African countries.

The diagnosis and management of CRF is standard. In many tropical countries, long-term dialysis is not available and only conservative

Table 22.2 Renal causes of renal failure (intrinsic, parenchymal damage)

Causes	Comments
1 Secondary to prerenal failure	Very common in the tropics
2 Acute renal failure	
(a) Postoperative	
(b) Obstetric causes	Two peaks in incidence: 8–16 weeks' gestation – related to abortion and sepsis 34–36 weeks' gestation – related to eclampsia, APH, PPH, puerperal sepsis
(c) Massive intravascular haemolysis	*Plasmodium falciparum* (see p. 340) *Salmonella typhi* (see p. 338) G-6-PD deficiency: drug ingestion or infection Snake venom (see p. 348) Incompatible transfusion
(d) Myoglobinuria	Major trauma Snake venom (see p. 348)
3 Infections	Gram-negative septicaemia *S. typhi* (see p. 338) Clostridial infections *Meningococcus* Diphtheria Trichinosis Leptospirosis (Trypanosomiasis)
4 Acute parenchymal disorders	
(a) Acute pyelonephritis	
(b) Acute glomerulonephritis	
(c) Acute interstitial nephritis	Drugs Infections Leptospirosis Scrub typhus Leprosy Toxins (see p. 347) Snake venom Bee, wasp, hornet stings
5 Nephrotoxins	Animal toxins (see p. 348) Snake, bee, wasp, hornet, spider, scorpion stings Cantharides

APH, Ante-partum haemorrhage; PPH, post-partum haemorrhage.

management is possible. The duration of survival of a patient in CRF living in his/her tropical home may be diminished for several reasons, which include:

1 Increased susceptibility to any infection.
2 Continuing exposure to *P. malariae*.
3 Ingestion of herbal remedies, which may be nephrotoxic.
4 Ingestion of over-the-counter drugs.
5 Limited supplies of appropriate drugs.

Table 22.3 Postrenal renal failure (renal tract obstruction)

Causes	Comments
1 Intrarenal	
2 Bilateral ureteric	*Schistosoma haematobium* (see p. 347) Neoplasia Squamous carcinoma of bladder (related to *S. haematobium* infestation) Carcinoma of cervix: occurs in young women, who often present with advanced disease
3 Urethral	Gonococcal urethral stricture

6 Paucity of medical facilities.
7 Long distances from available facilities and transport difficulties.

Glomerulonephritis

The following points emerge from several studies carried out in African countries, where patients with nephritis are common in medical wards.
1 There is an extremely high incidence of nephritis, 10 times greater than in temperate areas.
2 The minimal-change lesion in infants and children is rare, which may account for the apparently later onset of nephrotic syndrome in African children, the peak age being between 5 and 10 years.
3 In children, the onset of disease is rapid and the clinical presentation severe. There is a high incidence of proliferative, membranous and focal proliferative nephritides. Young adults may show more severe histological damage than older age-groups. These different clinical patterns may be attributable to several factors:
(a) Genetically determined susceptibility to nephritis.
(b) Nature of the causal antigens.
(c) Poor nutritional state.
(d) Concomitant viral or parasitic infections, which affect immune response.
4 There is little definitive evidence for any specific aetiological agents, although infection with a variety of organisms has been suggested. A survey from Zimbabwe reported that a quarter to a half of nephrotic patients had evidence of infection: predominantly streptococcal, HBV and syphilitic. The role of *P. malariae* infection in Nigeria and Uganda is well documented. Conflicting evidence exists regarding schistosomiasis, but it is generally accepted that a nephropathy occurs.

Hepatitis B-associated glomerulopathy has been reported from many centres. In Zimbabwe, an absolute consistency of the association of membranous nephropathy with HBV antigenaemia has been reported in nephrotic children, without a direct role for the HBV antigen. Transient glomerulonephritis may occur in the early phase of acute HBV infection, together with polyarthralgia and skin rashes. Immunization against HBV infection and its implication in renal disease have yet to be evaluated.

Glomerular lesions have also been reported with Epstein–Barr virus and in Burkitt's lymphoma, mumps, varicella, measles and dengue fever.

5 Much chronic infective illness is seen in tropical countries, which may account for the various types of infections that have been documented as responsible for acute nephritis: bacterial endocarditis, respiratory infections (mainly abscesses), chronic osteomyelitis, leprosy, *Treponema pallidum*, streptococcal infections of the skin and oropharynx, and filariasis.

Chronic infections, often bacterial, are prevalent and may be associated ultimately with the development of amyloid.

6 The use of skin-lightening creams is still widespread. These contain the nephrotoxin ammoniated mercuric chloride. Glomerulopathy occurs, usually as a minimal-change lesion but it may be proliferative or membranous. Resolution of the lesion usually follows withdrawal of use. Dimercaprol, penicillamine or ethylenediamine tetra-acetic acid may be useful. Steroids or cyclophosphamide are not indicated.

Clinical presentation, diagnosis and principles of management of these nephritides do not differ from standard practice in Western countries.

Acquired immune deficiency syndrome-related nephropathy

Studies of glomerular morphology in patients who have urinary abnormalities and who either are human immunodeficiency virus (HIV)-positive or have acquired immunodeficiency syndrome (AIDS) have yet to be completed. Sufficient renal biopsies have been performed to show that there is no uniform morphology in these African patients. Histological findings include minimal-change disease, mesangial proliferation, membranous mesangiocapillary and diffuse endocapillary morphologies. Focal and segmental glomerulosclerosis (FSGS) is conspicuous by paucity in numbers, although FSGS is not an uncommon morphology in Zimbabwe. One factor that differentiates these patients from those in American studies is that there is no intravenous drug abuse in Zimbabwe.

Urinary tract infection

The incidence of asymptomatic bacteriuria is much higher in the tropics than in Western countries. Various reasons are suggested:

1 Frequency of pelvic venereal disease.

2 Morbidity following obstetric trauma.

3 High incidence of urinary tract obstruction due to urethral stricture (venereal) and ureteric strictures (bilharzial).

In cases of sterile pyuria, the possibility of genitourinary tuberculosis is real: tuberculosis is increasingly widespread in the tropics. Early morning samples of urine may yield acid- and alcohol-fast bacilli on specific media. There is often evidence of tuberculosis in other organs.

Management of urinary infection in all other aspects is standard (see Chapter 7, p. 90, and Chapter 8, p. 108).

Tropical diseases

Typhoid fever

Typhoid fever is endemic in many tropical African countries. Renal involvement, which is not uncommon, ranges from mild to severe. There are four patterns of renal involvement.

Acute renal failure

The incidence of ARF varies from 14 to 20% of patients with typhoid. In typhoid ARF carries a mortality of up to 10%. Typhoid must be suspected in any case of ARF seen in a tropical environment or in a patient who has recently returned from the tropics, even if the patient is apyrexial at presentation.

Mechanisms include the following:

1 Hypovolaemia and Gram-negative septicaemia.

2 Intravascular haemolysis is well recognized and two groups of patients are affected: normal individuals and those who are G-6-PD-deficient. It may be that G-6-PD deficiency increases susceptibility to typhoid fever.

3 Myoglobinuria: severe rhabdomyolysis may occur and the resulting myoglobinuria may cause or contribute to ARF.

4 Haemolytic uraemic syndrome was documented in 12.5% of patients in one series. The probable pathogenesis is that the endotoxin of *S. typhi* causes a glomerular microangiopathy, which in turn leads to renal intravascular coagulation, red cell fragmentation and uraemia.

Early diagnosis and treatment is vital. Diagnosis is clinical and supported by culture of the organism from blood, urine or stool. The Widal test may be unreliable.

Acute nephritis

The incidence of acute nephritis is not known; it may be more frequent than is realized but overlooked in view of other severe acute symptomatology. Proteinuria, if present, is usually mild and rarely exceeds 1.2 g/24 hours. Renal function is usually normal.

Salmonella Vi antigen has been demonstrated in glomeruli, implying a possible causative relationship.

Acute nephritis resolves completely with antibiotic therapy of the typhoid fever.

Interstitial nephritis

Interstitial nephritis occurs in up to 1% of patients with typhoid. Clinical features include oedema, which may be protracted, hypertension, fever and splenomegaly. Renal functional impairment is variable: ARF may occur.

Antibacterial therapy, together with supportive and symptomatic treatment, results in resolution of the disease.

Association with Schistosoma haematobium

Typhoid is a fairly common complication of chronic *S. haematobium* infestation. It may also occur with *Schistosoma mansoni*. Schistosomal infestation seems either to impair host immunity or to affect the propensity of the *Salmonella* to invade tissue and cause disease.

Clinical features include a febrile illness, skin rash and hepatosplenomegaly. The majority of patients have nephrotic-range proteinuria.

Salmonella typhi (or *Salmonella paratyphi* A and C) is recoverable by blood and urine culture in two-thirds of patients.

Histologically, either an interstitial nephritis or a proliferative nephritis is found. The former is associated with minor proteinuria and no impairment of glomerular filtration rate. In those patients with nephritis, there is a short-lived period of functional impairment.

Complete resolution occurs on treatment of the underlying salmonellosis.

Treatment

Chloramphenicol remains the antibiotic of choice. The dose is 2 g daily orally (500 mg 6-hourly) for 7 days and then 1.5 g/24 hours for 14 days. Treatment may need to be commenced intravenously in severely ill patients. This regimen has been found to have a substantially lower rate of relapse than other regimens. Other antibiotics used are amoxycillin, ampicillin, co-trimoxazole and trimethoprim. All are used for 14–21 days but they are associated with a higher relapse rate.

Unfortunately, world-wide, multi-drug-resistant strains of *S. typhi* are increasingly becoming recognized. This is due to over-the-counter antibiotics, which are available in many developing countries and are taken for non-specific diarrhoeal conditions. In this circumstance, the quinolone, ciprofloxacin, is the antibiotic of choice, but it is very expensive and difficult to obtain outside the developed world.

For *S. typhi* and *S. paratyphi* infections, barrier nursing must be instituted. Supportive measures depend on the individual patient and complications are treated symptomatically.

Malaria

About 3% of patients with malaria develop a combination of serious cerebral, pulmonary and renal complications. The occurrence of complications is related to the capacity for red cell invasion by the different plasmodia:

1 *Plasmodium falciparum.* High parasite levels (15–20%) result from multiple invasions of erythrocytes of all ages.

2 *Plasmodium malariae.* Invades mature erythrocytes only. The parasitaemia rarely exceeds 1%. Chronic renal disease in endemic areas occurs.

3 *Plasmodium ovale* and *Plasmodium vivax.* Invade reticulocytes, causing parasite levels of not more than 2%. Renal damage is most infrequent.

Discussion of the renal complications will be limited to the first two species. Mention should be made, however, of a febrile proteinuria, which is a mild transient acute nephropathy ascribed to formation of *in situ* glomerular complexes. This occurs in up to a quarter of those with *P. falciparum* and *P. vivax* infection, but is most common with *P. malariae* (50%). Renal function remains normal. The proteinuria occurs in the second or third week after infection and resolves completely 4–6 weeks after treatment.

Plasmodium falciparum infection

The following renal clinical pictures are common with *P. falciparum*:

1 Acute renal failure.

2 Acute nephritis.

Acute renal failure

Acute renal failure is common and often worsened by dehydration and long distances to travel for treatment. A history of travel in a malarial endemic area will alert the clinician to the possibility of malaria, irrespective of the clinical presentation. The pathophysiology is complex. The following mechanisms may be involved:

1 Damage to capillary endothelium causes increased vascular permeability, which leads to impaired microcirculation. Hyperviscosity due to plugging of capillaries by deformed, parasitized erythrocytes contributes to renal ischaemia.

2 Intravascular haemolysis.

3 Immunological reaction to plasmodial antigen.

4 Hypotension, dehydration and hyponatraemia.

5 Coagulopathy: full-blown disseminated intravsacular coagulation (DIC) is extremely uncommon.

6 Pyrogens are released by rupture of erythrocytes.

Malarial ARF may be divided into the two categories of massive intravascular haemolysis and heavy parasitaemia without overt haemoglobinuria.

Massive intravascular haemolysis (blackwater fever) Haemolysis is induced by malaria infection alone, or by the use of antimalarials (chloroquine, quinine, pyrimethamine) in normal and G-6-PD-deficient individuals. Blackwater fever is thought to occur in non-immune persons or in residents of endemic areas who have partially lost their immunity through periods of absence from their homes. In the latter, an unusual sensitivity to reinfection appears to exist. The trigger factor for the massive haemolysis is not known. Acute tubular necrosis occurs. Hyperbilirubinaemia may further compromise renal function.

Clinical features vary from a mild febrile illness with malaise, loin pain and dark brown-black urine to a severe syndrome of high fever, vomiting, diarrhoea and 'blackwater'. Patients are anaemic; jaundice may be mild or severe, with concomitant hepatic damage. Renal failure may be hypercatabolic.

The prognosis is good with antimalarial therapy. If death occurs, it is invariably due to accompanying cerebral or pulmonary complications of the malaria. Haemodialysis is preferred to peritoneal dialysis, the efficiency of which may be precluded by the involvement of the microcirculation.

Heavy parasitaemia without overt haemoglobinuria This occurs in up to 90% of patients with malaria and ARF. These patients often have multiple complications and are severely ill. The histology is an acute tubular necrosis (ATN), with more prominent distal tubular necroses than proximal.

Clinical features are that patients are acutely ill and febrile and may be confused or comatose. Jaundice is variable; it is hepatocellular in nature. Renal failure is usually hypercatabolic. Pulmonary complications and DIC may supervene. Mild intravascular haemolysis may occur.

The prognosis depends on the severity of the complications and the early institution of specific and supportive therapy.

Acute nephritis

Mild proteinuria (less than 1 g daily) and abnormal urinary sediment occurs in 20–50% of patients. Renal dysfunction is unusual, as are oedema and hypertension. Acute renal failure is uncommon. Occasionally, frank clinical nephritis, with nephrotic proteinuria, occurs, which is considered to be an unusual host response and may be allied to prolonged infection or a chloroquine-resistant strain.

Glomeruli show proliferative lesions varying in severity and type. The capillary wall is thickened and may be 'plexiform' in appearance. IgM, IgG and C3 are found in the mesangial matrix. *P. falciparum* antigen has been detected in the granular deposits.

The histological changes resolve within 4–6 weeks of successful antimalarial therapy.

Treatment

It is often imperative to commence definitive treatment before receiving

Table 22.4 Treatment of malaria. Note that doses must be adjusted for children and infants and that quinidine in appropriate dose may be used if quinine is not available

	Drug	Dose	Route
Chloroquine-susceptible strains			
1 Uncomplicated			
(a) *Plasmodium falciparum*	Chloroquine	600 mg stat and day 2 (child: 10 mg/kg body-weight) 300 mg on 3rd day (child: 5 mg/kg)	Oral
(b) *Plasmodium vivax* *ovale* *malariae*	Chloroquine followed by primaquine	As above 15 mg daily × 14–21 days	Oral
2 Complicated			
P. falciparum	Chloroquine	Total dose 25 mg/kg SC, or 3.5 mg base/kg 6-hourly IM, or 0.83 mg base/kg hourly IV Change to oral chloroquine as soon as feasible	IV *Indications for IV use*: (a) ill patients (b) delay in diagnosis (3–4 days from onset of symptoms) (c) 5% of RBCs infested
Chloroquine-resistant strains			
1 Uncomplicated			
P. falciparum *P. vivax*	1 Quinine sulphate	600 mg tds × 7 days (child: 10 mg/kg)	Oral
	with pyrimethamine and sulfadoxine (Fansidar)	1500 mg } total dose 75 mg } 3 tablets as single dose at end of quinine course	Oral
	or tetracycline	250 mg gds × 7 days	Oral
	or		
	2 Mefloquine	20 mg/kg divided into 2 doses 6 hours apart (max. = 1500 mg)	Oral
	or		
	3 Halofantrine	500 mg 6-hourly for 3 doses (child: 8 mg/kg) Repeat course after 7 days	Oral
2 Complicated	Quinine dihydrochloride	20 mg/kg in 5% dextrose over 4 hours. Then, at 8-hourly intervals, 10 mg/kg 4-hourly. Use until patient can swallow, then oral quinine 10 mg/kg to complete 7 days of therapy	IV

Table 22.4 *Cont.*

	Drug	Dose	Route
	or		
	Quinidine gluconate	15 mg/kg over 4 hours. Then, after interval of 4 hours, give 7.5 mg/kg over 4 hours. Repeat 8-hourly until patient can swallow. Then use oral quinine as above	IV

Chloroquine is dispensed as sulphate or phosphate. Doses quoted refer to chloroquine base.
Mefloquine is contraindicated in pregnancy, patients taking β-blockers and if there is a history of psychiatric disease or epilepsy.
Halofantrine should probably not be used in pregnancy.
Quinine should never be given by bolus injection. For patients weighing >70 kg, dose should be calculated as for 70 kg.
Chloroquine resistance is increasingly widespread and there is increasing evidence of multiple-drug-resistant strains in highly endemic areas.
Quinine may induce severe hypoglycaemia, requiring 50% dextrose infusions repeatedly (Molyneux & Fox, 1993).

positive identification of the parasite on blood slides. If there is a high clinical index of suspicion, negative blood slides do not preclude the diagnosis.

1 Antimalarials – see Table 22.4.

2 Heparin and other viscosity-reducing agents have not been found to be of use.

3 Steroids are contraindicated and are harmful in the event of cerebral complications.

4 Haemodialysis and other supportive measures for ARF.

5 Exchange transfusion has been advocated for patients with >20% parasitaemia. There have been no controlled trials; the indications are not clearly defined and the benefits are not proven.

6 Appropriate treatment of pulmonary complications. Careful fluid balance is vital because fluid overload may precipitate acute pulmonary oedema.

7 If G-6-PD deficiency is suspected, it should be sought 3 months after the acute haemolytic episode.

If the diagnosis of malaria is made or suspected in a patient in Britain, it is prudent to seek telephonic advice from a member of staff of a school of tropical medicine. Chloroquine-resistant malaria is becoming increasingly widespread in many different countries: expert advice should be sought. Telephone numbers are quoted in the *British National Formulary.*

Plasmodium malariae infection

Acute malaria occurs but the chronic glomerulopathy caused by persistent, repeated infection is of greater importance. The exoerythrocytic cycle, with recycling of merozoites in hepatic cells, results in prolonged antigen release. This perpetuates the immune response, causing persistent glomerular lesions.

Nephrotic syndrome is the most frequent presentation in children, with a peak incidence at 7 years, corresponding with peak malaria infection. In adults, features of CRF may predominate and one-third are hypertensive. Children are usually normotensive. Fever is not a feature, although an occasional spike may be noted which coincides with mild non-specific symptoms – anorexia or lassitude. Growth retardation and under-nutrition occur. Proteinuria is usually marked and non-selective; microscopic haematuria is often present.

The natural history follows one of three courses:

1 Partial remission for months or years with no clinical features and stable renal function.

2 Short-lived remission with varying subsequent course.

3 Slow, intractable progression to CRF in adolescence or early adulthood.

Glomeruli sampled from nephritic patients with chronic *P. malariae* infection show chronic and progressive lesions resembling membranous or mesangiocapillary nephritides. The picture in adults is more severe and may resemble mesangiocapillary nephritis type III. Capsular adhesions occur late and crescents are rare. Intramembranous, subepithelial and subendothelial deposits containing IgM, IgG2, IgG3, complement and sometimes malarial, antigens occur.

Diagnosis

Diagnosis is usually straightforward:

1 *Children.* Although blood slides usually reveal *P. malariae*, often with a high parasite density, repeated examination may be necessary.

2 *Adults.* Parasites are often scanty, especially if antimalarials have been taken. IgM may be elevated in the 'active' phase and malarial antibodies found.

Treatment

Treatment of malarial nephropathy includes the following:

1 Malaria prophylaxis over some years may be beneficial in reducing activity of the nephropathy and promoting growth in children.

2 Radical antimalarial treatment has no effect.

3 Steroids have no effect.

4 Immunosuppressive drugs are reported to have a good response in patients with a coarse or mixed granular pattern of immunofluorescence but no effect in patients with a fine granular pattern of deposits.

5 Standard measures to treat oedema, CRF and hypertension.

Schistosomiasis

Human schistosomiasis is caused by infestation with four epidemiologically distinct parasites. *Schistosoma haematobium* inhabits venules around the bladder and pelvic plexus and affects the genitourinary tract. *Schistosoma mansoni*, *Schistosoma japonicum* and *Schistosoma intercalatum* inhabit pericolonic venules and primarily affect the gastrointestinal tract.

Man becomes infected through exposure to water contaminated by the intermediate freshwater snail host, which excretes cercariae, the infective form of the organism. Four stages occur in human infection:

1 Cercarial invasion of skin after immersion in contaminated water.

2 Maturation of schistosomes, migration to preferred intravascular anatomical site for pairing of worms and subsequent egg-laying.

3 Intensive egg-laying. Half of the eggs are excreted and those retained in the body cause a granulomatous reaction. There is a cell-mediated immune response to egg antigen.

4 Progressive fibrosis around existing granulomata.

Numbers 3 and 4 are responsible for the symptoms in genitourinary schistosomiasis. Disease severity depends upon egg load.

Clinical patterns

Clinical patterns include the following:

1 *Urethral involvement.* This may lead to stricture and fistulae ('watering-can scrotum').

2 *Bladder involvement.* Terminal haematuria, frequency, terminal dysuria and suprapubic pain result from granulomata, which may coalesce into 'pseudopolyps' and which are maximal in the trigone.

Fibrosis and healing may result in a distended atonic bladder and, in hyperendemic areas, further fibrosis results in a shrunken bladder of reduced capacity and bladder neck obstruction. The presence of bladder calcification on X-ray implies a heavy load of ova and not fibrosis. Some reversal of obstruction and hydronephrosis may occur with treatment. Squamous metaplasia may occur and carcinoma of the bladder is a late sequela.

3 *Ureteric involvement.* Inflammation and fibrosis lead to obstruction and stricture formation with functional impairment and vesicoureteric reflux. Hydroureter, hydronephrosis and obstructive uropathy occur above the stenosed segment of ureter.

4 *Renal involvement.* Granulomata may occur but this is unusual. Nephrotic syndrome is reported as a consequence of *S. mansoni* and *S. japonicum* infestation. Histology reveals mesangiocapillary, focal proliferative and focal sclerosing lesions. Pathogenesis of the glomerulopathy is not fully elucidated. The schistosomal gut antigen appears to be important. Nephropathy in *S. haematobium* infections appears to be related to concomitant chronic salmonellosis. Secondary amyloid has been reported with *S. haematobium* infestation.

Urine microscopy invariably shows a sterile pyuria, eosinophils predominantly.

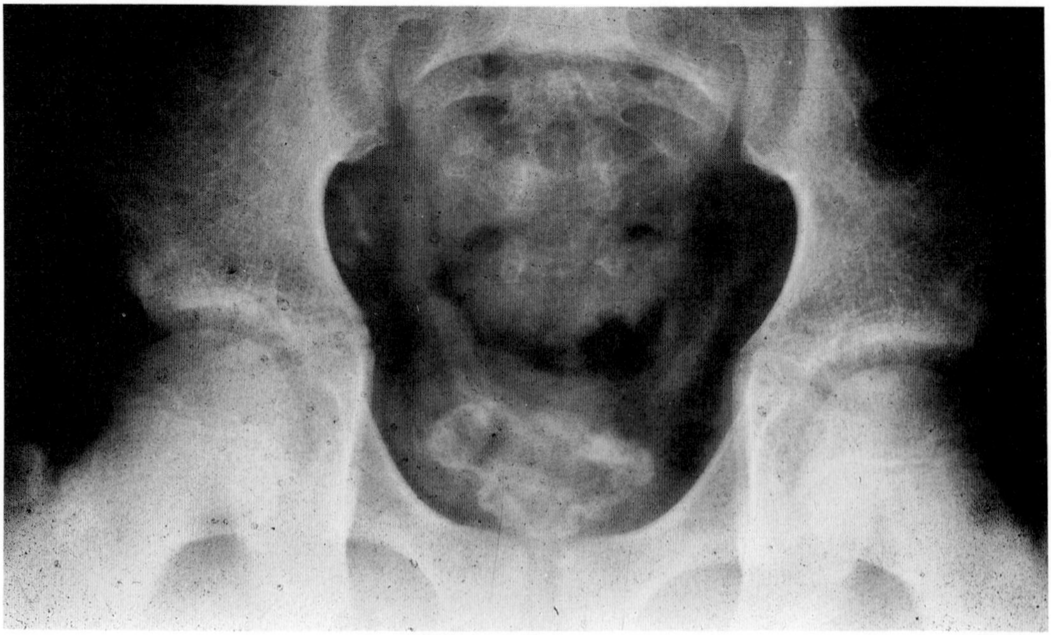

Fig. 22.1 A plain X-ray of the pelvis of a Shona boy aged 9 demonstrating extensive bladder and ureteric calcification due to schistosomal infestation.

Diagnosis

Diagnosis stems from the following:

1 Demonstration of ova in urine, stool, rectal biopsy or surgical specimens.

2 Serological: a variety of tests exist. A positive result for schistosomal antibodies should rarely, if ever, be taken as the sole criterion for infection. In the absence of demonstrable ova, a clear history of exposure to contaminated water plus two of the following 'minor criteria' are suggested for positive diagnosis:

(a) A proved diagnosis in a person who was accompanying the suspected patient at the time of exposure.

(b) Peripheral blood eosinophilia of $>4\%$.

(c) History of terminal haematuria.

(d) Bladder calcification on abdominal X-ray (Fig. 22.1).

(e) Presence of protein and red cells on urinalysis. In endemic areas, positive stick tests for protein and red cells correlate well with the finding of ova.

3 Intravenous urogram, ultrasound and isotope renography will provide additional information.

Treatment

In endemic areas, specific chemotherapy should be used, in addition to molluscicides, provision of safe water supplies, sanitation and health education. Drugs used may be effective against one or all species of schistosome (Table 22.5).

Patients living in or returning to endemic areas constitute a different population in terms of disease expression. The constant re-exposure and reinfection, especially in childhood, with heavy parasite loads will modify the chronic disease pattern. At the same time, many patients in endemic areas carry light, almost symptomless infections, which is a reflection upon the complex and ill-understood immune response.

Single-dose metriphonate (10 mg/kg) has been shown to reduce considerably the load of worms and therefore egg excretion, particularly in children with heavy infections. Mass treatment may be useful in the planning of *Schistosoma* control programmes in endemic areas, in order to reduce the numbers of eggs excreted into lakes, thereby reducing the probability of snail infection and transmission of disease.

Toxins

Snake bite

Renal lesions vary widely, depending on the type of snake. Reference to regional texts is recommended, providing the snake has been positively identified. Venoms may affect all parts of the nephron:

1 Glomeruli: a predominantly mesangial proliferative nephritis occurs.
2 Tubules: ATN occurs.
3 Interstitium: an acute interstitial nephritis is occasionally seen.
4 Vascular: a necrotizing arteritis, mainly involving interlobular

Table 22.5 Chemotherapy of schistosomiasis. Dosage expressed as mg/kg body-weight (praziquantel and metriphonate are not available on the UK market: seek expert advice)

Drug	Species	Dose and route	Side-effects
Praziquantel	*S. haematobium* or *S. mansoni*	40 mg/kg single oral dose	Usually transient and rarely require treatment
	Combined infection or heavy *S. mansoni*	50–60 mg/kg two divided oral doses over 24 hours	Fever, fatigue, urticaria, pruritus, mild gastrointestinal upset, headache, dizziness
	S. japonicum	20 mg/kg given orally three times on 1 day at 4-hourly intervals	
Metriphonate	*S. haematobium*	7.5–10 mg/kg given orally on three occasions at 2-weekly intervals	Rare. Cholinergic symptoms (the drug is an organophosphorus ester)
Oxamniquine	*S. mansoni*	New World: 15–20 mg/kg single oral dose	Rare. Headache, dizziness, hallucinations, fits, minor increase in serum transaminases
		Africa: 40–60 mg/kg given orally over 2–3 days	

arterioles, occurs, with renal infarction. Thrombophlebitis of arcuate veins has been shown. Bleeding may be worsened by a coagulation defect and thrombocytopenia.

5 Cortical necrosis: this occurs rarely.

The extent of the renal lesions varies widely. Renal function may remain normal or ARF may supervene rapidly. When ARF does occur, it is due not only to the nephrotoxicity of the snake venom, but to a combination of the following factors:

1 Intravascular haemolysis.
2 DIC.
3 Myoglobinuria.
4 Shock.
5 Hypovolaemia.

Therapy varies according to the type of snake and includes:

1 Specific antivenom.
2 Wound toilet.
3 Antitetanus toxoid.
4 Antibiotics.
5 General supportive measures, which may include haemodialysis and exchange transfusion.

Ideally, anyone accompanying the envenomed patient should find and kill the snake responsible so that it can be taken with the patient to hospital for positive identification. A specific antivenom can then be chosen.

Other animal stings

There may be a renal component to the envenomation by bees, hornets, wasps, spiders and scorpions. This is due to:

1 Hypotension causing ischaemic ARF.
2 Intravascular haemolysis.
3 Myonecrosis and myoglobinuria.

If ARF occurs, it is usually due to ATN: glomerular change, if present, is minimal.

Specific antivenoms must be used within 1–4 hours of the sting. Otherwise treatment is symptomatic and supportive.

Sickle-cell disease

Renal involvement includes the following:

1 *Haematuria.* This may be micro- or macroscopic and results from intrarenal vascular sickling, localized cortical infarction and tubular or papillary necrosis.

2 *Proteinuria.* This ranges from mild to nephrotic range. Histologically, mesangial proliferative or mesangiocapillary nephritides or FSGS are found.

3 *Tubular disorders.* Impaired concentrating ability is a constant feature of sickle-cell kidney, and it worsens with increasing age.

The pathogenesis of the above possible events is not fully elucidated. Evidence suggests that the abnormal renal haemodynamics lead to hyperfiltration and glomerular injury, with subsequent deterioration in renal function.

Summary

Acute renal failure is very common in the tropics, most often secondary to infection. Septic abortion is a common cause of ARF and is frequently worsened by nephrotoxic abortifacients and haemorrhage.

Typhoid must be considered in anyone who has recently returned from a tropical area and who develops ARF. Likewise, malaria can be incubated during a return journey: prophylactic agents do not give complete protection.

Acute nephritis occurs often. The peak age of onset of nephrotic syndrome is 5–10 years. Proliferative nephritides are common and minimal-change disease rare. *Plasmodium malariae* and HBV are probably the most important pathogens. There is a high incidence of CRF in tropical countries, the major causes being severe hypertension, chronic nephritis secondary to *P. malariae* or HBV and the obstructive uropathy due to schistosomiasis.

Further reading

1 Adu, D., Anim-Addo, Y., Foli, A.K. *et al.* (1976) Acute renal failure in tropical Africa. *Br. Med. J.* **1**, 890–2.
2 Allon, M. (1990) Renal abnormalities in sickle cell disease. *Arch. Intern. Med.* **150**, 505–10.
3 Andrade, Z.A. & Rocha, H. (1979) Schistosomal nephropathy. *Kidney Int.* **16**, 23–9.
4 Barsoum, R.S. (1990) Parasitic nephropathies. *Med. Forum* no. 35.
5 Boonpucknavig, V. & Sitprija, V. (1976) Renalr disease in acute *Plasmodium falciparum* infection in man. *Kidney Int.* **16**, 44–52.
6 Buka, I. & Coovadia, H.M. (1980) Typhoid glomerulonephritis. *Arch. Dis. Child.* **55**, 305–7.
7 Chugh, K.S. & Sakhuja, V. (1990) Glomerular disease in the tropics. *Am. J. Nephrol.* **10**, 437–50.
8 Davis, A. (1986) Recent advances in schistosomiasis. *Quart. J. Med.* **58**, 95–110.
9 Dukes, D.C. (1969) The schistosome and the kidney: a controlled clinical study. MD thesis, University of Birmingham.
10 Dukes, D.C., Dukes, H.M., Gordon, J.A., Mynors, J.M. & Weinberg, R.W. (1969) Acute renal failure in Central Africa: the toxic effects of traditional African medicine. *Central Afr. J. Med.* **15**, 71–8.
11 Editorial (1980) Nephrotic syndrome in the tropics. *Lancet* **ii**, 461–2.
12 Editorial (1985) Criteria for the recognition of schistosomiasis in the absence of demonstrable ova. *Central Afr. J. Med.* **21**, 37.
13 Giglioli, G. (1962) Malaria and renal Disease, with special reference to British Guiana. I – Introduction. II – The effect of malaria eradication on the incidence of renal disease in British Guiana. *Ann. Trop. Med. Parasitol.* **56**, 101–9 and 225–41.
14 Hutt, M.S.R. (1980) Renal disease in a tropical environment. *Trans. Roy. Soc. Trop. Med. Hygiene.* **74**, 17–21.

15 Kasilo, O. (1988) Current information on malaria – Part I. *Drug and Toxicology Information Service Bulletin* University of Zimbabwe Department of Pharmacy August, no. 13.
16 Kibukamusoke, J.W. (ed.) (1984) *Tropical Nephrology*. Citforge Pty Ltd., Canberra.
17 Lwanga, D. & Wing, A.J. (1970) Renal complications associated with typhoid fever. *East Afr. Med. J.* **47**, 146–52.
18 Molyneux, M. & Fox, R. (1993) Diagnosis and treatment of malaria in Britain. *Br. Med. J.* **306**, 1175–80.
19 Ngu, J.L. & Youmbissi, T.J. (1987) Special features, pathogenesis and aetiology of glomerular diseases in the tropics. *Clin. Sci.* **72**, 519–24.
20 Peters, W. & Hall, A.P. (1985) The treatment of severe falciparum malaria. *Br. Med. J.* **291**, 1146–7.
21 Phillips, R.E. & Gilles, H.M. (1988) Malaria. *Med. Int.* **54**, 2220–5.
22 Seggie, J., Davies, P.G., Ninin, D. & Henry, J. (1984) Patterns of glomerulonephritis in Zimbabwe: survey of disease characterised by nephrotic proteinuria. *Quart. J. Med.* **209**, 109–18.
23 Sitprija, V., Pipatanagul, V., Boonpucknavig, V. & Boonpucknavig, S. (1974) Glomerulonephritis in typhoid fever. *Ann. Intern. Med.* **81**, 210–13.
24 Sitprija, V., Vongsthongsri, M., Poshyachyachinda, V. & Arthachinta, S. (1977) Renal failure in malaria: a pathophysiologic study. *Nephron* **18**, 277–87.

Index

BOX N 1+1+1+1+1+1+1+1+1+1+1+1

BCO/CS 12+12+12+12+12+12+12+12+18+12+12+

=138

N - 48

5 Bks - 16/2/99 - 103

5 Bks - 18/8/98 - 064